MRI
The Basics

Third Edition

Ray Hashman Hashemi, M.D., Ph.D.

Director and CEO
Advanced Imaging Center, Inc.
Lancaster, California

William G. Bradley Jr, M.D., Ph.D., F.A.C.R.

Professor and Chairman
Department of Radiology
University of California, San Diego
San Diego, California

Christopher J. Lisanti, M.D., Col. (ret) USAF, MC, SFS

Chief, Body MRI
Department of Radiology
Brooke Army Medical Center
Fort Sam Houston, Texas

Wolters Kluwer | Lippincott Williams & Wilkins
Health

Philadelphia · Baltimore · New York · London
Buenos Aires · Hong Kong · Sydney · Tokyo

Acquisitions Editor: Charles W. Mitchell
Product Manager: Ryan Shaw
Vendor Manager: Bridgett Dougherty
Senior Manufacturing Manager: Benjamin Rivera

Senior Marketing Manager: Angela Panetta
Design Coordinator: Doug Smock
Production Service: Macmillan

Printed in China

Library of Congress Cataloging-in-Publication Data
Hashemi, Ray H.
  MRI: the basics/Ray Hashman Hashemi, William G. Bradley Jr., Christopher J. Lisanti. — 3rd ed.
    p.; cm.
  Includes bibliographical references and index.
  ISBN 978-1-60831-115-6
  1. Magnetic resonance imaging. I. Bradley, William G. II. Lisanti, Christopher J. III. Title.
  [DNLM: 1. Magnetic Resonance Imaging—Examination Questions. 2. Magnetic Resonance Imaging—Problems and Exercises. 3. Mathematics—Examination Questions. 4. Mathematics—Problems and Exercises. 5. Physics—Examination Questions. 6. Physics—Problems and Exercises. WN 18.2 H348m 2010]
  RC78.7.N83H44 2010
  616.07'548—dc22

                                                                                    2010001237

To purchase additional copies of this book, call our customer service department at (800) 638-3030 or fax orders to (301) 223-2320. International customers should call (301) 223-2300.

Visit Lippincott Williams & Wilkins on the Internet: at LWW.com. Lippincott Williams & Wilkins customer service representatives are available from 8:30 am to 6 pm, EST.

10 9 8 7 6 5 4 3 2 1

To my wonderful wife, Heidi Hame, DDS, MS, for her relentless support and love over the past fifteen years; our son Tristen for bringing more joy to our lives; and our parents for all their caring and generosity.

RHH

To my MRI fellows over the last quarter century who raised many of the questions answered in this book. At UCSD I now go through "The Basics" with the MRI fellows from cover to cover over the course of the year.

WGB

Soli Deo Gloria.

CJL

Preface to the First Edition

"Things should be made as simple as possible—but no simpler."
—ALBERT EINSTEIN

MRI has been called "the most important development in medical diagnosis since the discovery of the x-ray" 100 years ago. It has become one of the major new tools of radiology, now being applied to virtually every part of the body. So, one might ask, if this MRI is so wonderful, why are so many radiologists reluctant to "get into" it? In a word: "physics." The physics of MRI can be truly terrifying, particularly for those attempting to enter the explanation halfway through without a proper foundation in the basics. And without a proper understanding of the basics, any MR clinician is merely "faking it," not truly understanding the physical basis for the signal changes in the image. *MRI: The Basics* attempts to rectify that situation.

In this book we have attempted to present this complicated topic in a readable, understandable, and even entertaining fashion without sacrificing the fundamental concepts. The reader will find a comprehensive coverage of MRI physics, from basic principles to more advanced topics such as MR angiography and fast scanning techniques. Some of the latest MR techniques made possible with high performance gradients, e.g., echo planar imaging, are also discussed. Because most of the chapters arose from lectures given by the first author to radiology residents, the language used through most of the text is of an informal or conversational nature that makes it easy to follow.

While attempting to be thorough, this book does not get bogged down in the minor details. An introductory math chapter is designed to introduce the reader to the most fundamental mathematics used in MRI (no knowledge of calculus is required!). Considerable attention is paid to the process of image creation, including the concepts of gradients, signal/image processing, and k-space. One of the distinguishing features of this book is its introduction and treatment of signal/image processing. There are two chapters dedicated to image creation, two to k-space, one to Fourier transform, and one to signal processing, as well as several chapters on fast scanning (fast spin echo, gradient echo, fast gradient echo, and echo planar imaging). There are also chapters that deal in depth with flow and MR angiography as well as MRI artifacts.

More than 400 illustrations provide the reader with a clear visual tool to follow the text. *The key points* of each chapter are summarized at the end of that chapter. In addition, there is a set of *problem solving and multiple choice questions* at the end of each chapter (with answers at the end of the book) to test the reader's knowledge of that chapter. The material presented in smaller print may be skipped because it is intended for the mathematically oriented reader.

This book is intended primarily for radiologists and radiology residents and fellows as well as radiologic technologists. However, other physicians, medical students, scientists, and professionals dealing with MRI could also benefit from it. It is intended to provide the shortest learning path from the basics through the applications, avoiding the extraneous. This book can be used by radiology residents preparing for the physics portion of the American Board of Radiology exam and by MR technologists preparing for their MR certification exam.

In short, you can find in this book almost everything you always wanted to know about MR physics but were afraid to ask. In addition, this book may not only be read cover to cover as a textbook to learn about all aspects of MR basics, but also may be used as a reference for the fundamentals and advanced technological breakthroughs in MRI. We hope you'll enjoy reading it as much as we did writing it.

RHH
WGB

The first two editions of *MRI: The Basics* were well received, and we trust enhanced MRI knowledge and practical application. This current edition of the *The Basics* spans the gamut from basic physics to multiuse MR options to specific applications. Although MRI is a maturing technology, it, nevertheless, continues to challenge radiologists, residents, and technologists. More improvements and new features are constantly being developed and applied producing diagnostic images faster, with higher image quality and reproducibility. This power, however, invariably gives the MR user more options, and these various options must be sorted and thought through in order to give optimal results.

In response to advancements in MRI, we have updated the book and added completely new chapters addressing parallel imaging, cardiac MRI, and MR Spectroscopy. These areas are used with increasing regularity in MR imaging, and we hope that you will glean new insight into these features and applications in order to enhance your practice.

Again, we are pleased to present to you the third edition of *MRI: The Basics*, and hope that it will be a trusty companion during your MRI journey.

Ray Hashman Hashemi, MD, PhD
William G. Bradley Jr, MD, PhD, FACR
Col. (ret) Christopher J. Lisanti, MD

Acknowledgments

We would like to thank Robert Mulkern (Brigham and Women's Hospital) for helpful comments on the equations in Chapter 17. This generated an e-mail debate on the formula for signal-to-noise, which went on for a month and included MR giants such as Mark Haacke (Wayne State), John Mugler (UVa), Felix Wehrli (Penn), Gary Fullerton (UColo), and Mark Bydder (UCSD—Graeme's son and future giant).

Contents

Basic Concepts

Introduction

In this chapter, we review some of the basic mathematical concepts that are used in MR imaging. We don't want to scare you away so we keep things as simple as possible. An understanding of these basic concepts will help the reader a great deal to comprehend the subtleties of MR imaging and obtain the necessary tools for manipulating the scan parameters to improve the quality of the images.

It is not that important to memorize these mathematical formulas; what's crucial is the understanding of the **concepts** behind these formulas. In this chapter, we hope to emphasize the most important mathematical concepts of MRI physics.

Sinusoidals

Consider a **right triangle** (having a right angle) with sides a and b and hypotenuse c and angle x formed by a and c (Fig. 1-1). We can define sin x

Table 1-1

	0	$\pi/6$	$\pi/4$	$\pi/3$	$\pi/2$	π
x	0°	30°	45°	60°	90°	180°
sin x	0	1/2	$(\sqrt{2})/2$	$(\sqrt{3})/2$	1	0
cos x	1	$(\sqrt{3})/2$	$(\sqrt{2})/2$	1/2	0	−1
tan x	0	$1/(\sqrt{3})$	1	$(\sqrt{3})$	∞	0

(read *sine* of x), cos x (read *cosine* of x), tan x (read *tangent* of x), cotan x (read *co-tangent* of x), and arctan x (read *arc-tangent* of x) in terms of a, b, and c:

$$\sin x = b/c$$
$$\cos x = a/c$$
$$\tan x = \sin x/\cos x = b/a$$
$$\text{cotan } x = 1/\tan x = \cos x/\sin x = a/b$$
$$\arctan b/a = \arctan(\tan x) = x \quad \textbf{(Eqn. 1-1)}$$

The variable x can be represented in degrees, that is, 45°, 90°, and 180°, or it can be represented in radians, that is, $\pi/4$, $\pi/2$, and π, where $\pi = 180°$. Table 1-1 shows x versus. sin x, cos x, and tan x, where $\sqrt{2} \cong 1.4$ so $\sqrt{2}/2 \cong 0.7$ and $\sqrt{3} \cong 1.7$ so $\sqrt{3}/2 \cong 0.85$.

Let's plot x versus sin x (Fig. 1-2). This is called a sinusoidal function. What about cos x? (Fig. 1-3). Let's now draw cos x and sin x on a single graph (Fig. 1-4). We can appreciate the symmetry between sin x and cos x. The difference between the two functions is that sin x is shifted to the right of cos x by 90°. Later, when we talk about phase and phase shifts, this mathematical concept will become more important. We can think of sin x as being cos x with a phase difference of 90°.

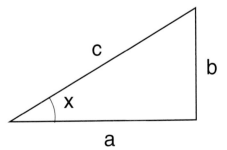

Figure 1-1. A right triangle with sides a and b and hypotenuse c and angle x formed by a and c.

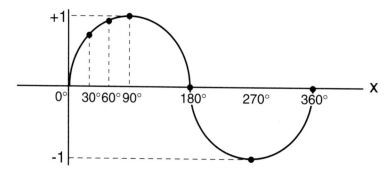

Figure 1-2. Graph of sin (*x*).

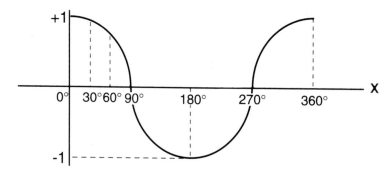

Figure 1-3. Graph of cos (*x*).

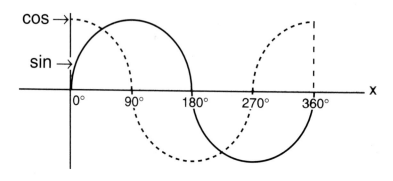

Figure 1-4. Sin (*x*) and cos (*x*) plotted on the same graph.

Now, let's go back to Figure 1-1. What is *c* in terms of *a*, *b*? According to the Pythagorean theorem:

$$c^2 = a^2 + b^2 \text{ or } c = \sqrt{(a^2 + b^2)}$$

By Equation 1-1

$$(\sin x)^2 + (\cos x)^2 = b^2/c^2 + a^2/c^2$$
$$= (a^2 + b^2)/c^2$$
$$= c^2/c^2 = 1$$

So

$$(\sin x)^2 + (\cos x)^2 = 1$$

If we go back to our graph of sin *x* and cos *x* (Fig. 1-4), we can see graphically that because

of the **phase difference** between the cos *x* and sin *x*, the sum of their squares will always equal 1. Another way of looking at *sine* and *cosine* is to consider a circle with a radius of 1 (Fig. 1-5). To understand this concept, it is necessary to bring up the concepts of vectors, imaginary numbers, and exponentials.

Vector. We'll designate a vector by using a letter such as **v** with an arrow above it ($\vec{v}$). This concept will become important later on in the understanding of resonance of spins and dephasing. A vector is a mathematical entity that has both a magnitude and a direction. For example, speed is not a vector—it only has magnitude.

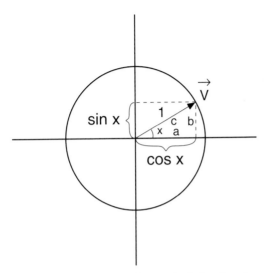

Figure 1-5. A vector **v** with magnitude 1 and angle x to the horizontal. cos x and sin x are the horizontal and vertical components of this vector, respectively.

Velocity, however, is a vector—it has both magnitude and direction. Another example of a vector is *force* that describes a magnitude (*weight*) and a direction (direction where the force is applied).

The vector that we've drawn in the circle (Fig. 1-5) has a magnitude of 1. The angle between the vector and the horizontal axis is denoted x. If we draw perpendiculars from the vector both horizontally and vertically, we'll get two components of the vector:

(a) The horizontal component of the vector would correspond to cos x. (Remember that the ratio a/c in Figure 1-1 is cos x.)

(b) The vertical component of the vector would correspond to sin x. (Remember that the ratio b/c in Figure 1-1 is sin x.)

Imaginary Numbers. A positive number n^2 has two square roots, $+n$ and $-n$. For example,

$$\left.\begin{array}{l} 3^2 = 9 \\ (-3)^2 = 9 \end{array}\right\} \text{ so (3) and } (-3) \text{ are the square roots of 9}$$

It is impossible to square a real number and have a negative product. Therefore, we shall make up an entity and call the number $\sqrt{-n}$ an imagi-

nary number. Any of the following would be imaginary numbers:

$$(\sqrt{-9}), (\sqrt{-37}), (\sqrt{-1}), (\sqrt{-18})$$

Imaginary numbers can be manipulated in the following way:

$$(\sqrt{-9}) = (\sqrt{[(9)(-1)]} = (\sqrt{9})(\sqrt{-1})$$

Any imaginary number can be written as a positive number times $(\sqrt{-1})$. The expression $(\sqrt{-1})$ is designated by the letter "*i*". (Mathematicians use the symbol *i* to denote an imaginary number, whereas engineers use the symbol "*j*" in lieu of *i* because *i* is reserved to symbolize electric current!) The symbol *i* is then known as the **imaginary unit**. In other words, $i \times i = -1$.

Example

$$\sqrt{-16} = \sqrt{(16)(-1)} = \sqrt{16}\sqrt{-1}$$
$$= i\sqrt{16} = 4i$$

So *i* is an *imaginary* number. It doesn't exist. When you take a square root of a number, it has to be a positive number. However, in this case, if we multiply *i* by *i*, we get (-1). Therefore, *i* is an imaginary number that doesn't exist.

Complex Numbers. A **complex** number is a number that has both a **real** and an **imaginary** component:

$$\text{Complex} = \text{real} + \text{imaginary}$$

Example

Let's say a complex number has two components: 2 and 3. The imaginary component is multiplied by (*i*), where $i = \sqrt{-1}$ is the imaginary unit. Then,

$$c = (2) + i(3)$$

If you draw this complex number on an $x - y$ plane (Fig. 1-6), the vector (2,3) illustrates the complex number $2 + 3i$. Usually you only care about the real part of a complex number, but it makes life easier to deal with the complex number and carry all the computations using complex numbers or vectors and then, at the end, just keep the real part.

Magnitude and Angle. Sometimes, however, the imaginary part is also helpful. For example, consider Figure 1-6. In this diagram, if we take

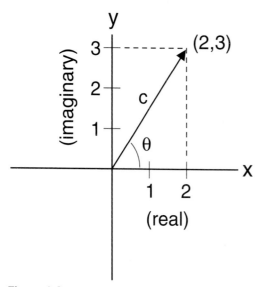

Figure 1-6. Representation of a complex number $2 + i\,3$ as a point in a two-dimensional (Cartesian) coordinate system and the relationship between a complex number, its angle θ, and its real and imaginary components.

the tangent of the **angle** between the vector and the x-axis, we get

$$\tan \theta = 3/2 = \text{imaginary/real}$$

In other words, the ratio of the imaginary part to the real part gives us the *tangent* of the **angle.** The **magnitude** of the vector (sometimes called the **modulus**) is given by the **Pythagorean theorem**

$$c = \sqrt{(a^2 + b^2)}$$

Thus,
vector magnitude

$$= \sqrt{[(\text{imaginary part})^2 + (\text{real part})^2]}$$
$$= \sqrt{[(3)^2 + (2)^2]} = \sqrt{13} \cong 3.6$$

When you're dealing with a complex number, if you take the ratio of the imaginary part to the real part, you get some sort of measure of the **angle** of the vector. If you sum the squares of the imaginary and real part, you get the **magnitude** of the vector (squared).

Function. A mathematical function, designated as $f(x)$, is an entity that varies with respect

to a variable, x. For example, $\sin x$ is a function that varies with respect to x in a sinusoidal manner, as we saw earlier in the chapter.

Signal. A signal is a time-varying function, that is, something that varies over time, usually millivolts versus time. If the x-axis is time, and the y-axis is magnitude, then a signal is a **waveform** that varies in magnitude with time.

In an electrical system, a signal is a time-varying current or voltage that can be measured. In MRI, the signal is just a current or voltage that is induced by an oscillating magnetic field. Some signals are periodic—they *repeat* themselves—as the *sine* wave or *cosine* wave repeats itself.

Frequency, Period, and Cycle. Let's now introduce the concepts of **frequency** and **period.** Every periodic function has a frequency, which we will call f. If we measure the time interval between two peaks (or where the signal crosses 0), this interval is called a **period,** and we'll denote this by T. Now, frequency = 1/period = 1/T:

$$f = 1/T$$

A **cycle** in a periodic function is any part of the function over one period. For example, let's say that we have three complete cycles occurring in 1 sec (Fig. 1-7). In this case,

$$3 \text{ periods take 1 sec}$$
$$3T = 1 \text{ sec}$$
$$T = 1/3 \text{ sec}$$
$$\text{Frequency} = f = 1/T = 3$$
$$\text{cycles per sec} = 3 \text{ Hz}$$

The unit we use to describe frequency is Hertz or Hz (for cycles per sec). There are 2π radians in one cycle. That is to say,

    f = frequency when we refer to **linear frequency** in cycles per sec

    ω = frequency when we refer to **angular frequency** in radians per sec; angular frequency (in radians/sec) = ω = (2π) × linear frequency (in Hz)

where $\pi = 3.1415927 \cong 3.14$. In short,

$$\boldsymbol{\omega = 2\pi f} \qquad \text{(Eqn. 1-2)}$$

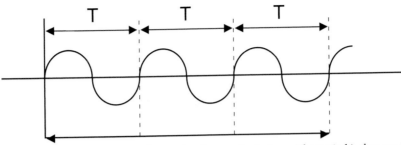

Figure 1-7. An example of a periodic signal spanning three cycles in 1 sec. The period is thus one third of 1 sec (1/3 sec).

Example

If the vector in the circle makes 3 revolutions/sec, then the vector has a frequency of 3 Hz. Therefore, $\omega = (2\pi)(3) = 6\pi = 18.85$ radians/sec.

Sometimes a signal (such as a sine wave) is represented in the following way:

$$S(t) = \sin(\omega t) = \sin(2\pi f t)$$

Here, we can say that the signal is a sine wave with a frequency of ω. So, frequency $= f = \omega/2\pi$.

Example

Draw the signal $\sin(\omega t)$ versus time t assuming $f = 1$ Hz (i.e., $T = 1$ sec or $\omega = 2\pi$ radians/sec). Thus, $\sin(\omega t)$ 5 $\sin(2\pi t)$. This equation is illustrated in Figure 1-8:

   when $t = 0$, then $\omega t = 0$, resulting in
   $\sin \omega t = \sin 0 = 0$;
   when $t = 1/4$, then $\omega t = (2\pi)(1/4) = \pi/2$,
   resulting in $\sin \omega t = \sin \pi/2 = 1$;
   when $t = 1/2$, then $\omega t = (2\pi)(1/2) = \pi$,
   resulting in $\sin \omega t = \sin \pi = 0$; etc.

Phase. Now, let's talk about **phase.** Consider two *sine* waves, with one shifted slightly compared with the other (Fig. 1-9). The two sinusoids

have the same frequency—they oscillate at the same rate—but one of them is **shifted** just a little from the other. Suppose they are shifted apart from each other by a time interval $= \tau = 1$ sec. Suppose further that the period of 1 cycle $= T = 4$ sec (Fig. 1-9).

$$T = 1 \text{ period} = 360° \text{ in 4 sec}$$
$$\tau = 1 \text{ sec} = 1/4 \text{ of the total time of 1 period}$$

Thus, 1/4 of $360° = 90°$. This measurement is the **phase offset** or **phase shift** of the two sinusoidals.

Example

What is $\sin(x + 90°)$?

Here we have the sine wave and a phase offset of 90°. Let's figure out what this looks like on a circle diagram (Fig. 1-10). If x is the angle, sine of vector x is the initial component perpendicular to vector. Take a phase offset of 90°. This offset causes the original vector to be rotated counterclockwise by 90°, as can be seen in Figure 1-10. Now, drop a vertical perpendicular from this new vector. Because the vertical component of a vector is equal to the sine of its angle, then the vertical component of the new vector (with its new angle $x + 90°$) is sine of ($x + 90°$). Now, by the law of congruent triangles, this new vertical component (which is longer than the horizontal component in Fig. 1-10) is equal to the longer horizontal component of the original angle x, which is, in fact, $\cos x$. In other words,

$$\sin(x + 90°) = \cos x \qquad \text{(Eqn. 1-3)}$$

From this, we see that *sine* and *cosine* of any given vector have a phase difference of 90°.

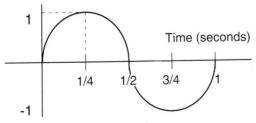

Figure 1-8. Graph of $\sin(2\pi t)$.

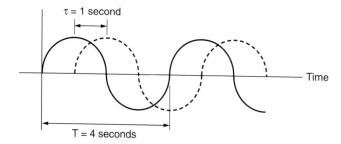

Figure 1-9. Two similar sinusoidal signals with a phase offset.

Exponentials

With **exponential functions** (e^x), the letter e is the base of the natural logarithm with a numerical value of

$$e = 2.7182818 \cong 2.72$$

First, let's consider the values of e^x for various values of x:

for $x = 0$, $e^0 = 1$ (anything to the power of $0 = 1$)

for $x = 1$, $e^1 = 2.72$

for $x = 2$, $e^2 = (2.72)(2.72) = 7.4$

for $x = \infty$, $e^\infty = \infty$

for $x = -1$, $e^{-1} = 1/e = 1/2.72 = 0.37$

for $x = -2$, $e^{-2} = 1/e^2 = 1/(2.72)(2.72)$
$= 0.14$

for $x = -3$, $e^{-3} = 0.05$

for $x = -\infty$, $e^{-\infty} = 0$

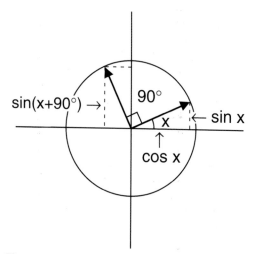

Figure 1-10. Two vectors with a phase difference of 90°. This difference demonstrates the relationship between cos (x) and sin ($x + 90°$).

If we graph e^x, we see that it is an exponentially growing function (Fig. 1-11). From this graph, we can see that the function e^x grows exponentially from $-\infty$ to $+\infty$.

Now let's consider a decaying function by drawing (e^{-x}) (Fig. 1-12):

for $x = 0$, $e^0 = 1$

for $x = 1$, $e^{-1} = 0.37$

for $x = 2$, $e^{-2} = 0.14$

for $x = 3$, $e^{-3} = 0.05$

for $x = \infty$, $e^{-\infty} = 0$

for $x = -1$, $e^{-(-1)} = e^1 = 2.72$

for $x = -2$, $e^{-(-2)} = e^2 = 7.4$

This represents an exponentially *decaying* function. Let's change x to t and look at a time-varying function e^{-t} (Fig. 1-13). This now becomes a decaying function of time. Table 1-2 shows the values of e^{-t} for various values of t.

How about a graph of $(1 - e^{-t})$?

for $t = 0$, $(1 - e^{-t}) = 1 - 1 = 0$

for $t = 1$, $(1 - e^{-t}) = 1 - 2.7^{-1}$
$= 1 - 1/2.7$
$= 1 - 0.37 = 0.63$

for $t = 2$, $(1 - e^{-t}) = 1 - (2.7)^{-2}$
$= 1 - 1/(2.7)(2.7)$
$= 1 - 0.13 = 0.86$

As t gets larger, e^{-t} gets much smaller, so that $(1 - e^{-t})$ approaches 1. Therefore, a graph of $1 - e^{-t}$ (Fig. 1-14) is the reverse of the exponential curve for e^{-t} (Fig. 1-13).

Time Constant or Decay Constant. In the graph of $(1 - e^{-t})$, the value gets close to 1 after about four to five **time constants**. Let's make the exponential function a little more complicated. Consider

$$e^{-t/\tau}$$

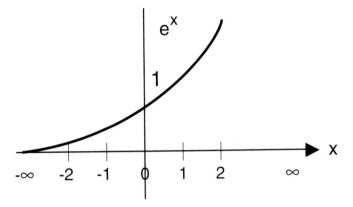

Figure 1-11. Graph of an exponentially growing function e^x.

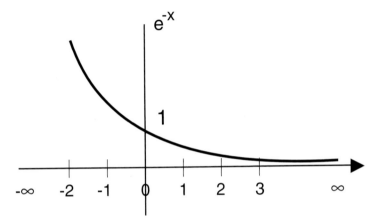

Figure 1-12. Graph of an exponentially decaying function e^{-x}.

where τ is a **time constant.** So when $t = \tau$, then

$$e^{-t/\tau} = e^{-1} = 0.37$$

If we draw a **tangent** at $t = 0$ (where the function equals 1 on the vertical axis) along the exponential decay curve $e^{-t/\tau}$, the point of intersection on the time line (i.e., the horizontal axis) is the time constant τ (Fig. 1-15). At this point, the value of $e^{-t/\tau} = e^{-1} = 0.37$ $\cong 1/3$. This means that at the time of one time constant, we have about one third of the original signal left. The other interesting thing about this decaying function is that after two time constants (2τ), we are left with one third of the signal that remained after one time constant, which is $(e^{-2}) = e^{-1} \times e^{-1} \cong 1/3 \times 1/3 = 1/9$.

The nice thing about this exponentially decaying function is that you can stop anywhere on the curve and the same equation will apply. No matter how many time constants you extend out along the decay curve, you still end up with a calculable percentage value of the original signal.

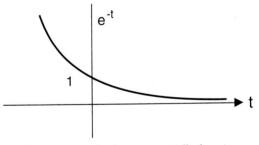

Figure 1-13. Graph of an exponentially decaying function of time e^{-t}.

Table 1-2								
t	0	1	2	3	4	5	...	∞
e^{-t}	1	.37	.14	.05	.02	.01	...	0
$1 - e^{-t}$	0	.63	.86	.95	.98	.99	...	1

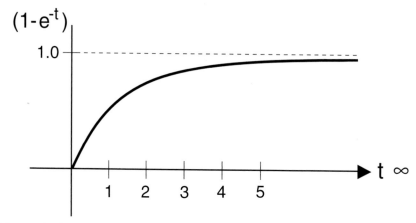

Figure 1-14. Graph of an exponentially growing function of time $1 - e^{-t}$.

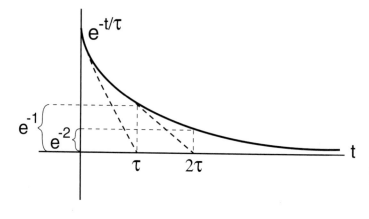

Figure 1-15. Graph of an exponentially decaying function $e^{-t/\tau}$, where τ is the time constant (decay rate).

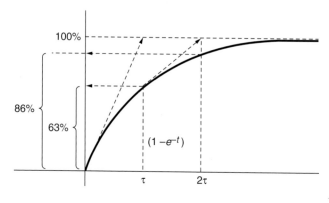

Figure 1-16. Graph of an exponentially growing function $1 - e^{-t/\tau}$, where τ is the time constant (growth rate).

On the recovery curve $(1 - e^{-t/\tau})$, things are just the opposite (Fig. 1-16). If you draw a tangent at the origin along the exponential recovery curve $(1 - e^{-t/\tau})$, the point of intersection on the maximum line corresponding to complete recovery occurs at one time constant (τ). At this point, we have recovered 63% of the original signal:

for $t = \tau$, $(1 - e^{-t/\tau}) = 1 - e^{-1} \cong 1 - 0.37$
$= 0.63$

At two time constants (2τ), we will have recovered 63% of the remaining signal, which comes to 86%.

Exponentially Decaying Sinusoidals

We've talked about a *sine* wave (sin ωt). We've also talked about an exponential function ($e^{-t/\tau}$). What happens if we multiply these functions together?

$$(e^{-t/\tau}) \cdot (\sin \omega t)$$

The first function is a decaying curve. The second function is a sinusoidal. If you multiply the two together, you'll get a graph, as in Figure 1-17. The sinusoidal function will have the same frequency but it's contained between the **"envelopes"** of the decaying exponential curve and its mirror image, causing the **magnitude** of the *sine* wave to decrease exponentially with time.

Sinc Function

There is another function that looks somewhat like Figure 1-17. It is called a *sinc* function and is expressed as (sin t)/t:

$$\sin(t)/t = \text{sinc}(t) \qquad \text{(Eqn. 1-4)}$$

Question: What is sinc t at time $t = 0$?

Answer: sinc $(0) = \sin(0)/0 = 0/0$, which is **indeterminate.** However, using the principles of differential equations and limits, it can be shown that sinc $(0) = 0/0 = 1$ (refer to Question 1-3, at the end). From here on, sinc (t) is an oscillating wave of t (Fig. 1-18). However, the envelope of this wave is not an exponential function. This is what a **Radio Frequency (RF) pulse** generally looks like. (The **frequency** or **Fourier transform [FT]**

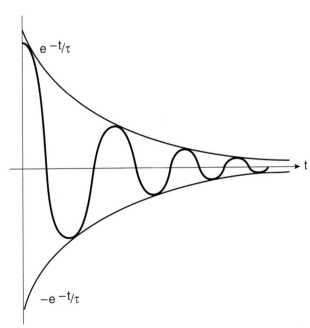

Figure 1-17. Graph of $e^{-t/\tau} \underline{x} \cos \omega t$. This is a sinusoidal with angular frequency ω whose "envelope" is given by $e^{-t/\tau}$ and $-e^{-t/\tau}$.

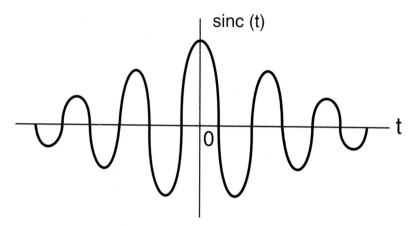

Figure 1-18. Graph of sinc $(t) = \sin(t)/t$.

of this pulse is a rectangle. More about this later.)

Having been introduced to the concepts of vectors, imaginary numbers, and exponentials, let's again go back to the vector in Figure 1-5 and introduce a new equation called **Euler's equation.** (The importance of this equation will become clear later when the concept of "spinning protons" is addressed.)

Euler's Equation

$$e^{i\theta} = \cos\theta + i\sin\theta \qquad \text{(Eqn. 1-5)}$$

This equation describes the vector that we saw in Figure 1-5 with an angle $= \theta$ and a magnitude $= 1$. The symbol i is the imaginary unit $\sqrt{-1}$.

Equation 1-5 expresses a complex exponential function of an imaginary number $(i\theta)$ in terms of the *sine* and *cosine* functions of the angle θ.

Now consider the Euler's equation for the complex signal $e^{i\omega t}$ (using ωt instead of θ):

$$e^{i\omega t} = \underbrace{\cos\omega t}_{\text{real}} + \underbrace{i\sin\omega t}_{\text{imaginary}}$$

This formula has a "real" part and an "imaginary" part. The real part (cos ωt) is what we are interested in because it corresponds to the measured signal. We use the imaginary part (sin ωt) because it makes the mathematics simpler (believe it or not!). At the end, we ignore the imaginary part and keep the real component corresponding to the actual signal.

Each value of $(e^{i\omega t})$ is a **vector** that spins around at an angular frequency of ω (Fig. 1-19). It is important to understand the concept of angular frequency because later, when we talk about proton precession, we'll see that the principle of precessional frequency (which is an angular frequency) is used frequently.

Logarithms

The logarithm (log) is sort of the inverse of an exponential, that is,

$$\log(e^x) = x$$

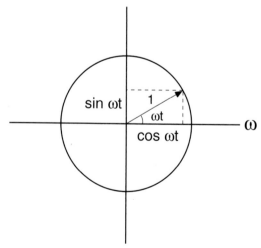

Figure 1-19. Representation of $e^{i\omega t}$ in terms of a rotating vector.

The base of log is usually 10. However, a logarithm can have any base. Let's say that the log of a number y with base a is equal to x:

$$\log_a y = x$$

Then, taking the exponential of both sides, we obtain

$$a^x = y$$

Thus,

$$\log_a y = x \Leftrightarrow a^x = y$$

That is, if the log of y with base a equals x, this implies that a to the power of x equals y.

Example

$$\log_2 8 = 3 \Rightarrow 2^3 = (2)(2)(2) = 8$$

The log of a number x to base e is also denoted as the ln of that number, or "the natural log" of x.

$$\log_e x = \ln x$$

(ln) is just the notation for log to the base e (e is the base of the natural logarithm, e = 2.71...).

$$\ln e = \log_e e = 1$$

This means log of e to its own base is 1.

Properties of Exponentials

Mathematical operations done with exponentials include (e^x is e to the power of x):

(a) Multiplying exponentials

$$(e^x) \cdot (e^y) = e^{x+y}$$

(b) Negative exponentials

$$(e^{-x}) = 1/e^x$$

(c) Dividing exponentials

$$e^x/e^y = e^{x-y}$$

Derivation
Equation (c) is derived from the first two Equations (a) and (b) in the following way: $e^x/e^y = (e^x)(e^{-y})$ derived from the statement about negative exponentials; $(e^x) \cdot (e^{-y}) = e^{x-y}$ derived from the statement about multiplying exponentials. Therefore, $e^x/e^y = (e^x)(e^{-y}) = e^{x-y}$.

Properties of Logarithms

(a) The logarithm of the product of two numbers (A and B) is equal to the sum of their logarithms.

$$\log (A \cdot B) = \log A + \log B$$

This holds for *any base*. So

$$\ln (A \cdot B) = \ln A + \ln B$$

(b) The log of x to a power a is

$$\log x^a = a \log x$$

This also holds for any base, so

$$\log_b x^a = a \log_b x$$
$$\ln x^a = a \ln x$$

Example
Let's solve the equation: $1/2 = e^{-t/T2}$ for t. (This would be the formula for finding the time t when a function [with a first-order decay constant T2] decays to half of its initial value.)

1. Take ln of both sides:

$$\ln (1/2) = \ln e^{-t/T2}$$

2. Remember that $1/2 = 2^{-1}$, so

$$\ln (1/2) = \ln (2^{-1}) = -\ln 2$$

3. Now from Equation (b)

$$\ln (e^{-t/T2}) = -t/T2 \ln (e)$$

so

$$-\ln 2 = -t/T2 \ln (e)$$

4. Remember that $\ln (e) = \log_e e = 1$ (log of a number to its own base = 1), so

$$-\ln 2 = -t/T2 \, (1) \text{ or}$$
$$-\ln 2 = -t/T2$$

5. Multiply both sides by -1:

$$\ln 2 = t/T2 \text{ or}$$
$$\log_e 2 = t/T2 \text{ or}$$
$$0.693 = t/T2 \text{ or}$$
$$t = 0.693$$

This formula also calculates the half-time (or $t_{1/2}$) in nuclear medicine.

Key Points

Understanding a few mathematical concepts will help you a great deal in understanding MRI physics.

1 Four sinusoidal functions were discussed:

$$\sin x, \cos x, \tan x, \text{cotan } x$$
$$\tan x = \sin x/\cos x$$
$$\text{cotan } x = 1/\tan x$$

2 The angle (or *arc*) on which the above sinusoidal wave is applied is defined as

arcsin, arccos, arctan, arccotan

For example,

$\arctan(\tan x) = x$, $\arcsin(\sin x) = x$, etc.

3 A *vector* possesses magnitude and direction. *Force*, for example, has magnitude (*weight*) and direction. Another example of a vector is *velocity*, which has a *speed* and a direction.

4 *Imaginary numbers* are represented by a *real* and an *imaginary* component:

$$c = a + ib$$

where i is the imaginary unit $\sqrt{-1}$.

5 A *function* f of a variable x is designated $f(x)$ and represents variations in f as x is varied.

6 A *signal* is a function of time.

7 A *periodic signal* is a function of time that repeats itself after a certain *period T*.

8 The (linear) *frequency* of a periodic signal is defined as $f = 1/T$, where T is the period.

9 The *angular frequency* ω is defined as $\omega = 2\pi f$.

10 A periodic signal over one period represents one cycle.

11 An example of a periodic signal is $\cos \omega t = \cos(2\pi f t)$.

12 *Phase* represents the offset between two periodic signals of the same frequency. For example, $\cos(\omega t)$ and $\cos(\omega t + \theta)$ have the same frequency (ω) but are *out of phase* by θ.

13 The function e^t is an *exponential* function of time. It is actually an exponentially *growing* function. It is 1 at $t = 0$ and ∞ at $t = \infty$. At $t = 1$, $e^1 = e = 2.7182818 \cong 2.72$.

14 The function e^{-t} is also an exponential function of time. It is an exponentially *decaying* function. It is 1 at $t = 0$ and 0 at $t = \infty$. At $t = 1$, $e^{-1} = 0.37$.

15 The function $e^{-t/\tau}$ is an exponentially decaying function with a *time constant* or *decay constant* τ. The value of the signal at time constant τ is 37% ($e^{-1} = 0.37$) of its previous value. The signal is practically zero after five time constants ($e^{-5} \cong 0$).

16 The function $e^{i\omega t}$ is given by *Euler's equation* as

$$e^{i\omega t} = \cos \omega t + i \sin \omega t$$

which represents a vector of radius 1 spinning at an angular frequency ω (in radians/sec).

17 The *sinc* function is defined as

$$\text{sinc } t = \sin t/t$$

which is 1 at $t = 0$. An ideal RF pulse is a sinc wave because its *Fourier transform* (as we will see later) has a perfect rectangular shape.

18 A *logarithm* (base 10) of a variable y is represented as $\log y$ and is related to an exponential as

$$\text{if } \log y = x \quad \text{then} \quad 10^x = y$$

19 The *natural logarithm* (base e) of y is designated $\ln y$. Therefore

$$\text{if } \ln y = x \quad \text{then} \quad e^x = y$$

Having understood the above mathematical concepts, the reader can now read and understand the remainder of this book with greater ease. As mentioned previously, it is not that important to memorize the formulas, but rather to understand the *concepts* behind them.

Questions

1-1 Draw the following functions versus x (from $-\infty$ to $+\infty$)

(a) $e^{-x} \cos x$ (b) $\sin x / x \equiv \mathrm{sinc}\,(x)$

1-2 Prove the following equalities

$\cos (x + y) = \cos x \cdot \cos y - \sin x \cdot \sin y$ and $\sin (x + y) = \cos x \cdot \sin y + \sin x \cdot \cos y$

Hint: Make use of the Euler equation $e^{ix} = \cos x + i \sin x$ and note that $i \times i = i^2 = -1$

1-3 It can be shown that for certain functions

$$f(0)/g(0) = \lim_{x \to 0} [\, f(x)/g(x)]$$
$$= \lim_{x \to 0} [\, f'(x)/g'(x)]$$

where f and g are functions of x and f' and g' are their derivatives, that is, $[f'(x) = d/dx \cdot f(x)]$; "lim" denotes the "limit" as x approaches 0.

Using the above fact, show that

$$\mathrm{sinc}(0) = \frac{\sin(0)}{0} = \lim_{x \to 0} \frac{\sin x}{x} = 1$$

Hint: $d/dx\,(\sin x) = \cos x$ and $d/dx\,(x^n) = n \cdot x^{n-1}$ (n = any integer)

1-4 **(a)** What is the value of an exponential function $e^{-t/T}$ at one time constant T?

(b) How about at two time constants 2T?

(c) What is the ratio of (b) to (a)?

1-5 Take the exponentially decaying function $f(t) = A \cdot e^{-t/T}$ as shown in Figure 1-20A. Prove that if a tangent is drawn at point A, it will cross the t-axis at $t = T$ (T = decay constant).

Hint: The derivative $d/dt\,(e^{\alpha t}) = \alpha \cdot e^{\alpha t}$ where α = a constant.

1-6 Solve the equation $e^x = 8$ for x. Note: ln 2 = 0.693.

1-7 What is (a) sin (0°); (b) sin (30°); (c) sin (90°); (d) sin (180°); (e) cos (0°); (f) cos (60°); (g) cos (90°); (h) cos (180°)?

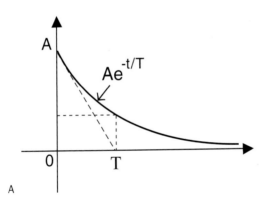

A

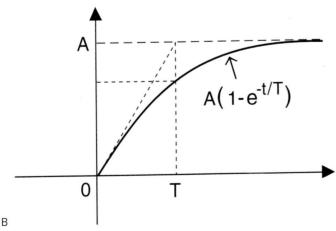

B

Figure 1-20. A–B

Basic Principles of MRI

Introduction

In this chapter, we will discuss the basic principles behind the physics of *magnetic resonance imaging* (MRI). Some of these principles are explained using **Newtonian physics,** and some using **quantum mechanics,** whichever can convey the message more clearly. Although this might be confusing at times, it seems to be unavoidable. In any case, we'll try to keep it straightforward.

Nuclear magnetic resonance (NMR) is a chemical analytical technique that has been used for over 50 years. It is the basis for the imaging technique we now call MRI. (The word *nuclear* had the false connotation of the use of nuclear material; thus, it was discarded from the MR lexicon, and "NMR tomography" was replaced by the phrase *magnetic resonance imaging* [MRI].)

Electromagnetic Waves

To understand MRI, we first need to understand what an electromagnetic wave is. Table 2-1 demonstrates the characteristics of a variety of electromagnetic waves, including X-ray, visible light, microwaves, and radio waves. All electromagnetic waves have certain fundamental properties in common:

1. They all travel at the speed of light $c = 3 \times 10^8$ m/sec in a vacuum.
2. By Maxwell's wave theory, they all have two components—an electric field E and

Table 2-1 The Electromagnetic Spectrum Illustrating the Windows for Radio waves, Microwaves, Visible Light, and X-Rays

	Frequency (Hz)	Energy (eV)	Wavelength (m)
Gamma rays and X-rays	10^{24}	10^{10}	10^{-16}
	10^{23}	10^{9}	10^{-15}
	10^{22}	10^{8}	10^{-14}
	10^{21}	10^{7}	10^{-13}
	10^{20}	10^{6} (1 MeV)	10^{-12} (1 pm)
	10^{19}	10^{5}	10^{-11}
	10^{18}	10^{4}	10^{-10}
Ultraviolet	10^{17}	10^{3} (1 keV)	10^{-9} (1 nm)
	10^{16}	10^{2}	10^{-8}
Visible light	10^{15}	10^{1}	10^{-7}
Infrared	10^{14}	10^{0} (1 eV)	10^{-6} (1 μm)
	10^{13}	10^{-1}	10^{-5}

Table 2-1 (*continued*)

Microwaves	10^{12}	10^{-2}	10^{-4}
	10^{11}	10^{-3}	10^{-3} (1 mm)
	10^{10}	10^{-4}	10^{-2} (1 cm)
	10^{9} (1 GHz)	10^{-5}	10^{-1}
MRI	10^{8} (100 MHz)	10^{-6}	10^{0} (1 m)
	10^{7}	10^{-7}	10^{1}
Radio waves	10^{6} (1 MHz)	10^{-8}	10^{2}
	10^{5}	10^{-9}	10^{3} (1 km)
	10^{4}	10^{-10}	10^{4}
	10^{3} (1 kHz)	10^{-11}	10^{5}
	10^{2}	10^{-12}	10^{6}

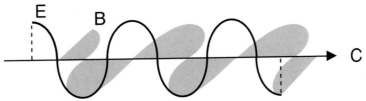

Figure 2-1. Two components of an electromagnetic wave, the electric component E and the magnetic component B. These two components are perpendicular to each other, are 90° out of phase, and travel at the speed of light (c).

a magnetic field B—that are perpendicular to each other (Fig. 2-1). We will designate the sinusoidal wave, which is drawn in the plane of the paper, the electrical field E. Perpendicular to it is another sinusoidal wave, the magnetic field B. They are perpendicular to each other and both are traveling at the speed of light (c). The electric and magnetic fields have the same frequency and are 90° out of phase with each other. (This is because the change in the electric field generates the magnetic field, and the change in the magnetic field generates the electric field. For this reason, electromagnetic waves are self-propagating once started and continue out to infinity.)

3. If we think in terms of vectors, the vectors **B** and **E** are perpendicular to each other, and the propagation factor C is perpendicular to both (Fig. 2-2). Both the electrical and magnetic components have the same frequency ω. So what we get is a vector that is spinning (oscillating) around a point at angular frequency ω. Remember,

the angular frequency ω is related to the linear frequency f:

$$\omega = 2\pi f$$

4. We are interested in the magnetic field component—the electric field component is undesirable because it generates heat.

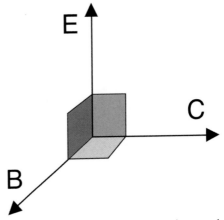

Figure 2-2. The vector representation of **B**, **E**, and **C**.

Table 2-2

	Frequency	Energy	Wave Length
X-ray	$1.7–3.6 \times 10^{18}$ Hz	30–150 keV	80–400 pm
Visible light (violet)	7.5×10^{14} Hz	3.1 eV	400 nm
Visible light (red)	4.3×10^{14} Hz	1.8 eV	700 nm
MRI	3–100 MHz	20–200 MeV	3–100 m

Table 2-3

AM radio frequency	0.54–1.6 MHz
	(540–1600 kHz)
TV (Channel 2)	Slightly over 64 MHz
FM radio frequency	88.8–108.8 MHz
RF used in MRI	3–100 MHz

Table 2-2 summarizes the important electromagnetic windows in nature. In this table, the following notations are used:

$$keV = 10^3 \, eV = \text{kilo-electron-volts}$$
$$pm = 10^{-12} \, m = \text{picometer}$$
$$nm = 10^{-9} \, m = \text{nanometer}$$
$$MHz = 10^6 \, Hz = \text{megahertz}$$
$$MeV = 10^{-3} \, eV = \text{million electron volts}$$

In MRI, we deal with much lower energies than X-ray or even visible light. We also deal with much lower frequencies. (The energy of an electromagnetic wave is directly proportional to its frequency, $E = hv$.) The wave lengths are also much longer in the radio frequency (RF)

window. Table 2-3 contains a few examples of frequency ranges in the electromagnetic spectrum.

This is why the electromagnetic pulse used in MRI to get a signal is called an RF pulse—it is in the **RF** range. It belongs to the RF *window* of the electromagnetic spectrum.

Spins and Electromagnetic Field

One of the pioneers of NMR theory was Felix Bloch of Stanford University, who won the Nobel Prize in 1946 for his theories. He theorized that any **spinning charged particle** (like the hydrogen nucleus) creates an **electromagnetic field** (Fig. 2-3). The magnetic component of this field causes certain nuclei to act like a **bar magnet,** that is, a magnetic field emanating from the south pole to the north pole (Fig. 2-4).

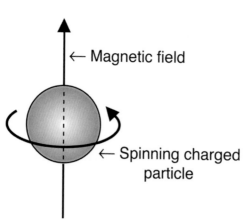

Figure 2-3. A spinning charged particle generates a magnetic field.

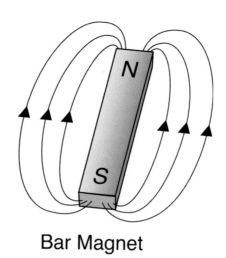

Bar Magnet

Figure 2-4. A bar magnet with its associated magnetic field.

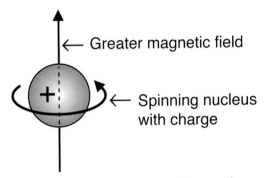

Figure 2-5. A spinning charged hydrogen nucleus (i.e., a proton) generating a magnetic field.

In MRI, we are interested in **charged nuclei,** like the **hydrogen nucleus,** which is a single, positively charged proton (Fig. 2-5).

The other thing that we know from quantum theory is that atomic nuclei each have specific **energy levels** related to a property called **spin quantum number S.** For example, the hydrogen nucleus (a single proton) has a spin quantum number **S** of 1/2:

$$S(^{1}H) = 1/2$$

The number of energy states of a nucleus is determined by the formula:

$$\text{Number of energy states} = 2S + 1$$

For a proton with a spin $S = 1/2$, we have

$$\text{Number of energy states} = 2 \, (1/2) + 1$$
$$= 1 + 1 = 2$$

Therefore, a hydrogen proton has two energy states denoted as $-1/2$ and $+1/2$. This means that the hydrogen protons are spinning about their axis and creating a magnetic field. Some hydrogen protons spin the opposite way and have a magnetic field in just the opposite direction. The pictorial representation of the direction of proton spins in Figure 2-6 represents the two energy states of the hydrogen proton. Each one of these directions of spin has a different energy state.

Other nuclei have different numbers of energy states. For example,

$$^{13}Na \text{ has a spin } S = 3/2$$
$$\text{Number of energy states of } ^{13}Na = 2 \, (3/2) + 1$$
$$= 4$$

The four energy states of ^{13}Na are denoted as $(-3/2, -1/2, 1/2, 3/2)$.

The important fact about all this is that in the hydrogen proton, we have one proton with two energy states that are aligned in opposite directions, one pointing north (parallel), and the other pointing south (antiparallel). (If there were an **even** number of protons in the nucleus, then every proton would be *paired*: for every proton spin with magnetic field pointing up, we'd have a paired proton spin with magnetic field pointing down (Fig. 2-7). The magnetic fields of these paired protons would then cancel each other out, and the net magnetic field would be zero.) When there are an **odd** number of protons, then there always

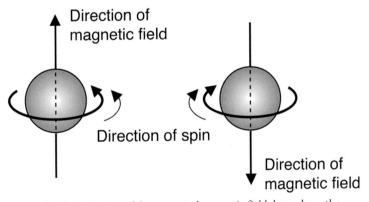

Figure 2-6. The direction of the generated magnetic field depends on the direction of rotation of the spinning protons.

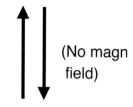

(No magn field)

Paired protons

Figure 2-7. The magnetic fields of paired protons (rotating in opposite directions) cancel each other out, leaving no net magnetic field.

Table 2-4

Nucleus	Spin Quantum Number (S)	Gyromagnetic Ratio (MHz/T)
^{1}H	1/2	42.6
^{19}F	1/2	40.0
^{23}Na	3/2	11.3
^{13}C	1/2	10.7
^{17}O	5/2	5.8

spins of all the other nuclei with odd numbers of protons.

Magnetic Susceptibility

All substances get magnetized to a degree when placed in a magnetic field. However, the degree of magnetization varies. The **magnetic susceptibility** of a substance (denoted by the Greek symbol χ) is a measure of *how* magnetized they get. In other words, χ is the measure of magnetizability of a substance.

exists one proton that is *unpaired*. That proton is pointing either north or south and gives a net magnetic field (Fig. 2-8) or a **magnetic dipole moment** (MDM) to the nucleus. Actually, an MDM is found in any nucleus with an *odd* number of protons, neutrons, or both. **Dipole–dipole interactions** refer to interactions between two protons or between a proton and an electron.

The nuclei of certain elements, such as hydrogen (^{1}H) and fluorine (^{19}F), have these properties (Table 2-4). Every one of these nuclei with an **odd** number of protons or neutrons can be used for imaging in MR. However, there is a reason why we stay with hydrogen. We use *hydrogen* for imaging because of its *abundance*. Approximately 60% of the body is *water*. We find hydrogen protons (^{1}H), for example, in water (H_2O) and fat ($-CH_2-$). Later on we'll find out how we use the spin of the hydrogen proton and avoid the

To develop a mathematical relationship between the applied and induced magnetic fields, we first need to address the confusing issue regarding the differences between the two symbols encountered when dealing with magnetic fields: B and H. We caution the reader that the following discussion is merely a simplification; an advanced physics textbook will have details on the theory of electromagnetism. The field B is referred to as the **magnetic induction field** or **magnetic flux density,** which is the net magnetic field effect caused by an external magnetic field. The field H is referred to as the **magnetic field intensity.** These two magnetic fields are related by the following:

$$B = \mu H \quad \text{or} \quad \mu = B/H$$

where μ represents the **magnetic permeability,** which is the ability of a substance to concentrate magnetic fields. The magnetic susceptibility χ is defined as the ratio of the induced magnetic field (M) to the applied magnetic field H:

$$M = \chi H \quad \text{or} \quad \chi = M/H$$

Furthermore, χ and μ are related by the following:

$$\mu = 1 + \chi$$

making sure that the units used are consistent.

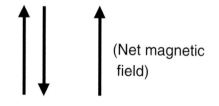

(Net magnetic field)

Unpaired protons

Figure 2-8. Unpaired protons yield a net magnetic field.

Three types of substances—each with a different magnetic susceptibility—are commonly dealt with in MRI: paramagnetic, diamagnetic, and ferromagnetic. These are described below.

Paramagnetism, Diamagnetism, and Ferromagnetism.

1. **Diamagnetic** substances have no unpaired orbital electrons. When such a substance is placed in an external magnetic field B_0, a weak magnetic field (M) is induced in the *opposite* direction to B_0. As a result, the effective magnetic field is *reduced*. Thus, diamagnetic substances have a small, negative magnetic susceptibility χ (i.e., $\chi < 0$ and $\mu < 1$). They are basically nonmagnetic. The vast majority of tissues in the body have this property. An example of diamagnetic effect is the distortion that occurs at an air–tissue interface (such as around paranasal sinuses).

2. **Paramagnetic** substances have unpaired orbital electrons. They become magnetized while the external magnetic field B_0 is on and become demagnetized once the field has been turned off. Their induced magnetic field (M) is in the *same* direction as the external magnetic field. Consequently, their presence causes an *increase* in the effective magnetic field. They, therefore, have a small positive χ (i.e., $\chi > 0$ and $\mu > 1$) and are weakly attracted by the external magnetic field. In such substances, **dipole–dipole** (i.e., proton–proton and proton–electron) interactions cause T1 shortening (bright signal on T1-weighted images). The element in the periodic table with the greatest number of unpaired electrons is the rare earth element **gadolinium** (Gd) with seven unpaired electrons, which is a strong paramagnetic substance. Gd is a member of the **lanthanide** group in the periodic table. The rare earth element **dysprosium** (Dy) is another strong paramagnetic substance that belongs to this group. Certain breakdown products of hemoglobin are paramagnetic: deoxyhemoglobin has four unpaired electrons, and methemoglobin has five. Hemosiderin, the end stage of hemorrhage, contains, in comparison, more than 10,000 unpaired electrons. Hemosiderin belongs to a group of substances referred to as **superparamagnetic,** which have magnetic susceptibilities 100 to 1000 times stronger than paramagnetic substances.

3. **Ferromagnetic** substances are strongly attracted by a magnetic field. They become *permanently* magnetized even after the magnetic field has been turned off. They have a large positive χ, even larger than that of superparamagnetic substances. Three types of ferromagnets are known: iron (Fe), cobalt (Co), and nickel (Ni). Examples include aneurysm clips and shrapnel.

As stated earlier, most tissues in the body are diamagnetic. For example, bulk water is diamagnetic. This may be surprising to hear because the protons that make up the water are the basis for NMR. It is true that the individual protons in a water molecule exhibit a magnetic moment (referred to as a **nuclear magnetic moment** or **nuclear paramagnetism**), but bulk water is diamagnetic, and its net induced magnetization is in the direction opposite to the main magnetic field. This has to do with the fact that NMR depends on nuclei (protons and neutrons), whereas bulk magnetism depends on electrons.

How Do We Actually Perform MR Imaging?

Let's review a few examples of different types of imaging.

(a) In **photography,** there is an object and a light source that emits light. The light is reflected off the object and is then received by a photographic plate within a camera (Fig. 2-9). This, of course, is utilization of the visible light window of the electromagnetic spectrum. Visible light does not penetrate the object, but instead is reflected off of it.

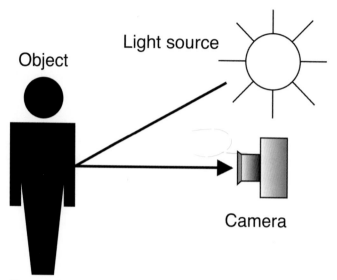

Figure 2-9. In photography, light is reflected off the object and is received by a photographic plate in a camera.

(b) In **X-ray** imaging, we have an X-ray source that emits radiation that penetrates the object. This penetrating radiation is then received by a photographic (X-ray) plate (Fig. 2-10).

(c) In **MRI,** low-frequency radio waves penetrate the tissue and reflect back off magnetized spins within the object (Fig. 2-11).

RF and MR Signal. If spinning, unpaired protons are placed in an external magnetic field, they will line up with that magnetic field.

If an RF wave of a very specific frequency is then sent into the patient, some spins will change their alignment as a result of this new magnetic field. After the RF pulse, they generate a signal as they return to their original alignment. This is the MR signal that we measure (Fig 2-12).

Spatial Encoding. If we generate a signal from the entire body, how do we differentiate whether the signal is coming from the head or the foot of the patient? This is the process of **spatial encoding,** which is used to create an image.

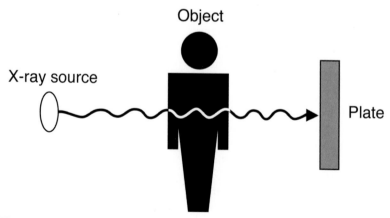

Figure 2-10. In X-ray, radiation penetrates the object and reaches a photographic plate behind the object.

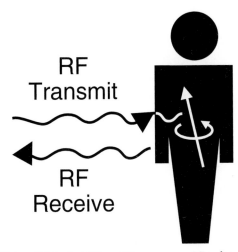

Figure 2-11. In MRI, an RF wave, or an RF pulse, is transmitted into the patient, and a signal is received from magnetized spins (protons) in the body.

It requires the use of gradient coils, which will be discussed later in this chapter.

B_0 **Field.** The external magnetic field is denoted B_0. In MRI, B_0 is on the order of 1 Tesla (1 T). One Tesla is equal to 10,000 Gauss. To appreciate the strength of this field, the earth's magnetic field, in comparison, is only about 0.5 Gauss (30,000 times weaker than a 1.5-T scanner!). This field is not uniform in reality. These nonuniformities are usually caused by improper shimming or environmental distortions. The required standard for magnetic uniformity is on the order of 6 to 7 ppm (parts per million). Proper **shim coils** (see later text) can help minimize this problem.

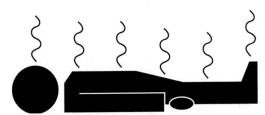

Figure 2-12. After the RF pulse, spins in the patient generate a signal, which can be measured by a receiver.

Types of Magnets

First of all, magnets can be categorized in terms of their field strength; five types exist:

1. Ultrahigh field (4.0 to 7.0 T); mainly used for research
2. High field (1.5 to 3.0 T)
3. Midfield (0.5 to 1.4 T)
4. Low field (0.2 to 0.4 T)
5. Ultralow field (<0.2 T)

Next, we can categorize magnets in terms of their design; three main types exist:

1. Permanent magnets
2. Resistive magnets
3. Superconducting magnets

1. **Permanent magnets** (mainly seen with OPEN MRI scanners such as Hitachi AIRIS) always stay on and cannot be turned off. They have the advantage of lower cost and lower maintenance (they require no cryogens for cooling).
2. **Resistive magnets** (such as the 0.23 T Philips Panorama and the Fonar 0.6 T Standup) are based on the electromagnetic principle that electric current running through a coil produces a magnetic field. These magnets can be turned off and on.
3. **Superconducting magnets** are a form of electromagnets. These magnets operate near absolute zero temperature (e.g., 4.2 K or −270°C). Consequently, there would be almost no resistance in their wires. This, in turn, allows us to use very strong electric currents to generate a high magnetic field without generating significant heat (hence the name superconducting). To achieve these ultralow temperatures, cryogens (such as liquid nitrogen and/or liquid helium) are required (which are very expensive). Most of the scanners available today are superconducting magnets.

Magnetic Dipole Moment

From now on, we will just talk about protons of hydrogen nuclei. We won't discuss any other nuclei. Let's take a number of protons. They all

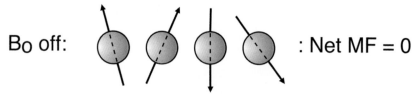

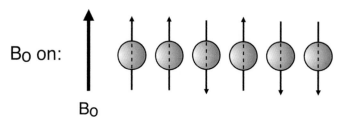

Figure 2-13. In the absence of an external magnetic field B_0, net magnetization is produced.

Figure 2-14. In the presence of an external magnetic field B_0, net magnetization is produced.

have their own small magnetic fields and they are all spinning about their own axes. Each one of the magnetic fields is called an MDM and is denoted by the symbol μ. The axes of the MDMs are arranged in a random way, and they all cancel each other out. If we add up all the dipole moments, the **net** magnetic field will be zero (Fig. 2-13). This result occurs in the absence of any external magnetic field (B_0).

What happens if we turn on an external magnetic field? What would happen to the proton spins? They will act like bar magnets and line themselves up with the large magnetic field, much like compass needles in the earth's magnetic field (Fig. 2-14). However, they don't all line up in the same direction. Approximately half point north and half point south. Eventually, enough extra spins point north (about one in a million[1]) to make the net magnetization point in the direction of B_0.

Let's examine how this happens. At time $t = 0$, proton spins are distributed randomly and the net magnetic field at $t = 0$ is zero. Immediately after being placed in a magnetic field, half the spins are lined up in the direction of the magnetic field and half are lined up in the reverse

direction. Over time, more spins line up in the direction of the magnetic field, creating net magnetization (Fig. 2-15). If we graph the net magnetization versus time, it will look like the curve in Figure 2-16. This increase in magnetization follows an *exponentially growing* curve that we talked about earlier (see Chapter 1). The time constant of this curve depends on the following:

1. The kind of tissue we are imaging
2. The strength of the magnet

T1 Relaxation Time

The time constant of the curve in Figure 2-16 is denoted T1. Therefore, the growth of magnetization M occurs with a time constant T1

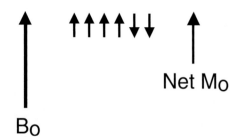

Figure 2.15. Vector representation of net magnetization M_0 a certain amount of time after introduction of the external magnetic field B_0.

---

[1]This number might appear insignificant. However, according to Avogadro's law, there are over 10^{23} molecules per gram of tissue. Thus, in each gram of tissue, there will be 10^{17} (i.e., $10^{23}/10^6$) excess hydrogen protons pointing north.

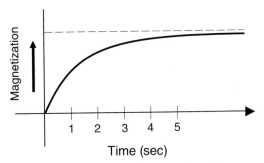

Figure 2-16. The graphic representation of net magnetization over time, which turns out to be an exponential function.

described by the expression $1 - e^{-t/T1}$. Usually, when we talk about T1, we're talking about **recovery** of magnetization along the axis of the B_0 field. As time goes by, more and more spins are going to line up with the external magnetic field. The net magnetization keeps growing exponentially until it reaches a limit (Fig. 2-17). Remember how with an exponential growth curve we would draw a tangent at the beginning of the curve to establish T1, and then we would draw a tangent from the curve at that time to establish 2 T1? After about four or five T1 times, we almost reach the plateau of the exponential growth curve.

If we were to change the *strength* of the magnetic field, what would happen to T1? If B_0 decreases, the T1 of the tissue also decreases:

$$\downarrow B_0 \rightarrow \downarrow T1$$

For instance, biologic tissues have shorter T1 values at 0.5 T than at 1.5 T.

Proton (Spin) Density

Magnetization also depends on the *density* of the protons (or **spins**), that is, how many protons per unit volume there are in the tissue. Certain tissues have more protons per unit volume than other tissues. For example, air doesn't have a large number of protons in it, so it has a very small **proton density (spin density)**. We denote proton density or spin density by $N(H)$. It isn't just the *absolute number* of protons in the tissue that's important; it is also the number of protons that are **mobile** enough to be able to change direction and line up with the external magnetic field.

$$N(H) = \text{density of } \textbf{mobile protons}$$

The **net magnetization** at a particular time is based both on the T1 of the tissue and on the mobile proton density:

$$\text{Magnetization} \propto N(H)(1 - e^{-t/T1})$$

If we redraw the T1 growth curve, the x-axis would be time, and the y-axis would be

$$M = N(H)(1 - e^{-t/T1})$$

Precession

When a proton is placed in a large magnetic field, it begins to "wobble" or **precess**. When we take a single proton spinning about its axis, but

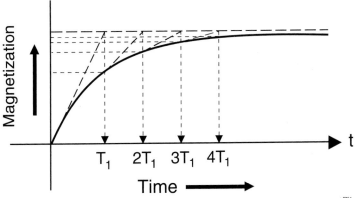

Figure 2-17. Net magnetization is described by the recovery curve $1 - e^{-t/T1}$, where T1 is the time constant (recovery rate).

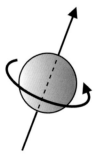

Figure 2-18. In the absence of an external magnetic field B_0, a proton rotating about its own axis generates a magnetic field.

not in an external magnetic field, it will generate its own small magnetic field (Fig. 2-18). When we turn the external magnetic field *on*, the proton behaves like a spinning top, which not only spins about its own axis but also **wobbles** about the vertical axis as a result of gravity (Fig. 2-19). The proton, likewise, not only spins about its own axis, but also rotates or "precesses" about the axis of the external magnetic field (B_0).

Each proton spins much faster about its own axis than it rotates or precesses around the axis of the external magnetic field.

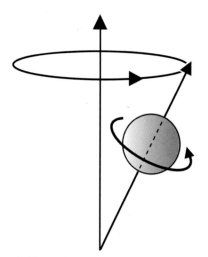

Figure 2-19. In the presence of an external magnetic field B_0, a proton not only rotates about its own axis but also "wobbles" about the axis of B_0.

Larmor Equation

The rate at which the proton precesses around the external magnetic field is given by an equation called the **Larmor equation:**

$$\omega = \gamma B_0 \qquad \text{(Eqn. 2-1)}$$

where ω is the angular precessional frequency of proton, γ the gyromagnetic ratio, and B_0 the strength of external magnetic field.

The angular frequency ω can be expressed in Hertz (Hz) or radians per second, depending on the units used for γ. If γ is in terms of MHz/T, then ω (or, actually, the linear frequency f) is expressed in terms of MHz. The gyromagnetic ratio γ is a proportionality constant that is fixed for the nucleus with which we're dealing. For hydrogen protons, $\gamma(H) = 42.6$ MHz/T.

Example

If the magnetic field strength is 1 T, the precessional frequency of hydrogen is

$$(42.6)(1) = 42.6 \text{ MHz}$$

As the external magnetic field strength increases, the precessional frequency of the hydrogen proton also increases, that is, at 1.5 T the precessional frequency of hydrogen is

$$(42.6)(1.5) = 64 \text{ MHz}$$

Remember that MRI involves the RF portion of the electromagnetic spectrum, in the range of 3 to 100 MHz. This range is caused by the precessional frequency ranges of the hydrogen protons for the magnetic field strengths we use clinically, that is,

$$\text{for } B_0 \text{ from } 0.2 \text{ T} \rightarrow 3\text{T,}$$
$$\omega = 8.5 \text{ MHz} \rightarrow 128 \text{ MHz}$$

Coils

A coil is an electrical device generally composed of multiple loops of wire (Fig. 2-20) that can either generate a magnetic field (**gradient coil**) or detect a changing (oscillating) magnetic field as an electric current induced in the wire (**RF coil**). Several types of coils are used in MRI, including the following:

1. Gradient coils
   (a) Imaging gradient coil
   (b) Shim coil

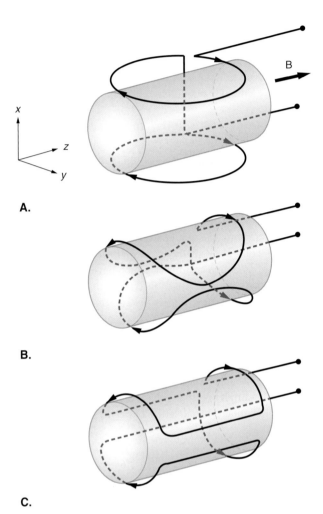

A.

B.

C.

Figure 2-20. A: "Ideal" loops of coils positioned perpendicular to changing transverse magnetization rotating in x–y plane. This changing magnetization induces a voltage in the coils, which causes current to flow (*arrows*). **B and C:** Loops of coils gradually molded to fit inside bore of magnet while retaining sensitivity to changing transverse magnetization.

2. Transmit and/or receive RF coils
    (a) Single phase or quadrature (receive or transmit)
    (b) Surface or volume (Helmholtz or solenoid)
    (c) Single or phased array

Transmit/Receive Coil. A transmitter coil sends or transmits an RF pulse. A receiver coil receives an RF pulse. Some coils are both transmitters and receivers (such as body coils and head coils). Others are just receivers (e.g., surface coils). These coils act in much the same way as do radio or television antennas.

The body coil is a fixed part of the magnet that surrounds the patient and is used in a variety of applications as a transmitter and/or receiver. A head coil is a helmetlike device that surrounds

the patient's head and may act as both a transmitter and receiver or just as a receiver. There are a variety of surface coils (e.g., coils used in imaging the joints) that serve as receivers, with the body coil employed as the transmitter. Even when a surface coil is placed over the area of interest, the received signals come from the entire body (this situation again differs from computed tomography [CT] imaging); however, the signals received in the region of the surface coil have a higher magnitude, that is, a higher signal-to-noise ratio (SNR). In other words, surface coils improve SNR in the region of interest.

Gradient Coils. Gradient coils cause an intentional *perturbation* in the magnetic field homogeneity (usually in a linear fashion), which allows one to decipher *spatial information* from the

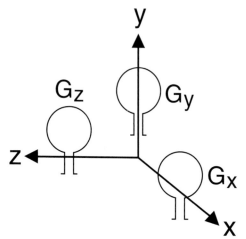

Figure 2-21. The gradient coils exist in MRI, one along each direction (x, y, and z).

received signal and localize it in space. This perturbation or variation in magnetic field is several orders of magnitude smaller than the external magnetic field but is significant enough to allow spatial encoding. To achieve this, three orthogonal gradient coils are used (Fig. 2-21) corresponding to the axes x, y, and z in a three-dimensional coordinate system. This then allows encoding (or deciphering) of data in three coordinates. These gradients are referred to as

1. The **slice-select** gradient
2. The **phase-encoding** gradient
3. The **frequency-encoding** or **readout** gradient

For an axial image, these would correspond to G_z, G_y, and G_x, respectively. They are discussed at length in chapters to come.

Shim Coils. These coils are used to create a more uniform external magnetic field B_0. Keep in

mind that inhomogeneities in the external field are undesirable and can cause artifacts, especially when a gradient-echo or a chemical fat suppression technique is used. Shim coils help to minimize (although not totally eliminate) such variations.

Quadrature Coils. In quadrature coil design, two receivers are present 90° to one another, capable of distinguishing *real* and *imaginary* components of the received signal. This design can increase the SNR by a factor of $\sqrt{2}$.

Solenoid Coils. These coils can be wrapped around the patient and increase SNR. These coils are usually used in lower field magnets (e.g., open scanners), which have a vertical magnetic field orientation (rather than a horizontal orientation in higher field scanners).

Phased-Array Coils. These coils contain multiple small surface coils that are positioned on either side of the anatomy of interest. These coils allow faster scanning with finer details. An example is the pelvic array coil that allows exquisite visualization of pelvic structures.

Plane of Imaging

Selection of the gradient coils along x-, y-, or z-axis is arbitrary. Imaging in different (axial, sagittal, coronal, or oblique) planes in MRI is different from CT and is possible simply by appropriate assignment of the gradient coils while the patient is always positioned in the magnet with his or her long axis along the long axis of the scanner (Fig. 2-22). For instance, assuming the z-axis to be along the long axis of the magnet in the craniocaudal (CC) direction, the y-axis to be in the posteroanterior (PA) direction, and the x-axis to be from right to left

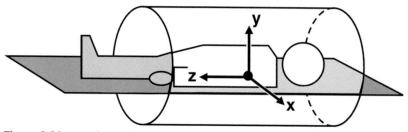

Figure 2-22. An arbitrary designation of x, y, and z for a patient in the scanner.

(R–L),[2] then axial images are obtained by allowing the slice-select gradient to be along the z-axis. The possibilities are summarized in Table 2-5. **Oblique** planes are obtained by combining the previously mentioned gradients in a linear fashion.

Table 2-5			
	Slice-Select Gradient	Phase-Encoding Gradient	Frequency-Encoding Gradient
Axial	z	y	x
Sagittal	x	y	z
Coronal	y	x	z

---

[2]This is in fact the convention used throughout this book for simplicity.

Key Points

In this chapter, we have discussed the basic principles behind MR. We have talked about electromagnetic waves, proton spins, external magnetic fields, and longitudinal magnetization. We briefly introduced the parameter T1 that is an inherent property of a tissue. Let's summarize:

1 Electromagnetic waves (as the name applies) have two components: an electric component (E) and a magnetic component (H or B). These two components are perpendicular to each other and 90° out of phase.

2 The propagation component C is perpendicular to both the E and B components, all traveling at the speed of light ($c = 3 \times 10^8$ m/sec).

3 In MRI, it is the magnetic component that interests us. The electric component merely generates heat.

4 Electromagnetic waves are periodic functions of time, oscillating at a frequency of

$$\omega = 2\pi f$$

where ω is the angular frequency (in radians per second) and f is the linear frequency (in cycles per second or Hz).

5 Many types of electromagnetic waves exist throughout the electromagnetic spectrum: X-rays, visible light, microwaves, radiofrequencies, and so on.

6 The frequencies used in MRI fall in the RF range (3 to 100 MHz). They are therefore called RF pulses.

7 Spinning charged particles generate an electromagnetic field.

8 An example of the previous point in the body is the hydrogen proton (^{1}H).

9 The magnetic components of hydrogen protons behave like bar magnets. This behavior is referred to as a magnetic dipole moment (MDM).

10 In general, all particles with an *odd* number of electrons in their covalent orbit have this property (i.e., they can generate a magnetic field).

11 Although many different protons exist in the body, hydrogen protons are dealt with in MRI because they are the most prevalent in the body (particularly in H_2O, which comprises 60% of the body).

12 The main magnetic field in MRI is denoted B_0.

13 When a patient is placed in a magnetic field B_0, some of the protons are aligned parallel to B_0 and some antiparallel to it, but more are parallel than antiparallel, producing a net magnetization (longitudinal magnetization).

14 These protons also oscillate or *precess* about the axis of the external magnetic field.

15 The frequency of precession of protons is described by the *Larmor equation*

$$\omega_0 = \gamma B_0$$

where γ is the gyromagnetic ratio (in MHz/T). Therefore, the stronger the magnetic field, the faster the protons precess about it.

16 Magnetic susceptibility refers to the ability of a substance to get magnetized when placed in a magnetic field.

17 Three types of substances with different magnetic susceptibility effects were discussed: diamagnetic, paramagnetic, and ferromagnetic.

18 There are five types of magnets based on field strength: ultralow field, low field, midfield, high field, and ultrahigh field.

19 There are three types of magnets based on design: permanent magnets, resistive magnets, and superconducting magnets.

20 Most existing scanners are high-field, superconducting magnets (these require liquid cryogens like liquid helium and nitrogen for cooling).

21 Most "open"-type MR scanners are permanent or resistive magnets; they require no cryogens and thus have low maintenance. However, they usually have lower field strengths and thus generate less signal.

22 To create an image, RF pulses are transmitted into the patient. These pulses flip the longitudinal magnetization and generate a signal from the patient.

23 RF pulses flip the longitudinal magnetization M_z away from the z-axis: 90° pulses flip M_z by 90°; 180° pulses by 180°; and partial RF pulses by α, which is less than 90°.

24 The received signal has no spatial information. Three types of gradient coils (slice-select, readout or frequency-encoding, and phase-encoding gradients) are employed for the purpose of spatial discrimination.

25 Different types of coils are used: body coil, head coil, and surface coil.

26 Surface coils are used for smaller body parts (e.g., joints) to increase the signal and reduce the noise (thus increasing the signal-to-noise ratio).

27 The rate at which the longitudinal magnetization recovers from the transverse plane (after having been flipped by a 90° pulse) is given by the time parameter T1. This parameter also describes the rate at which protons are magnetized when they are placed in an external magnetic field.

28 The equation for this recovery at any time t is given by

$$1 - e^{-t/T1}$$

which is an exponential growth curve.

What do we need to create an image from the information received from the patient? This process is initiated by the use of an RF pulse and is discussed in the next chapter.

Questions

2-1 Calculate the Larmor frequency of a proton at the following magnetic field strengths:

(a) 0.35 T   **(b)** 0.5 T   **(c)** 1 T
(d) 1.5 T   **(e)** 2 T   **(f)** 3 T

(the gyromagnetic ratio, γ, of a proton $\cong$ 42.6 MHz/T).

2-2 T/F The rate at which protons are magnetized when placed in a magnetic environment is the same as the rate of recovery of longitudinal magnetization.

2-3 T/F Proton density represents the density of *all* the protons in the tissue.

2-4 T/F When placed in a magnetic field, protons will line up with that field immediately.

2-5 T/F The T1 of a tissue is larger at a stronger magnetic field environment.

2-6 T/F Electromagnetic waves travel at the speed of sound.

2-7 T/F The main purpose of x, y, and z gradients is for slice selection and spatial encoding.

2-8 T/F The rate at which protons precess about the main magnetic field is faster than that about their own axes.

2-9 T/F When placed in a magnetic field, *all* the protons in the body will line up with the field.

2-10 T/F Hydrogen protons are used in MRI because of their abundance.

2-11 T/F In MRI, the imaging plane is determined by proper assignment of the x, y, and z gradients.

Radio Frequency Pulse

Introduction

In the last chapter, we discussed the concept of longitudinal magnetization. However, we have not yet addressed the issue of receiving a signal from the patient. We can only transmit and receive signals that oscillate (like an AC voltage). In addition, we're only sensitive to oscillations along certain axes. Because the longitudinal magnetization is *not* an oscillating function (like a DC voltage), it cannot be read by a receiver. In addition, we're not sensitive to oscillations along the z-axis. Consequently, this magnetization needs to be "flipped" into the transverse x–y plane (where it can oscillate or "precess" about the z-axis) to generate a readable signal. This is the purpose of the radio frequency (RF) pulse.

RF Pulse

Suppose that a patient is in the magnet. Then we transmit an **RF pulse.** What happens? Remember that an **RF pulse** is an **electromagnetic wave.** Initially, all the spins are lined up along the axis of the external magnetic field B_0 about which they are precessing (Fig. 3-1). Then we transmit an RF pulse. In a three-dimensional (x, y, z) coordinate

system, the direction of the external magnetic field always points in the z direction. Thus, the net magnetization vector M_0 will also point in the z direction (Fig. 3-2).

One point of clarification about the **magnetization vector M_0**: even though all of the individual spins are precessing around the external magnetic field axis, the **net magnetization** (which is made up of the *vector sum* of all the individual spins) does *not* precess. The reason for this is that all the individual spins are precessing, but they are all *out of phase* with each other. Therefore, if we add them all up, they'll have a large component along the z-axis; however, because of their phase differences, they all cancel each other out and are left with no component along the x- or y-axis (Fig. 3-3). (Note that in Fig. 3-3B, while the two protons are precessing at the same rate, one is pointing toward the right and the other is pointing toward the left.) Thus, the *net vector* of *magnetization* does not precess (at least initially—it only precesses in response to the RF pulse—see later text).

Now, let's transmit an RF pulse along the x-axis *perpendicular* to the magnetization vector M_0, that is, the axis of B_0. (The RF pulse would be along the axis "C" in Fig. 2-2.) Any proton

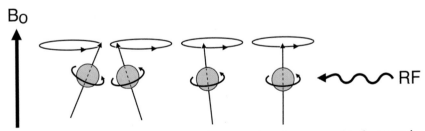

Figure 3-1. An RF pulse is transmitted after the protons have been exposed to the external magnetic field B_0.

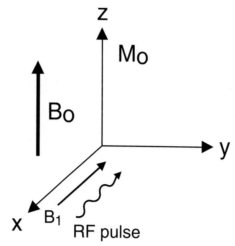

Figure 3-2. The net magnetization vector $\mathbf{M}_0$ has the same direction as the external magnetic field B_0.

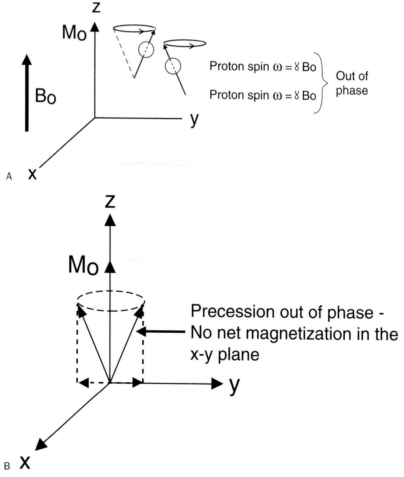

Figure 3-3. Two protons rotating out of phase **(A)** will lead to a net longitudinal magnetization but no component in the x–y plane **(B)**.

that is subjected to any sort of magnetic field starts to precess about the axis of that magnetic field at a frequency ω_0 given by the Larmor equation ($\omega = \gamma B$), where B is the strength of that magnetic field. Protons precess about the axis of B_0 at a frequency $\omega_0 = \gamma B_0$. Now we introduce a magnetic field (namely, the magnetic component of the RF pulse) into the system with a direction along the x-axis. The protons that were previously aligned with the external magnetic field B_0 in the z direction will now also begin to *precess* about the x-axis, that is, about the axis of the new (RF) magnetic field.

At what rate will these protons precess around this new magnetic field? The new precessional frequency will be

$$\omega_1 = \gamma B_1 \qquad \text{(Eqn. 3-1)}$$

where B_1 is the weaker magnetic field associated with the RF pulse.

> **We are now dealing with two different magnetic fields:**
>
> B_0 = a very strong external magnetic field (e.g., 1.5 T)
>
> B_1 = a very weak magnetic field generated by the RF pulse (e.g., 50 mT)

B_0 is a *fixed* magnetic field (much like a DC voltage). B_1, however, is an **oscillating** magnetic field (much like an AC voltage). It oscillates because it is derived from the magnetic component of an oscillating electromagnetic wave.

Because the magnetic field strength of B_1 is much weaker than the external magnetic field B_0, the frequency of precession ω_1 of the spins around the axis of B_1 is much *slower* than the precessional frequency ω_0 of the spins around the axis of the external magnetic field B_0.

So, since $B_1 \ll B_0$,
then $\omega_1 \ll \omega_0$.

The protons are precessing about the B_0 field (z-axis) at frequency ω_0 and about the B_1 field (x-axis) at frequency ω_1 at the same time. This results in a **spiral motion** of the net magnetization vector from the z-axis into the x–y plane. This spiral motion is called **nutation.**

Another thing to remember about the RF pulse is that, referring back to Chapter 1, the RF pulse has a cos (ωt) waveform. The frequency ω of the RF pulse should be identical to the Larmor frequency of the precessing protons. Otherwise, the protons will not precess around the B_1-axis of the RF pulse. This point might be clarified if we first discuss the concept of *resonance.*

Resonance. If the frequency ω of the RF pulse *matches* the frequency of precession of the protons, then **resonance** occurs. Resonance results in the RF pulse adding energy to the protons. A simple example of resonance is the frequency of a child on a swing. Based on the length of the swing and the weight of the child, a natural mechanical resonance frequency exists. If the child is pushed faster or slower from this frequency, the effort will be inefficient. If the child is pushed at his or her resonance frequency, energy is added and he or she swings higher. Similarly, if the proton precesses at frequency ω_0 and the frequency of the RF pulse is not ω_0 (say it is ω_2 instead), then the magnetic field B_1 is oscillating at a different frequency than the protons, and the two frequencies won't be matched. If the RF frequency does not match the precessional frequency of the spins, the system won't resonate and no energy will be added.

Consider this in the x–y plane. The protons are spinning at frequency ω_0. If we then have the B_1 magnetic field oscillating at a frequency $= \omega_2$ different from the proton precessional frequency ω_0, then the system won't resonate, that is, the protons won't "flip" into the x–y plane. A point of clarification: the RF pulse is characterized by two parameters, strength (B_1) and frequency (ω_2). The *frequency* of the RF pulse must match the proton precessional frequency ω_0 in order for resonance to occur— and for the RF pulse to have any effect on the protons at all. If the frequency ω_2 is correct, then the *strength* of the RF pulse (B_1) results in precession of protons about the x-axis at frequency ω_1 (according to the Larmor equation $\omega_1 = \gamma B_1$).

If ω_0 and ω_2 match (i.e., $\omega_2 = \omega_0$), then the system resonates and the protons flip into the x–y plane. In doing so, the protons precess around the axis of the B_1 magnetic field at a much lower frequency (ω_1), corresponding to the Larmor frequency associated with the RF magnetic field B_1 and not with the larger magnetic field B_0.

Another point of clarification: remember that before the RF pulse, the protons precess about the z-axis but they are **out of phase** and hence have no net transverse component. After the RF pulse, the protons are introduced to a *new* magnetic field B_1 (also oscillating at frequency ω_0). Consequently, they will also tend to line up with the *new* magnetic field and will then be **in phase.** This, in effect, creates transverse magnetization. As more and more protons line up, **phase "coherence"** increases, as does transverse magnetization. Simultaneously, as previously discussed, the B_1 field also causes a spiral downward motion of the protons. These two factors explain the process of flipping.

Going back to the three-dimensional coordinate system (Fig. 3-4), the vector $\mathbf{M}_0$ (the net magnetization in the direction of the protons aligned along the external magnetic field) begins to precess about the x-axis in the z–y plane. Depending on the *strength* of the RF pulse B_1, and its *duration* τ, we can determine the **flip angle** (i.e., the fractional angle of a single precession):

$$\theta = \gamma B_1 \tau \qquad \text{(Eqn. 3-2)}$$

According to Equation 3-2, the flip angle is proportional to

1. $\tau =$ the duration of the RF pulse
2. $B_1 =$ the strength of the RF magnetic field, that is, the strength of the RF pulse
3. $\gamma =$ the gyromagnetic ratio

We could have a very strong RF pulse applied over a short period of time, or we could have a weak RF pulse applied over a longer time, and still attain the same **flip angle.** The relationship between the flip angle (θ) and frequency (ω_1) is

$$\theta = (\omega_1)(\tau) \qquad \text{(Eqn. 3-3)}$$

Thus,

flip angle = (frequency of RF precession) $\times$ (duration of RF pulse)

Rotating Frame of Reference

To simplify the concept of "flipping," consider a new reference frame that rotates at the Larmor frequency ω_0. (If you wanted to study the motion of someone riding a carousel, wouldn't it be easier to be *on* the carousel than to watch it from outside?)

Suppose there were someone who was not in this coordinate system, but rather on the *outside* looking in (Fig. 3-5). To this person, the protons would be precessing simultaneously about the z-axis of the B_0 field at frequency ω_0, and about the x-axis of the B_1 field at frequency ω_1. This outside observer would witness a rapid

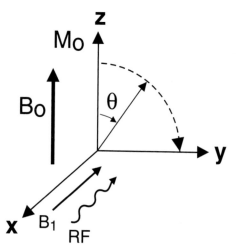

Figure 3-4. A certain amount of time after the application of the RF pulse, the magnetization vector is partially "flipped" toward the x–y plane, forming an angle θ with the z-axis.

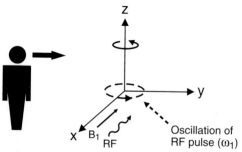

Figure 3-5. An outside observer looking at the coordinate system sees rapid precession of protons and B_1 about the z-axis.

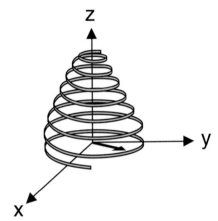

Figure 3-6. The observer outside the coordinate system sees a spiral motion of the magnetization vector toward the x–y plane.

precession around the z-axis that would slowly spiral down into the x–y plane (Fig. 3-6). This nutational motion is the result of the two precessional motions happening simultaneously.

If, however, the observer is located within the rotating coordinate system, and moving at the same frequency as one of the oscillating systems (B_1 or B_0), then she will see *only* the movement of the second system. If, for example, she is rotating at the oscillation frequency of the spins in the external magnetic field ω_0, then she will only notice the slow precession of the protons from the z-axis into the x–y plane as if they were moving in a simple arc (Fig. 3-7). The above occurs if and only if $\omega_0 = \omega_2$, that is, when the RF pulse frequency ω_2 matches the precessional

frequency of the protons ω_0. This condition will put the system in *resonance*.

If we go back for a moment to the spiral motion of the protons seen from an outside observation point (Fig. 3-6), the consecutive circles around the z-axis represent the oscillation frequency ω_0 of the spins in response to the external magnetic field B_0, and the slow downward progress of the spiral to the x–y plane represents the oscillation frequency of the spins in response to the magnetic field of the RF pulse, B_1. If the observer herself is oscillating within the system at a frequency $= \omega_0$, then all she will see is the slow downward arc of the protons precessing in response to the RF pulse. Because the magnetic field created by the RF pulse (B_1) is much smaller than the fixed external magnetic field (B_0), the precessional frequency around the z–y plane is much slower than is the precessional frequency around the z-axis.

90° RF Pulse. In response to a strong magnetic field in the z direction, the spins line up. This results in net magnetization, $\mathbf{M}_0$. Next, we apply an external RF pulse that **flips** the magnetization vector 90° into the x–y plane. When the **magnetization vector** is in the x–y plane, we call this $\mathbf{M}_{xy}$.

$$\mathbf{M}_{xy} = \text{component of } \mathbf{M}_0 \text{ in the x–y plane}$$

If the entire vector flips into the x–y plane, then the **magnitude** of $\mathbf{M}_{xy}$ equals the magnitude of the vector $\mathbf{M}_0$. This is called a **90° flip** (Fig. 3-8). The pulse that causes the 90° flip is called a **90° RF pulse.**

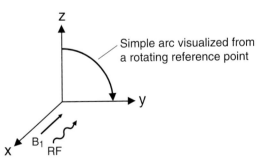

Figure 3-7. If the observer stands within the coordinate system, she would then see a simple arc motion rather than a spiral motion.

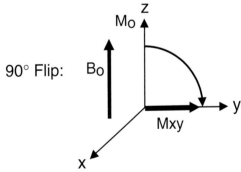

Figure 3-8. When the entire magnetization vector is flipped into the x–y plane, it is called a 90° flip.

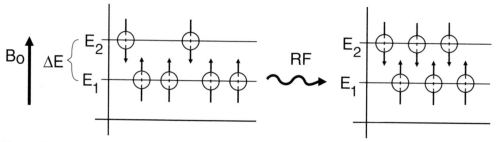

Figure 3-9. When placed in a magnetic field B_0, protons will fall into one of two energy states: in the lower energy state, protons are lined parallel to B_0, whereas in the higher energy state they are antiparallel to it.

The protons that are aligned with the external magnetic field are in two energy states (Fig. 3-9). Those in the lower energy state (E_1) are lined up with (i.e., parallel to) the magnetic field B_0, and those in the higher energy state (E_2) are aligned in the opposite direction. After a 90° RF pulse, some of the protons from the lower energy state are boosted to the higher energy state. This happens only at the **Larmor frequency.**

or, alternatively,

$$f = (2\mu/h)B_0$$

With

$$\gamma = 2\mu/h \text{ (in Hz/T)}$$

where

$$\hbar = h/2\pi \quad \text{and} \quad f = v = \omega/2\pi$$

MATH: The Larmor equation can be derived from the following principle. The energy difference between E_1 and E_2, denoted ΔE, is given by

$$\Delta E = E_2 - E_1 = (2\boldsymbol{\mu})(B_0) \quad \text{(Eqn. 3-4a)}$$

where μ is the **magnetic dipole moment** (MDM). In other words, to go from one energy state to another, the energy required depends on the magnetic dipole moment of the proton and the strength of the magnetic field B_0. By Planck's law:

$$E = hc/\lambda = hv = hf = \hbar\omega \quad \text{(Eqn. 3-4b)}$$

where $v = f$ denotes the linear frequency (in cycles per second or Hz), ω denotes the angular frequency (in radians per second), h is the Planck's constant (6.62×10^{-34} J/sec or 4.13×10^{-18} keV/sec), and $\hbar = h/2\pi$. Then, combining Equations 3-4a and 3-4b, we can deduce that

$$\hbar\omega = 2\mu B_0 = E$$

and thus,

$$\omega = (2\mu/\hbar)B_0$$

which is the Larmor equation, with

$$\gamma = 2\mu/\hbar \text{ (in rad/T)}$$

At equilibrium after the protons are placed in the magnetic field, the number of protons in the low energy state (north-pointing) is greater than the number in the high energy state (south-pointing), resulting in the longitudinal magnetization vector $\mathbf{M}_0$ (Fig. 3-10A). As energy is added by the RF pulse to flip the north-pointing protons to the higher energy state, the number of protons in both states can be equalized. When this occurs, a measurable longitudinal magnetization vector no longer exists. In addition, the RF pulse causes the spins to begin precessing *in phase* with each other. The vector sum of the in-phase north- and south-pointing precessing protons lies in the transverse plane (Fig. 3-10B). This transverse magnetization precesses at the Larmor frequency.

The angular frequency at which the protons rotate 90° about the x-axis is given by the Larmor equation:

$$\omega_1 = \gamma B_1$$

where, again, B_1 is the magnetic field associated with the RF pulse. As stated previously, the phase, that is, the number of degrees of

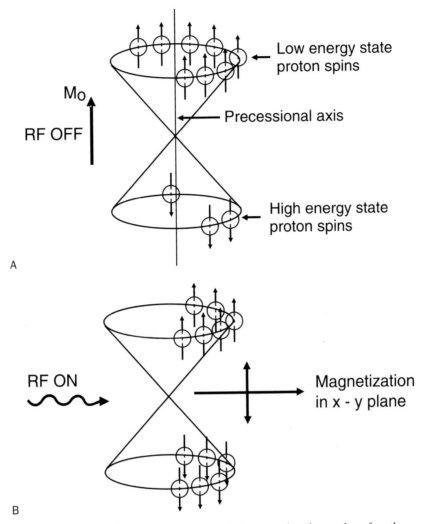

Figure 3-10. The application of the RF pulse (**B**) can equalize the number of north- and south-pointing protons (**A**).

precession, is related to the frequency ω_1 and the duration τ of the RF pulse:

$$\theta = \omega_1\tau = \gamma B_1\tau \qquad \text{(Eqn. 3-5)}$$

From this, we can calculate the time τ it would take to precess the protons 90° ($\pi/2$), that is, the time it would take for an RF pulse to "flip" the spins 90° into the x–y plane at a given RF strength B_1. Setting

$$\theta = 90° = \pi/2 = \gamma B_1\tau_{\pi/2}$$

then we obtain

$$\tau_{\pi/2} = (\pi/2)/\gamma B_1 \qquad \text{(Eqn. 3-6)}$$

This equation shows that if we keep the RF pulse on for time $\tau_{\pi/2}$, the magnetization vector is flipped 90°.

180° Pulse

A 180° pulse has twice the power (or twice the duration) of a 90° pulse, as shown in Equation 3-5. After a 180° RF pulse, the longitudinal magnetization vector is inverted, and the spins begin to recover from $-\mathbf{M}_0$. After a 180° RF pulse, the excess north-pointing spins are boosted from the low energy state to the high energy state.

A 180° pulse exactly reverses the equilibrium northward-pointing excess without inducing phase coherence, that is, transverse magnetization.

Using Equation 3-5, we can calculate the RF time duration required for a 180° RF pulse at a given RF strength B_1

$$180° = \pi = \gamma B_1 \tau_\pi$$

resulting in

$$\tau_\pi = \pi / \gamma B_1$$

To recapitulate, to obtain a 180° RF pulse, we can use either an RF pulse having the same strength as the 90° pulse but twice as long in duration, or an RF pulse that's twice as strong for the same duration.

Partial Flip

In the case of a **partial flip** (<90°), the component of magnetization ending up in the x–y plane (i.e., M_{xy}) is less than the magnitude of the original magnetization vector M_0 (Fig. 3-11).

In fact,

$$M_{xy} = M_0 \sin \theta$$

A partial flip is achieved by decreasing either the strength or the duration of the RF pulse, according to Equation 3-5. Such flip angles are common in **gradient echo** (GRE) imaging, as will be discussed in later chapters.

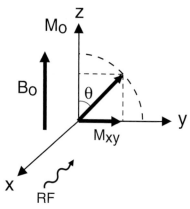

Figure 3-11. In a partial flip, transverse magnetization is smaller than the original longitudinal magnetization. In fact, $M_{xy} = M_0 \sin \theta$.

Auto RF (Prescan)

Prescan is the process of preparing the scanner for a specific patient. This process is done via an **auto RF pulse,** which automatically does the following:

1. It sets transmit gain (which determines the RF power and thus the flip angle). In fact, the flip angle α is proportional to the square root of the transmit power:

$$\alpha \propto \sqrt{\text{power}}$$

2. It sets the receive gain.
3. It sets the optimum ω_0.

Key Points

1   An RF (radio frequency) pulse is a brief electromagnetic burst with frequencies in the radio frequency spectrum.

2   Like all electromagnetic waves, an RF pulse has associated magnetic and electric fields. We are interested in the magnetic component B_1. (The electric component causes tissue heating.)

3   The purpose of the RF pulse in MRI is to flip the longitudinal magnetization.

4   This flip is done by first causing the protons to precess *in phase* about the axis

of the external field (B_0), as well causing them to precess about the axis of the RF field (B_1). The result is a *spiral* motion of spins toward the x–y plane, called *nutation.*

5   The flip angle is a function of the RF strength (B_1) and its duration (τ) and could be 180°, 90°, or a fraction thereof (i.e., a *partial flip* <90°), depending on the clinical application.

Questions

3-1 **T/F** The flip angle is determined by the duration of the RF pulse and its power.

3-2 **T/F** The function of the RF pulse in MRI is to magnetize the protons.

3-3 **T/F** The immediate action of the RF pulse is to cause the protons to precess in phase.

3-4 **T/F** An RF pulse has a magnetic component.

3-5 **T/F** An RF pulse stands for radio frequency pulse, which is a form of an electromagnetic wave with frequencies in the radio frequency spectrum.

3-6 **T/F** A 180° pulse has 10 times the power of a 90° pulse.

3-7 **T/F** A partial flip has an angle between 0° and 90°.

Introduction

We have already introduced relaxation times T1, T2, and T2*. In this chapter, we discuss the physical properties behind them and see what conditions cause them to be increased or decreased. As we have discussed before, T1 and T2 are *inherent* properties of tissues and are thus fixed for a specific tissue (at a given magnetic field strength). The parameter T2*, however, also depends on inhomogeneities in the main magnetic field, but again is fixed for a specific tissue within a given external magnetic environment.

T1 Relaxation Time

The term **relaxation** means that the spins are relaxing back into their lowest energy state or back to the equilibrium state. (Equilibrium by definition is the lowest energy state possible.) Once the **radio frequency** (RF) pulse is turned **off**, the protons will have to realign with the axis of the B_0 magnetic field and give up all their excess energy.

T1 is called the **longitudinal** relaxation time because it refers to the time it takes for the spins to realign along the longitudinal (z)-axis. T1 is also called the **spin-lattice** relaxation time because it refers to the time it takes for the *spins* to give the energy they obtained from the RF pulse back to the surrounding *lattice* in order to go back to their equilibrium state.

T1 = longitudinal relaxation time
T1 = thermal relaxation time
T1 = spin–lattice relaxation time

Immediately after the 90° pulse, the magnetization $\mathbf{M}_{xy}$ precesses within the x–y plane, oscillating around the z-axis with all protons rotating *in phase* (Fig. 4-1). After the magnetization has been flipped 90° into the x–y plane, the RF pulse is turned off. A general principle of thermodynamics is that every system seeks its lowest energy level. Therefore, after the RF pulse is turned off, two things will occur:

1. The spins will go back to the lowest energy state.
2. The spins will get out of phase with each other.

These events result from two simultaneous but separate processes occurring after the RF pulse is turned off (Fig. 4-2):

1. The $\mathbf{M}_{xy}$ component of the magnetization vector decreases rapidly.

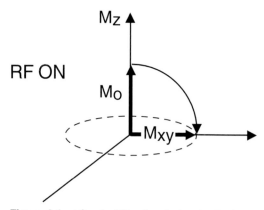

Figure 4-1. After the RF pulse, the longitudinal magnetization vector is flipped into the x–y plane.

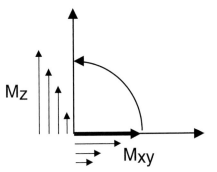

M_z

M_{xy}

Figure 4-2. Once the RF is turned off, the transverse magnetization vector begins to decay while the longitudinal component begins to recover.

2. The M_z component slowly recovers along the z-axis.

Question: What time constant characterizes the rate at which the M_z component recovers its initial magnetization M_0?

Answer: The T1 relaxation time.

When we first discussed magnetization, we said that the protons start to line up with the external magnetic field at a rate given by T1. (Because T1 is a time [in sec], the rate is 1/T1 [in sec^{-1}].) The same phenomenon occurs when we flip the magnetization M_0 away from the longitudinal z-axis and then allow it to realign with the main magnetic field after an RF pulse. The rate at which M_z recovers to M_0 is also given by T1.

Immediately after a 90° pulse, all magnetization is in the x-y plane. The M_z component then starts to grow at a rate characterized by T1 (Fig. 4-3):

$$M_z(t) = M_0(1 - e^{-t/T1}) \qquad \text{(Eqn. 4-1)}$$

T2 Relaxation Time

Figure 4-2 also shows rapid decay of the M_{xy} component after the RF pulse is turned off.

Question: What time constant characterizes the rate at which the M_{xy} component decays?

Answer: The T2 relaxation time.

As the longitudinal magnetization vector M_z recovers, the transverse vector M_{xy} decays at a rate characterized by T2 (Fig. 4-4):

$$M_{xy}(t) = M_0 e^{-t/T2} \qquad \text{(Eqn. 4-2)}$$

Realize that the recovery of magnetization along the z-axis and the decay of magnetization within the x-y plane are two independent processes occurring at two different rates (Fig. 4-5). Take a simple exponential process. We would expect the rate at which this process decays in the x–y plane to be the same as that at which it grows along the z-axis (Fig. 4-6). This is *not* the same in the MR system we are discussing because this system involves a much more complicated process. T2 decay occurs 5 to 10 times more rapidly than T1 recovery (Fig. 4-7). To understand this, we need to understand the concept of dephasing.

Dephasing. After the 90° **RF** pulse is turned **off,** all spins are **in phase;** they are all lined up in the same direction and spinning at the same frequency ω_0. There are two phenomena that will make the spins get out of phase: interactions between spins and external field inhomogeneities.

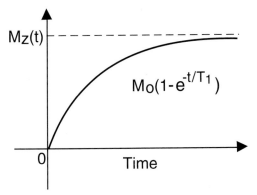

$M_z(t)$

$M_0(1-e^{-t/T_1})$

0   Time

Figure 4-3. The graph of recovery of longitudinal magnetization with the growth rate of T1.

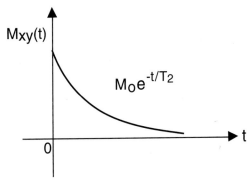

$M_{xy}(t)$

$M_0 e^{-t/T_2}$

0   t

Figure 4-4. The graph of transverse magnetization with the decay rate of T2 and RF off.

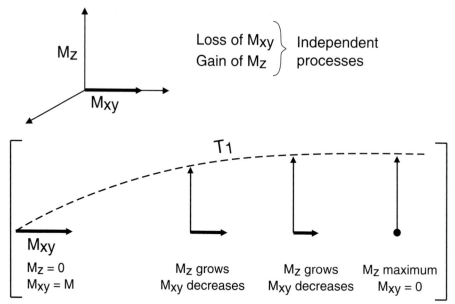

Figure 4-5. The recovery of longitudinal magnetization and the decay of transverse magnetization occur at the same time but are independent of each other with the RF off.

1. **Interactions Between Individual Spins**

   When two spins are next to each other, the magnetic field of one proton affects the proton next to it. Assume one proton is aligned with the field and the other is against it (Fig. 4-8). The proton aligned with B_0 creates a slightly higher magnetic field for its neighbor so that proton #1 is exposed to the magnetic field B_0 plus a small magnetic field created by the other proton (ΔB). The precessional frequency of the proton then will increase slightly as

$$\omega(\text{proton} \#1) = (B_0 + \Delta B)$$

   On the other side, the other proton is exposed to a slightly weaker magnetic field

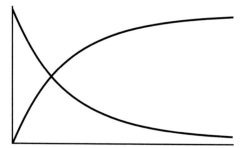

Figure 4-6. The rate of growth and decay of a simple exponential process is expected to be similar.

because the other proton points against B_0. Therefore, its overall magnetic field strength exposure will be slightly less. The precessional frequency of proton #2 then will decrease slightly as

$$\omega(\text{proton} \#2) = (B_0 - \Delta B)$$

   The difference in the magnetic environment created by these proton–proton interactions may be very small, but it makes a difference in the overall homogeneity of the magnetic field to which the spins are exposed. Thus, the first cause of dephasing is *inherent* in the tissue. It is called a **spin–spin interaction.** This interaction is an inherent property of every tissue and is measured by T2.

T2 = transverse relaxation time
T2 = spin–spin relaxation time

2. **External Magnetic Field Inhomogeneity**

   This is the second phenomenon that makes spins get out of phase. No matter how good a system we have, no matter how stable the external magnetic field is, some variation in the homogeneity of the mag-

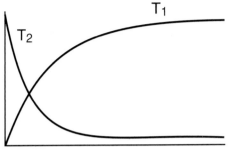

T1 — Growth of magnetization in z axis

T2 — Decay of magnetization in x-y plane

Figure 4-7. Contrary to the previous figure, the rate of decay of transverse magnetization is several times that of the recovery of longitudinal magnetization.

netic field still exists (usually measured in parts per million).

External magnetic field inhomogeneity makes protons in different locations precess at different frequencies because each spin is exposed to a slightly different magnetic field strength. These varying frequencies are very close to each other and very close to the true Larmor frequency; however, these tiny differences in frequency result in spin **dephasing.**

The two causes of spin dephasing:
1. **Spin–spin interactions (internal inhomogeneities)**
2. **External magnetic field inhomogeneities**

These two phenomena together cause protons to spin at slightly different frequencies. Imagine that we have three protons:

1. One is precessing at the true Larmor frequency $= \omega_0$.
2. One, exposed to slightly higher magnetic fields, is precessing at a frequency slightly faster than the Larmor frequency $= \omega_0^+$.
3. One, exposed to slightly weaker magnetic fields, is precessing at a frequency slightly slower than the Larmor frequency $= \omega_0^-$.

If we wait long enough, the three protons in the x–y plane will get completely out of phase. The net magnetic field within the x–y plane will then go to 0.

Therefore, at time $t = 0$, all spins are in phase, and their vector sum will be at maximum magnitude. As the spins begin getting out of phase with each other, their summation vector will become smaller and smaller. When all the spins are completely out of phase with each other, their vector sum will be zero. The effect of spin–spin interaction depends to a degree on the proximity of the spins to each other. For example, in water (H_2O), the protons are separated more widely than they are in a solid tissue. Hence, the dephasing effect of spin–spin interaction might not be as prominent in H_2O as it is in a solid tissue.

The Received Signal

Let's go back to the x–y plane with the RF aligned along the x-axis. The RF coil (e.g., head or body coil) is often both a **transmitter** and a

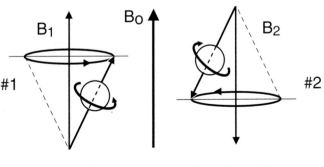

$B_1 = B_0 + \Delta B$

$B_2 = B_0 - \Delta B$

Figure 4-8. Two adjacent protons, one aligned with the field and the other against it.

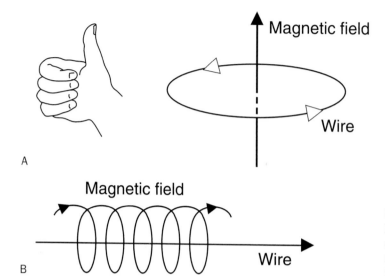

A

B

Figure 4-9. A, B: The right-hand rule determines the direction of generated magnetic field by an electric current in a wire.

receiver. The signal is received at the same location at which it is transmitted. Remember that a moving charged particle generates a magnetic field. The reverse is also true. A magnetic field causes movement of charged particles, that is, electrons. If we have a wire with electrons running in one direction (away from us), the direction of the magnetic field (according to the right-hand rule) can be determined (in this case, it is pointing up; Fig. 4-9A). Similarly, if we have a straight wire, and we have an oscillating magnetic field about this wire, the magnetic field will induce a voltage and current in the wire (Fig. 4-9B).

The measured current is what we mean by a **signal.** Remember that after a 90° pulse, the magnetization rotates in the x–y plane at frequency ω_0. This magnetization reflects a group phenomenon of multiple precessing protons. Associated with each proton is a magnetic field that is also precessing. Immediately after a 90° pulse, the protons precess in phase. When the magnetic field of each spin (or each group of spins) is in the same direction as the RF coil receiver, a very large signal is induced in the RF receiver coil.

Thus, at time $t = 0$ (in Fig. 4-10A), all the protons are lined up in the direction of the RF coil. As the spins rotate 90° at time $t = t1$, there will be no component of the magnetization vector along the x direction. All magnetization points in the y direction. However, this RF coil can only detect the component of magnetization along the x-axis. So at time t1, there is no signal. After another 90° rotation (at time t2), a signal exists, but it is the negative of the original signal. At time t3, there is again no magnetization in the x direction, and, therefore, no signal. At time t4, spins are again lined up with the receiver coil and signal is maximal. A graph of the received signal will then look like a sinusoidal curve (Fig. 4-10B). The frequency of the received signal is ω_0 because the protons are spinning at frequency ω_0.

However, is this really the received signal, or is there more to it?

Free Induction Decay

In an ideal situation, if we had a perfectly uniform magnetic field, the received signal would, in fact, have looked like Figure 4-10B. However, this is not what's really happening. What really happens is the following (Fig. 4-11): We start at time $t = 0$ in the x direction. However, because of spin **dephasing** (namely, spin–spin interactions and external magnetic field inhomogeneities), by the time the spins reach t4, they will have dephased slightly and the signal coming from the spins will be slightly less than it was originally. The signal becomes weaker and weaker as time goes by, and it spirals to the center of the x–y plane.

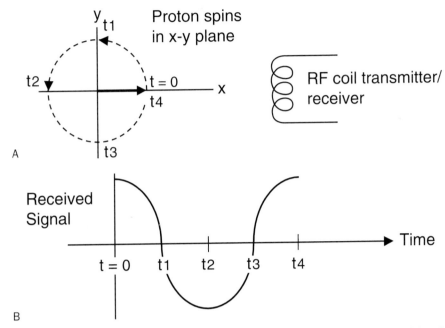

Figure 4-10. The relationship between transverse magnetization (**A**) and the received signal (**B**) at different points in time.

The signal vector is continuously decaying in magnitude as it is precessing around the x–y plane. How would the signal look to the RF receiver? The answer lies in Figure 4-12. This figure shows the shape of the signal picked up by the receiver; it is an oscillating, decaying signal. It is called a **free induction decay (FID)** because after we turn off the RF pulse:

1. The spins begin to precess *freely.*
2. The signal starts to *decay* with time.
3. The spins *induce* a current in the receiver coil.

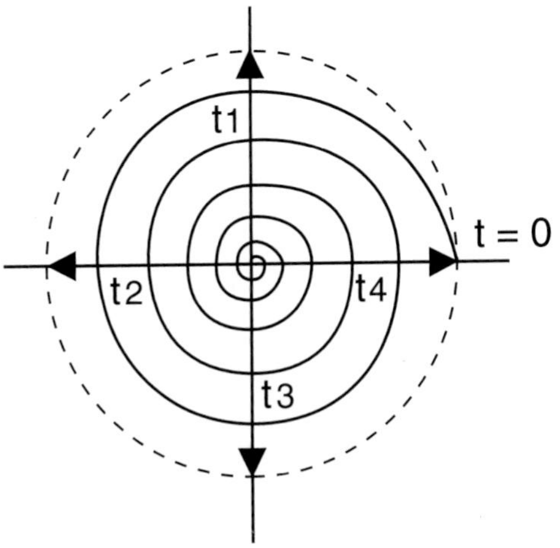

Thus, the FID results from an oscillating magnetic field generated by the oscillating spins, which induces a current in a receiver coil. This decaying oscillating signal is described mathematically as

$$M_{xy}(t) = M_0 e^{-t/T2^*}(\cos \omega_0 t) \quad \textbf{(Eqn. 4-3)}$$

We've seen these terms before (refer to Chapter 1):

1. $(\cos \omega_0 t)$: This is the formula for an oscillating wave, with a frequency of ω_0.
2. $(e^{-t/T2^*})$: Because the signal is decaying we have to include an exponential function. The time constant of this exponential function is given by T2*.

Therefore, the general form of the received signal is based on:

1. An *oscillating signal*, which varies as $\cos \omega_0 t$

Figure 4-11. The spiral-like decay of transverse magnetization.

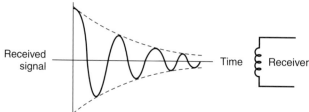

Figure 4-12. The decaying sinusoidal waveform of the received signal (the FID).

2. A *decaying signal,* which decays with time constant T2* as given by the exponential $e^{-t/T2^*}$

Differences Between T2 and T2*. T2* decay depends on both

1. External magnetic field
2. Spin–spin interactions

T2 decay depends primarily on

1. Spin–spin interactions[1]

T2 of a tissue, because it depends only on spin–spin interactions, is *fixed*—we have no control over what the spins do to each other. T2* depends on the homogeneity of the external magnetic field, so it is *not fixed.* It varies depending on how uniform the main magnet is. T2* is always less than T2. T2* decay is always faster than T2 decay (Fig. 4-13). The following equation relates the two together:

$$1/T2^* = 1/T2 + \gamma\Delta B \qquad \text{(Eqn. 4-4)}$$

The term *1/T* is the **relaxation rate** with units of $\sec^{-1}$ (recall that *1/T* is a frequency).

The relaxation rate (1/T2*) depends on the relaxation rate of the tissue (1/T2) plus the magnetic field inhomogeneity of the external magnet. If we have a perfect magnet that does not introduce any inhomogeneity, then $\Delta B = 0$ and T2* = T2. The newer systems have less magnetic field inhomogeneity, thus making the T2* effects less strong; however, complete homogeneity is not possible. Hence, there will always be some T2* effect.

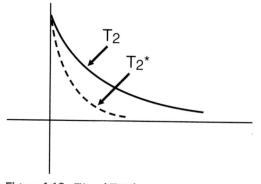

Figure 4-13. T2 and T2* decay curves.

Key Points

1. The rate of recovery of the longitudinal magnetization is given by T1.

2. The rate of decay of the transverse magnetization is given by T2.

3. The rate of decay of the FID is given by T2*.

4. T1 is 5 to 10 times greater than T2.

5. T2* is always less than T2.

6. T2 is a result of spin–spin interactions (internal tissue inhomogeneities), whereas T2* is dependent on **both** internal and external (main magnetic field) inhomogeneities.

7. FID is produced by a rotating magnetic field, which induces an electric current in a stationary coil.

---

[1]T2 also depends on **diffusion** (i.e., how rapidly spins spread out and leave the lattice); however, this is a minor factor in comparison with spin-spin interactions.

Questions

4-1 True/false questions:
- (a) T2* depends on the external magnetic field inhomogeneity.
- (b) T2 depends on the external magnetic field inhomogeneity.
- (c) T2 depends on T2*.
- (d) T2* depends on T2.

4-2 The recovery of longitudinal magnetization is proportional to
- (a) $e^{-t/T1}$
- (b) $1 - e^{-t/T1}$
- (c) $1 - e^{-t/T2}$
- (d) $e^{-t/T2}$
- (e) none of the above

4-3 The decay of transverse magnetization is proportional to
- (a) $e^{-t/T1}$
- (b) $1 - e^{-t/T1}$
- (c) $1 - e^{-t/T2}$
- (d) $e^{-t/T2}$
- (e) none of the above

4-4 T/F The rate of decay of the FID is given by T2.

4-5 Which one of the following equations is correct?
- (a) T2 > T2* > T1
- (b) T2* > T2 > T1
- (c) T1 > T2 > T2*
- (d) T1 > T2* > T2

4-6 Match the following: (i) T1; (ii) T2 with
- (a) recovery of longitudinal magnetization
- (b) decay of transverse magnetization

5

TR, TE, and Tissue Contrast

Introduction

In previous chapters, we discussed the roles of T1 and T2, longitudinal and transverse magnetization, and the radio frequency (RF) pulse. Obviously, by doing the procedures described in the previous chapters only once, we won't be able to create an image. To get any sort of spatial information, the process must be repeated multiple times, as we shall see shortly. This is where TR and TE come into play. The parameters TR and TE are related intimately to the tissue parameters T1 and T2, respectively. However, unlike T1 and T2, which are inherent properties of the tissue and therefore fixed, TR and TE can be controlled and adjusted by the operator. In fact, as we shall see later, by appropriate setting of TR and TE, we can put more "weight" on T1 or T2, depending on the type of clinical application.

How do we actually measure a signal? With the patient in a large magnetic field (Fig. 5-1A),

we apply a 90° RF pulse, and the magnetization vector flips into the x–y plane (Fig. 5-1B). Then, we turn off the 90° RF pulse, and the magnetization vector begins to grow in the z direction and decay in the x–y plane (Fig. 5-1C). By *convention*, we apply the RF pulse in the x direction, and for that reason, in a rotating frame of reference, the vector ends up along the y-axis (Fig. 5-1B).

After a 90° RF pulse, we have decaying transverse magnetization M_{xy} (which is the component of the magnetization vector in the x–y plane) and recovering longitudinal magnetization M_z (which is the component of the magnetization vector along the z-axis). Remember that the received signal can be detected only along the x-axis, that is, along the direction of the RF transmitter/receiver coil. The receiver coil only recognizes oscillating signals (like AC voltage) and not nonoscillating voltage changes (like DC voltage). Thus, rotation in the x–y plane induces a signal in the RF coil, whereas changes along the z-axis do not.

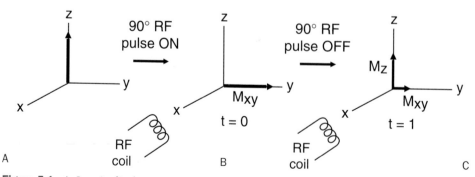

Figure 5-1. A: Longitudinal magnetization before the RF pulse. **B:** Immediately after the RF pulse, the magnetization vector is flipped into the x–y plane. **C:** After a certain time period, M_z has recovered by a certain amount while M_{xy} has decayed by a different amount.

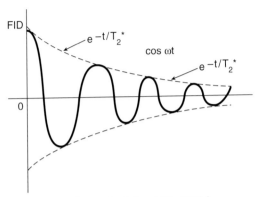

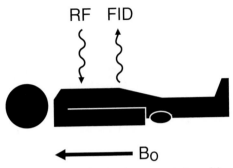

Figure 5-4. Immediately after transmission of the RF pulse, an FID is formed.

Figure 5-2. The received signal (the FID) has a decaying sinusoidal waveform.

At time $t = 0$, the signal is at a maximum. As time goes by, because of dephasing (see Chapter 4), the signal becomes weaker in a sinusoidal manner (Fig. 5-2). The decay curve of the signal is given by the following term:

$$e^{-t/T2^*}$$

The sinusoidal nature of the signal is given by the equation

$$\cos \omega t$$

Therefore, the decaying sinusoidal signal is given by the product

$$(e^{-t/T2^*})(\cos \omega t)$$

When $t = 0$:

$$\cos \omega t = \cos \omega(0) = \cos 0 = 1$$
$$e^{-t/T2^*} = e^0 = 1$$

When $t = 0$, $(e^{-t/T2^*})(\cos \omega t) = 1$. Thus, at time $t = 0$, the signal is maximum (i.e., 100%). As time increases, we are multiplying a sinusoidal function ($\cos \omega t$) and a decaying function ($e^{-t/T2^*}$), which eventually decays to zero (Fig. 5-3).

When we put a patient in a magnet, he or she becomes temporarily magnetized as his or her protons align with the external magnetic field along the z-axis. We then transmit an RF pulse at the Larmor frequency and immediately get back a free induction decay (FID; Fig. 5-4). This process gives one signal—one FID—from the entire patient. It doesn't give us any information about the location of the signal. The FID is received from the **ensemble** of all the different protons in the patient's body with *no* spatial discrimination. To get spatial information, we have to specify somehow the x, y, and z coordinates of the signal. Here, **gradients** come into play. The purpose of the **gradient coils** is to **spatially encode** the signal.

To spatially encode the signal, we have to apply the RF pulse multiple times while varying the gradients and, in turn, get multiple FIDs or other signals (e.g., spin echoes). When we put all the information from the multiple FIDs together, we get the information necessary to create an image. If we just apply the RF pulse once, we only get one signal (one FID), and we

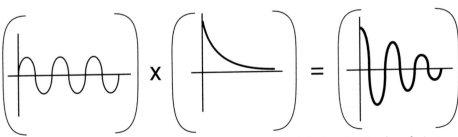

Figure 5-3. The product of a sinusoidal signal and an exponentially decaying signal results in a decaying sinusoidal signal.

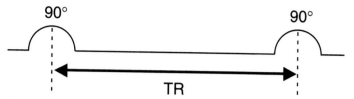

Figure 5-5. The time interval between two successive 90° RF pulses is denoted TR.

cannot make an image from one signal. (An exception to this statement is echoplanar imaging [EPI], which is performed after one RF pulse—see Chapter 22.)

TR (The Repetition Time)

After we apply one 90° pulse (the symbol we'll use for a 90° RF pulse is in Fig. 5-5), we'll apply another. The time interval between applications is called TR (the repetition time).

What happens to the T1 recovery curve during successive 90° pulses (Fig. 5-6)?

1. Immediately before time $t = 0$, the magnetization vector points along the z-axis. Call this vector $\mathbf{M}_0$ with magnitude $\mathbf{M}_0$.
2. Immediately after $t = 0$, the magnetization vector $\mathbf{M}_{xy}$ lies in the x–y plane, without a

component along the z-axis. $\mathbf{M}_{xy}$ has magnitude $\mathbf{M}_0$ at $t = 0^+$.

3. As time goes by and we reach time $t = $ TR, we gradually recover some magnetization along the z-axis and lose some (or all) magnetization in the x–y plane. Let's assume at time TR the transverse magnetization $\mathbf{M}_{xy}$ is very small. What happens if we now apply another 90° RF pulse? We flip the existing longitudinal magnetization vector $(\mathbf{M}_z)$ back into the x–y plane. However, what is the magnitude of the magnetization vector $\mathbf{M}_z$ at the time TR? Because

$$\mathbf{M}_z(t) = \mathbf{M}_0(1 - e^{-t/T1})$$

then at $t = $ TR,

$$\mathbf{M}_z(\text{TR}) = \mathbf{M}_0(1 - e^{-\text{TR/T1}}) \quad \textbf{(Eqn. 5-1)}$$

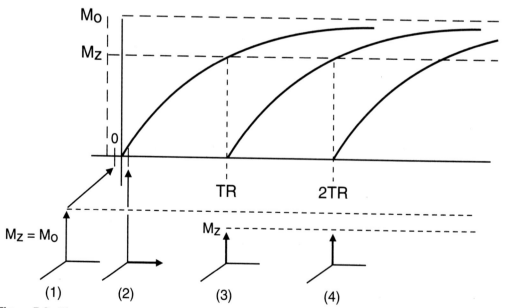

Figure 5-6. The recovery curves after successive RF pulses.

4. As we see in the T1 recovery curve, the magnetization vector ($\mathbf{M}_z$) at time TR is less than the original magnetization vector $\mathbf{M}_0$ because the second 90° RF pulse was applied before complete recovery of the magnetization vector $\mathbf{M}_z$.

5. After the magnetization vector is flipped back into the x–y plane, it will begin to grow again along the z-axis (according to the T1 recovery curve) until the next TR, when it will again be flipped into the x–y plane. We now have a *series* of exponential curves that never reach full magnetization.

Received Signal

Let's now take a look at the signal we are receiving (S). Because we are only applying a series of 90° pulses, the signal will be a series of FIDs:

1. At time $t = 0$, the initial signal will be a strong FID similar to that shown in Figure 5-7A.
2. At time $t = $ TR, the signal will be slightly less in magnitude but will also be an FID (Fig. 5-7B).
3. At time $t = $ 2TR, the signal will be equal in magnitude to that in Figure 5-7B (Fig. 5-7C).

Because the T1 recovery curve is given by the formula $1 - e^{-t/T1}$, if we could measure the signal immediately after the RF pulse is given with no delay, then each FID signal would be proportional to

$$1 - e^{-TR/T1}$$

(This cannot really happen in practice.) Up to now, the signal S is given by the formula

$$S \propto 1 - e^{-TR/T1}$$

Remember that the word "signal" is really a relative term. The signal that we get is a number without dimension, that is, it has no units. If we are dealing with a tissue that has many mobile protons, then, regardless of what the TR and T1 of the tissue are, we'll get more signals with more mobile protons (see Chapter 2). Thus, when considering the signal, we must also consider the number of **mobile protons** $N(H)$.

$$S \propto N(H)(1 - e^{-TR/T1}) \qquad \text{(Eqn. 5-2)}$$

For a given tissue, the T1 and the proton density are constant, and the signal received will be according to the above formula. If we measure the FID at time TR immediately after the application of the second 90° RF pulse, it will measure maximal and be equal to $N(H)(1 - e^{-TR/T1})$. Therefore, the FIDs that are acquired at TR intervals (i.e., 1TR, 2TR) are maximal if they can be measured right after the 90° pulse, that is, right at the beginning of the FID. However, in reality, we have to wait a certain period until the system electronics allows us to make a measurement.

TE (Echo Delay Time or Time to Echo)

TE stands for **echo delay time** (or time to echo). Instead of making the measurement immediately after the RF pulse (which we could not do anyway), we wait a short period of time and *then* make the measurement. This short time period is referred to as TE.

Let's go back to the T2* decay curve and see what happens. In the x–y plane, the FID

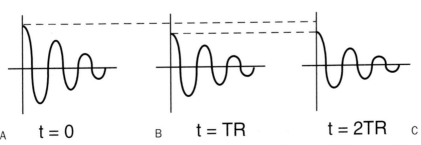

A $\quad t = 0$ B $\quad t = $ TR $t = $ 2TR   C

Figure 5-7. The FIDs after successive RF pulses: **A:** at $t = 0$; **B:** at $t = $ TR; **C:** at $t = $ 2TR.

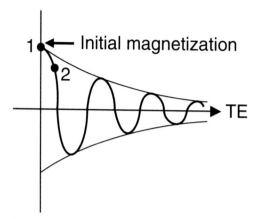

Figure 5-8. The value of the FID at time 0 is $\mathbf{M}_0$, whereas at time TE it is $\mathbf{M}_0 \cdot e^{-TE/T2^*}$.

signal decays at a very rapid rate because of two factors:

1. External magnetic field inhomogeneities
2. Spin–spin interactions

The signal decays at rate T2* according to the decay function

$$e^{-t/T2^*}$$

From this we see that if we take the signal measurement right away, before there is any chance for signal decay, the signal will be equal to the original magnetization ($\mathbf{M}_0$) flipped into the x–y plane (point 1 in Fig. 5-8). However, if we wait a short time period (TE) before we make a measurement, the signal will look like point 2 in Figure 5-8.

$$\mathbf{M}_0(e^{-TE/T2^*}) \qquad \text{(Eqn. 5-3a)}$$

Now we have to put the two curves together because both T1 recovery and T2 decay processes are occurring simultaneously (Fig. 5-9).

Let's go back to the T1 recovery curve. After the 90° RF pulse, the spins are flipped into the x–y plane. After a time interval TR, the amount of received longitudinal magnetization is

$$\mathbf{M}_0(1 - e^{-TR/T1}) \qquad \text{(Eqn. 5-3b)}$$

Superimposed on this T1 recovery curve, we'll draw another curve, which is the T2* decay curve, with two new axes. The T2* decay curve starts out at the value of $\mathbf{M}_0 (1 - e^{-TR/T1})$ on the T1 recovery curve and then decays very quickly. The decay rate of the new curve is given by T2* according to the formula

$$e^{-t/T2^*}$$

After a period of time TE, we can measure the signal. The value of the signal at TE will be a fraction of the maximum signal intensity on the T1 recovery curve. In other words, it will be the product of Equations 5-3a and 5-3b:

$$\text{Signal} = S \propto \mathbf{M}_0(1 - e^{-TR/T1})(e^{-TE/T2^*})$$

The confusing thing about the diagram is that there are two sets of axes (Fig. 5-9):

1. The first set of axes is associated with TR.
2. The second set of axes is associated with TE.

If we draw them to scale, the T2 decay curve (time scale TE) will be decaying much faster than the T1 curve is recovering (time scale TR). However, the graph does give us a visual concept of what the final signal intensity is going to be.

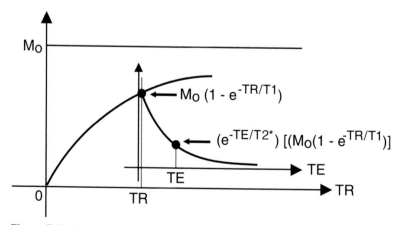

Figure 5-9. The recovery and decay curves plotted on the same graph.

Because the initial longitudinal magnetization M_0 is proportional to the number of mobile protons, that is,

$$M_0 \propto N(H)$$

then, in general, the signal intensity we measure is given by

$$\text{Signal Intensity} = \text{SI} \propto N(H)(e^{-\text{TE}/\text{T2}^*})$$
$$(1 - e^{-\text{TR}/\text{T1}}) \qquad \textbf{(Eqn. 5-4)}$$

(The difference between T2 and T2* is the correction for external magnetic field inhomogeneity achieved with spin-echo techniques.)

Tissue Contrast (T1 and T2 Weighting)

Let's see what happens when we deal with two different tissues. So far we have been dealing with a single tissue, but now we'll consider two tissues: tissue A and tissue B.

Question: Of the two tissues in Figure 5-10A, which one has the longer T1?

Answer: *Tissue A has the longer T1 (it takes longer to recover).*

If we draw just a tangent along each curve at the origin, tissue A has a longer T1 than tissue B. However, just by looking at the curves, it takes tissue A longer to reach equilibrium than tissue B. Let's say we have two different TRs:

1. Short TR = TR_1
2. Long TR = TR_2

Question: Which one of the TRs in Figure 5-10B gives better tissue contrast?

Answer: *TR_1 gives the better contrast.*

Let's go back to Equation 5-4 and see if this answer makes sense:

$$\text{SI} = N(H)(e^{-\text{TE}/\text{T2}^*})(1 - e^{-\text{TR}/\text{T1}})$$

where SI stands for signal intensity. If TR goes to infinity, then $1 - e^{-\text{TR}/\text{T1}}$ becomes 1. If TR $\rightarrow$ ∞, then $1 - e^{-\text{TR}/\text{T1}} \rightarrow 1$ and SI $\rightarrow N(H)$ $(e^{-\text{TE}/\text{T2}^*})$. If TR is very long, we can get rid of the T1 component in the equation. What this means in practice is that we eliminate (or, more realistically, reduce) the T1 effect by having a very large TR.

Long TR reduces the T1 effect.

We can't really achieve a long enough TR in practice to eliminate totally the T1 effect 100%, but we can certainly *minimize* the T1 effect with a TR of 2000 to 3000 msec (in general, if TR is <u>four to five times</u> T1, then the T1 effect becomes negligible). Let's go back to Figure 5-10B and see what happens at TR = TR_1. At this point, the TR is not long enough to eliminate the T1 term in the equation $(1 - e^{\text{TR}/\text{T1}})$. So we have:

$$\text{signal intensity (tissue A)} /$$
$$\text{signal intensity (tissue B)}$$
$$= (1 - e^{-\text{TR}_1/\text{T1(tissue A)}})/(1 - e^{-\text{TR}_1/\text{T1(tissue B)}})$$

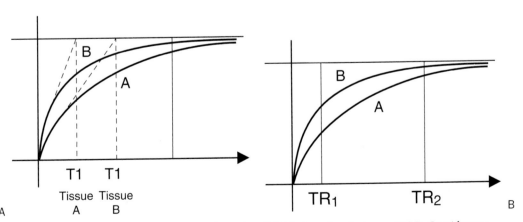

Figure 5-10. A: Two tissues A and B with different T1s. Which tissue has the longer T1? **B:** Consider two different TRs on a recovery curve. Which TR provides better tissue contrast between A and B?

Because the T1s of tissue A and tissue B are different, the short TR brings out the difference in contrast between tissue A and tissue B. Thus, for short TR, the two tissues can be differentiated on the basis of different T1s. In other words, we get T1 tissue contrast with short TR.

Short TR enhances the T1 contrast.

We don't want TR to be very long when we're evaluating T1 because, as we've already learned, when TR $\rightarrow \infty$, then $(1 - e^{-TR/T1})$ approaches 1, thus eliminating the T1 effect. However, we also don't want TR to be too short. If TR is close to 0, then

$$e^{-0/T1} = e^0 = 1$$

and

$$1 - e^{-TR/T1} = 1 - 1 = 0$$

In this situation, with very short TR, we end up with no signal. Ideally, we would like to have a TR that is not much different from the T1 of the tissue under study.

T2* Tissue Contrast

Let's consider T2* contrast between two tissues.

Question: In Figure 5-11A, which tissue has a longer T2?*

Answer: Again, if we graphically draw a tangent at t = 0 for each curve, we see that tissue A has a longer T2. Put differently, it takes the signal from tissue A longer to decay than that from tissue B.*

Let's pick two different TEs (Fig. 5-11B). Here we have two TEs:

1. Short TE = TE_1
2. Long TE = TE_2

Question: Which one of the TEs in Figure 5-11B results in more tissue contrast between tissue A and tissue B?

Answer: TE_2 gives us more contrast.

Let's again look at the formula for signal intensity (Equation 5-4):

$$SI = N(H)(e^{-TE/T2*})(1 - e^{-TR/T1})$$

If TE is very short (close to zero), then $e^{-TE/T2*}$ approaches 1.

$$TE \rightarrow 0 \Rightarrow e^{-TE/T2*} \rightarrow e^0 = 1$$

Then

$$\begin{aligned} signal\ intensity &= N(H)(1)(1 - e^{-TR/T1}) \\ &= N(H)(1 - e^{-TR/T1}) \end{aligned}$$

This means that, with a very short TE, we get rid of the T2* effect in the equation. Therefore, we eliminate (or, again, in reality, reduce) the T2* effect by having a very short TE.

Short TE reduces the T2* effect.

We can see this graphically from the graph (Fig. 5-11B) and mathematically from the equation (Equation 5-3). When we have a long TE, we enhance T2* contrast between tissues. Even though the signal-to-noise ratio is low (because there is greater signal decay for a longer TE), the tissue contrast is high.

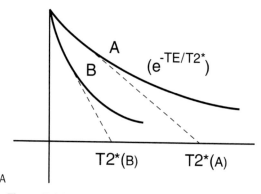

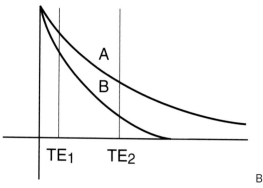

A   B

Figure 5-11. A: Two tissues A and B with different T2*s. Which tissue has the longer T2? **B:** Consider two different TEs on a decay curve. Which TE provides better tissue contrast between A and B?

Key Points

1 Long TR reduces T1 effect.

2 Short TR enhances T1 effect.

3 Short TE reduces T2* (T2) effect.

4 Long TE enhances T2* (T2) effect.

Questions

5-1 In the graph in Figure 5-12, the T1 and T2 curves are plotted simultaneously for convenience. Assume the following values for T1 and T2:

for white matter (WM): T1 = 500, T2 = 100 msec

for cerebrospinal fluid (CSF): T1 = 2000, T2 = 200 msec

Also assume a spin density N = 100 for both WM and CSF.

(a) For a TR = 2000 msec, find the relative signal intensities for WM and CSF (i.e., points A and B on the graph).

(b) Calculate the crossover TE where WM and CSF have identical T2 weighting (point C).

(c) Now, calculate the signal intensities of WM and CSF for TE = 25 (first echo) and TE = 100 msec (second echo), and the ratio CSF/WM.

(d) Repeat (a) to (c) for TR = 3000 msec and observe how one gets more T2 weighting in the second echo (higher ratio CSF/WM).

(e) Now, calculate the signal intensities for TR = 3000 and TE = 200 msec.

Notice that despite relative loss of signal for both WM and CSF, the ratio CSF/WM actually increases, indicating more T2 weighting (i.e., CSF gets brighter on the images).

The following values may be helpful for those of you without a sophisticated calculator:

$$e = 2.27, e^{-1} = 1/e = 0.37,$$
$$e^{-2} = 1/e^2 = 0.14, e^{-3} = 0.05,$$
$$e^{-4} = 0.02, e^{-5} = 0.01, e^{-6} \cong 0,$$
$$e^{-0.5} = 0.61, e^{-1.5} = 0.22, e^{-0.13} = 0.88;$$
$$\ln 0.64 = \log_e 0.64 = -0.45,$$
$$\ln 0.78 = -0.25$$

5-2 Suppose that at 1.0 T, the approximate T1 and T2 values for the following tissues are as follows.

Tissue	T1 (msec)	T2 (msec)
H_2O	2500	2500
Fat	200	100
CSF	2000	300
Gray matter	500	100

(a) Calculate the *signal intensity ratios* for

1. H_2O/fat
2. CSF/gray matter

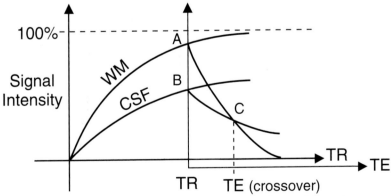

Figure 5-12. T1 and T2 curves are plotted simultaneously. Use this graph to answer the questions.

for the following pulse sequences:

1. T1WI/SE with TR = 500,
   TE = 25 msec
2. T2WI/SE with TR = 2500,
   TE = 100 msec

Note: Assume similar spin densities for these tissues.

(b) Demonstrate the above graphically.

Hint: $e^{-1} = 0.37$, $e^{-5} = 0.01$, $e^{-0.04} = 0.96$, $e^{-1.25} = 0.29$, $e^{-12.5} \cong 0$ $e^{-2.5} = 0.08$, $e^{-0.25} = 0.78$, $e^{-0.2} = 0.82$, $e^{-0.01} = 0.99$, $e^{-1/3} = 0.72$, $e^{-0.25/300} = 0.92$.

5-3 A longer TR
(a) increases T1 weighting
(b) reduces T1 weighting
(c) increases T2 weighting
(d) reduces T2 weighting

5-4 A longer TE
(a) increases T1 weighting
(b) reduces T1 weighting
(c) increases T2 weighting
(d) reduces T2 weighting

5-5 Calculate the signal $N(H)(1 - e^{-TR/T1}) e^{-TE/T2}$ for the following theoretical situations:
(a) TR = ∞
(b) TE = 0
(c) TR = ∞ and TE = 0

5-6 Match the following: (i) reduces T1 effect, (ii) enhances T1 effect, (iii) reduces T2 effect, (iv) enhances T2 effect with
(a) short TR
(b) long TR
(c) short TE
(d) long TE

6

Tissue Contrast: Some Clinical Applications

Introduction

In the previous chapter, we talked about T1 and T2 weighting in terms of the time parameters TR and TE. Now let's discuss the T1 and T2 characteristics of the following tissues and see what physical properties affect them:

1. H_2O
2. Solids
3. Fat
4. Proteinaceous material

T2 Characteristics

The T2 characteristics of a tissue are determined by how fast the proton spins in that tissue dephase. If they dephase rapidly, we get a short T2. If they dephase more slowly, we get a longer T2.

H_2O. Because of the structure of the water molecule (H–O–H) and because of the sparsity of these molecules, spin–spin interaction among the hydrogen protons is minimal. Therefore, dephasing occurs at a much slower rate in water compared with other tissues. The T2 relaxation time for H_2O is, therefore, long. Remember that T2 decay is caused either by external magnetic field inhomogeneities or by spin–spin interactions within or between molecules. In H_2O, the effect of one hydrogen proton on another is relatively small. The distance between hydrogen protons both within each molecule and between adjacent molecules is relatively large, so there is little spin–spin interaction and, therefore, less dephasing.

Solids. The molecular structure of solids is opposite to that of pure water. It is a very compactly structured tissue, with many interactions between hydrogen protons. This large number of spin–spin interactions results in more dephasing. Thus, the T2 for solids is short.

Fat and Proteinaceous Material. The structure of these materials is such that there is less dephasing than in solids but more dephasing than in water. Therefore, T2 for proteinaceous material or fat is intermediate.

T1 Characteristics

The T1 of a tissue has to do with the way the protons are able to give off their energy to the surrounding lattice, or to absorb the energy from the lattice. It turns out that the most efficient energy transfer occurs when the **natural motional frequencies**[1] of the protons are at the **Larmor frequency** (ω_0). Recall that the Larmor frequency is proportional to the strength of the magnetic field:

$$\omega_0 = \gamma B_0$$

For hydrogen, γ = 42.6 MHz/Tesla

In other words, the precessional frequency of a hydrogen proton is 42.6 MHz in a 1-Tesla

---

[1]Translation, rotation, and vibration.

57

magnetic field. However, the *natural motional frequency* of hydrogen protons depends on the physical states of the tissue. It is influenced by the atoms to which they are attached or to which they are proximal.

H₂O. Hydrogen protons in the small H_2O molecule have higher natural motional frequencies than, for example, hydrogen protons in a solid structure. The natural motional frequency of hydrogen protons in water is also much faster than the Larmor frequency for hydrogen.

$$\omega\,(H_2O) \gg \omega_0$$

Solids. Hydrogen protons in solids have lower natural motional frequencies than do water protons. The natural motional frequencies of hydrogen protons in solids are somewhat slower than the Larmor frequency for hydrogen.

$$\omega\,(solids) < \omega_0$$

Fat. Hydrogen protons in fat have natural motional frequencies that are almost equal to the Larmor frequencies used for MRI.

$$\omega\,(fat) \approx \omega_0$$

This result is caused by the rotational frequency of the carbons around the terminal C–C bond. Because this frequency is near the Larmor frequency, the *efficiency of energy transfer* from the protons to the lattice or from the lattice to the protons is increased, thus decreasing T1.

Proteinaceous Solutions. The foregoing discussion on the T1 and T2 characteristics of fluids such as water applies only to *pure* water (or **bulk phase water**). However, most of the water in the body is not in the pure state but is **bound** to a **hydrophilic macromolecule** such as a protein.

Such water molecules form hydration layers around the macromolecule and are called **hydration layer water** (Fig. 6-1). These bound H_2O molecules lose some of the freedom in their

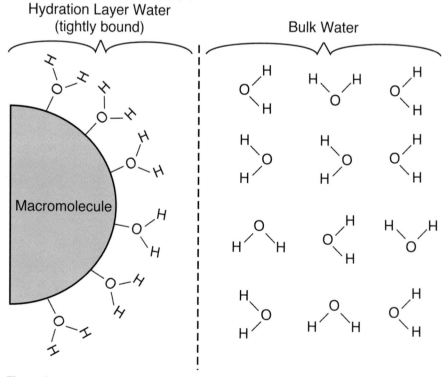

Figure 6-1. Hydration layer water.

motion. As a result, the natural motional frequencies of the H_2O molecules get closer to the Larmor frequency, thus yielding a more efficient energy transfer. The net result is a shortening in the T1 relaxation. Therefore, proteinaceous fluids, that is, hydration layer water, are brighter than pure water on T1-weighted images.

If the protein content is high enough, hydration layer water can cause some T2 shortening. This shortening is generally seen in gels and in **mucinous** fluids. Such proteinaceous fluids may be darker than pure fluids on T2-weighted images.

For H_2O and solid tissue, the energy transfer is not efficient, and the T1 for H_2O and solid tissue is long. Also, the T1 for H_2O is longer than the T1 for solid tissue because the difference between the Larmor frequency and the natural motional frequencies of hydrogen protons in H_2O is much greater than the difference between the Larmor frequency and the motional frequencies of hydrogen protons in solid tissue.

Let's now draw the T1 and T2 curves for these different tissues (Fig. 6-2):

1. **Fat** has the shortest T1 and will have the steepest T1 recovery curve.
2. **Proteinaceous fluid** also has a short T1.
3. **H_2O** has the longest T1 and will have the slowest T1 recovery curve.
4. **Solid** tissue has intermediate T1.

For the sake of argument, we'll assume that they all have the same proton density. Actually, the proton density of H_2O is higher because there are more hydrogen protons per volume in water than either fat or solid tissue, and intensity is based not only on T1 and T2 but also on the proton density $N(H)$:

$$SI \propto N(H)\,(e^{-TE/T2})\,(1 - e^{-TR/T1})$$

At a time TR, we transmit another radio frequency (RF) pulse. Let's superimpose the T2 decay curve on the T1 recovery curve (Fig. 6-3):

1. **H_2O** has a very long T2, so it will have a very shallow T2 decay curve.
2. **Solid** tissue has short T2 and will thus decay fairly rapidly.
3. **Fat** has an intermediate T2.
4. **Proteinaceous fluid** may have a short or intermediate T2 depending on the protein content.

Therefore, we see that if we pick a long enough TE (TE_3) in Figure 6-3, the signals that we measure from each tissue show the following:

1. **H_2O** has the highest signal intensity (point a, Fig. 6-3).
2. **Solid** tissue has the lowest signal intensity.
3. **Fat** has an intermediate signal intensity.
4. **Proteinaceous fluid** has an intermediate or low signal intensity depending on its protein content.

If we take a shorter TE (TE_2), we might pick a point where fat and H_2O might have the same signal intensity. This is a crossover effect (point b, Fig. 6-3).

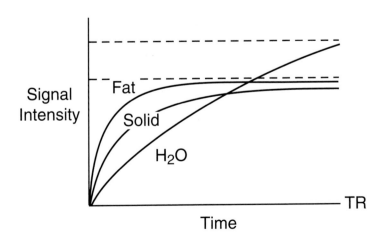

Figure 6-2. T1 recovery curves of fat, water, and a solid tissue.

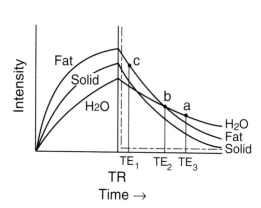

Figure 6-3. T2 decay curves of fat, water, and a solid tissue.

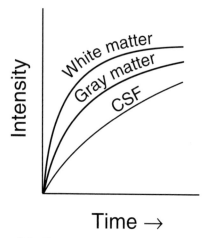

Figure 6-4. T1 recovery curves of CSF, white matter, and gray matter.

If the TE is really short (TE_1), we just get a T1 or proton density effect (it depends on the TR), where

1. **Fat** has the highest intensity (point c, Fig. 6-3).
2. **Proteinaceous fluid** also has high intensity similar to fat.
3. **Solid** tissue has intermediate intensity.
4. **H_2O** has the lowest intensity.

So, we can see from the curve that

1. If TR and TE are short, we get T1 weighting.
2. If TR and TE are long, we get T2 weighting.
3. If TR is long and TE is short, we get proton density weighting.

Let's now look at three different tissues in the brain: (i) gray matter, (ii) white matter, and (iii)

cerebrospinal fluid (CSF; Fig. 6-4). On a T1 recovery curve:

1. **White matter** is bright. The myelin sheath acts like fat; with more efficient energy exchange, it has a shorter longitudinal relaxation than does gray matter.
2. **Gray matter** is intermediate: without myelin, it acts more like a typical solid tissue.
3. **CSF** is dark: like water, it has inefficient energy exchange and thus the same long longitudinal relaxation, T1.

Let's add the T2 decay curves to the T1 recovery curves (Fig. 6-5):

1. **CSF**, like H_2O, has the least dephasing, and thus the longest T2.

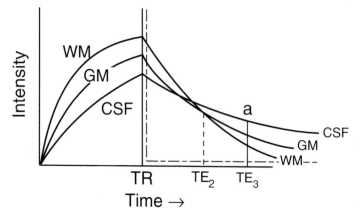

Figure 6-5. T2 decay curves of CSF, white matter, and gray matter.

2. **White matter** has a slightly shorter T2 than **gray matter**.

If we use a long TE (TE_3), then we'll get a typical T2-weighted image. Therefore, at TE = TE_3, we have (Fig. 6-6):

$$@TE = TE_3 \begin{cases} \text{CSF is \textbf{bright} (point a, Fig. 6-5)} \\ \text{Gray matter is intermediate \textbf{(gray)}} \\ \text{White matter is \textbf{dark}} \end{cases}$$

Let's pick a shorter TE = TE_2 (Fig. 6-6). At this point, white matter and CSF are isointense (crossover point). We want to achieve this isointensity on a proton density image. We can see the advantages by considering what tumors and demyelinating plaques do on a T1 recovery curve, or on a T2 decay curve. Most pathologic lesions have a slow T1 recovery curve because of their **vasogenic edema** (which contains H_2O). However, their T1 recovery curve is not as slow as pure water. Most pathologic lesions (e.g., tumor, edema, multiple sclerosis [MS] plaque) also have a long T2 but not as long as that of CSF.

In Figure 6-6, we've included a T1 recovery curve and a T2 decay curve for a pathologic lesion. If we are looking for MS plaques, let's first look at a T2-weighted image (long TE = TE_3 in the graph):

1. White matter is dark.
2. CSF is bright.
3. MS plaque is also bright.

Even though brightness may be different between the CSF and MS plaque, the ratio is not great enough to discern a difference (e.g., the lesion is adjacent to a lateral ventricle).

If we now look at the intensities at a shorter TE (TE_2) corresponding to the CSF and white matter crossover point, then CSF and white matter will be isointense.

The pathologic lesion (e.g., MS plaque) will be brighter than both CSF and white matter, and it can thus be detected more easily. Remember also that if we choose a long TR and a very short TE (TE_1 on the graph), the TE occurs before the crossover points of either CSF, gray matter, or white matter, resulting still in a proton density–weighted image.

This is a good time to bring up the proton density factor: $N(H)$. We've been, to a certain extent, ignoring it. We've talked about T1 and T2, and we've been assuming that all the tissues have almost the same proton density. However, in Table 6-1, we can see the differences in the proton densities of various tissues. Also, T1 is defined as the time when 63% of the longitudinal magnetization has recovered (with $3T1 = 95\%$ recovery), whereas T2 is defined as the time when 63% of the transverse magnetization has decayed (with $3T2 = 95\%$ decay).

For instance, if the CSF has a proton density of 1 (or 100%), then white matter has a proton density of 0.61 (61% of CSF) and edema has a proton density of 0.86 (86% of CSF). How does this difference in proton density affect the

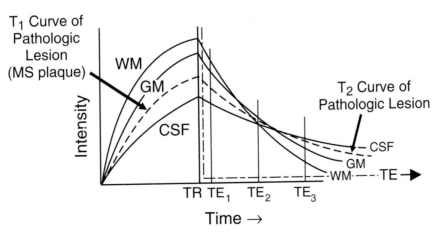

Figure 6-6. Recovery and decay curves of CSF, WM, GM, and a lesion.

Table 6-1	T1, T2, and proton density of brain tissues at 1.5 T[a]		
	T1 (msec)	**T2 (msec)**	**N(H)**
White matter	510	67	0.61
Gray matter	760	77	0.69
Edema	900	126	0.86
CSF	2350	180	1.00

[a] Stark and Bradley, p.44.

graphs of T1 and T2? Let's talk about two different tissues (Fig. 6-7):

1. CSF
2. White matter

CSF has a higher proton density than white matter, so it has a higher maximum limit on the T1 recovery curve. White matter has a lower proton density than CSF, but its T1 is shorter. The two recovery curves cross at the point where white matter and CSF have the same intensity (TR ≈ 2500 msec).

For the mathematically interested reader, this TR is the solution to the following equation:

$$1.0 \, (1 - e^{-TR/2650}) = 0.61 \, (1 - e^{-TR/510})$$

or

$$e^{-TR/2650} - 0.61 \, e^{-TR/510} - 0.39 = 0$$

using the T1 and N(H) values for white matter and CSF from Table 6-1, resulting in a TR of approximately 2500 msec (2462 msec to be exact!).

Let's now consider two situations:

1. Short TR
2. Long TR

1. First, draw the T1 recovery curves for white matter and CSF (Fig. 6-8). Now consider a **short TR** (say, 300 msec). White matter is initially brighter than CSF because of its shorter T1. However, CSF has a longer T2 than white matter. Therefore, after the T2 crossover point, CSF will become brighter than white matter (e.g., at TE_2). Thus, at long TE, we get T2 contrast. If we pick a short TE (TE_1), we get T1 contrast. Thus, with a short TR, which maximizes T1 contrast, we want to choose as short a TE as possible to maximize the T1 contrast.

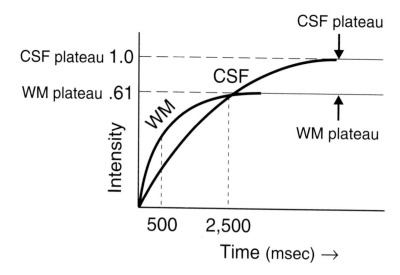

Figure 6-7. The plateau of the recovery curve of a tissue is determined by the proton density of that tissue N(H). For instance, N(CSF) is larger than N(WM).

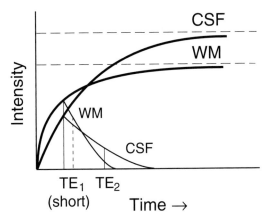

Figure 6-8. Recovery and decay curves for WM and CSF for a short TR.

T1W: Short TR/Short TE

2. Now, draw the T1 and T2 curves again and this time pick a **long TR**. Remember that CSF has a greater proton density than white matter, so it will have a higher plateau value than white matter, which is brought out by the long TR (Fig. 6-9). Then draw the T2 decay curves, keeping in mind that CSF has a longer T2 than white matter. If we now pick a very short TE (TE$_1$), the two signals are driven by

their respective proton densities: CSF will have greater intensity than white matter (i.e., 39%; Table 6-1). At this point, the difference in intensity reflects their (*true*) proton density differences (assuming a very short TE).

PDW: Long TR/Short TE

If TE is long (TE$_2$), increase the signal intensity differences between white matter and CSF. This increased intensity difference reflects the T2 difference.

T2W: Long TR/Long TE

Let's now introduce an abnormality—namely, edema—and incorporate it with CSF and white matter (Fig. 6-10). We know that the T1 recovery curve for edema is in between CSF and white matter—it has a shorter T1 than CSF and a longer T1 than white matter. We also know that the plateau for edema is less than that for pure CSF, but more than that for white matter. Again, if we choose a TR that is long enough for white matter to reach its plateau, and then choose a TE that is short (either at or

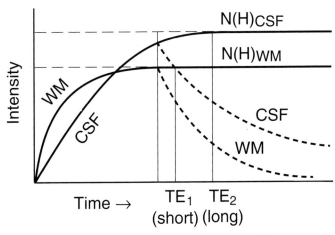

Figure 6-9. Recovery and decay curves of WM and CSF for a long TR.

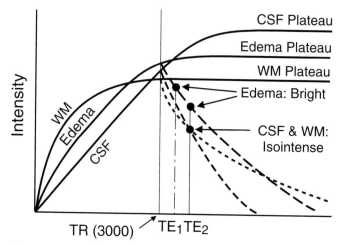

Figure 6-10. Recovery and decay curves of WM, CSF, and edema for a long TR.

before the crossover point for CSF and white matter T2 decay), then edema has the highest signal intensity.

Therefore, for "proton density" images (long TR/short TE):

1. Edema is bright.
2. CSF and white matter are isointense.

Now, pick a TR at the point of intersection of the T1 recovery curves for CSF and white matter—a point at which white matter has almost reached its peak intensity, but CSF has not (similar to the previous graphs, but TR is now longer in order to reach the crossover point; Fig. 6-11). Now, apply the 90° pulse, and follow the T2 decay curves. With a short TE, CSF is brighter than white matter. With a long TE, CSF is still brighter than white matter, but the difference in brightness gets magnified. On the long TR/short TE image, the difference in intensity reflects only the differences in proton densities between the two tissues, whereas the long TR/long TE image incorporates both proton densities and T2 differences between the two tissues.

Parenthetically, in a **true** protein density image (as in Fig. 6-9), CSF or H_2O has the highest signal (because water has more protons than

any other tissue). Therefore, to minimize the T1 and T2 influences on what should be a **true** proton density–weighted image, we need to make the TR long enough to allow the T1 recovery curves to reach their plateaus and then make the TE short enough to minimize T2 decay. (Actually, this may not be a desirable image because lesions and normal fluid may be indistinguishable.)

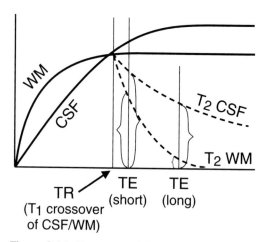

Figure 6-11. Recovery and decay curves of WM and CSF for a TR corresponding to the crossover point of CSF and WM.

Key Points

Table 6-2 summarizes the T1 and T2 properties of three tissues: water, solids, and fat/proteinaceous material. Table 6-3 contains the relative T1 and T2 values (short, intermediate, or long) for several tissues. Figures 6-12 through 6-20 show examples of tissue contrast.

Table 6-2 T1 and T2 as a function of natural motional frequencies (ω) vs. the Larmor frequency (ω_0) for different tissues

	H$_2$O/Fluids	Solids	Fat and Proteinaceous Material
T1	$\omega \gg \omega_0$ Inefficient energy transfer **Very Long T1**	$\omega < \omega_0$ Inefficient energy transfer **Long T1**	$\omega \approx \omega_0$ Efficient energy transfer **Short T1**
T2	Less dephasing **Long T2**	Most dephasing **Short T2**	Intermediate dephasing **Intermediate T2**

Table 6-3 Relative T1 and T2 values for several tissues[a]

	Long T1 (low SI)	Intermediate	Short T1 (high SI)
Long T2 (high SI)	Water/CSF Pathology Edema		**d (EC metHgb)**
Intermediate		Muscle GM **a (oxyHgb)** WM	
Short T2 (low SI)	Air Cortical bone Heavy Ca^{++} **b (deoxyHgb)** **e (hemosiderin)** Fibrosis Tendons		Fat Proteinaceous solution **c (IC met Hgb)** Paramagnetic materials (Gd, etc.)

[a] **a–d** represent breakdown products of hemoglobin (**a,** oxyhemoglobin; **b,** deoxyhemoglobin; **c,** intracellular methemoglobin; **d,** extracellular methemoglobin; **e,** hemosiderin). Abbreviations: GM, gray matter; WM, white matter; SI, signal intensity; Hgb, hemoglobin; IC, intracellular; EC, extracellular.

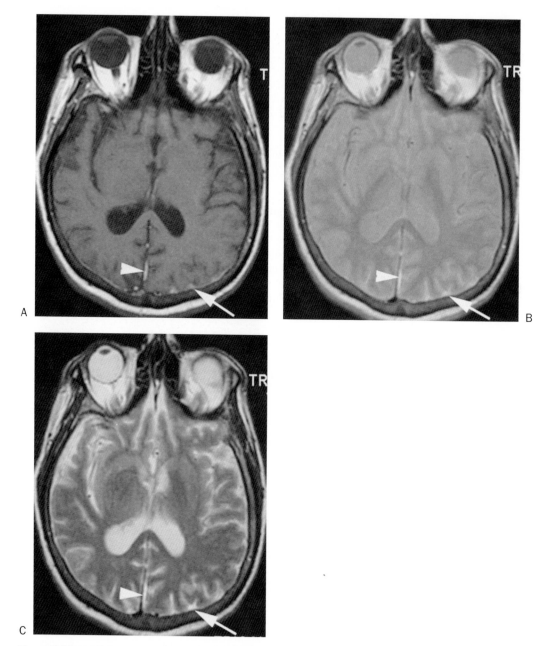

Figure 6-12. Axial T1 (**A**), proton density (**B**), and fast spin echo T2 (**C**) images of the brain. Note that on the T1 image the white matter is brighter than the CSF due to the shorter T1 of white matter. However, the CSF is brighter on the proton density image due to its higher proton density. The white matter becomes even darker on the T2 compared with the CSF secondary to additional T2 differences. The *arrow* points to a subarachnoid hemorrhage, whereas the *arrowhead* points to a small subdural hemorrhage. Note that the hemorrhage is isointense to CSF on the T2 due to a crossover point being achieved, whereas the hemorrhage is brighter on the T1 and on the proton density–weighted images due to the shorter T1 versus CSF.

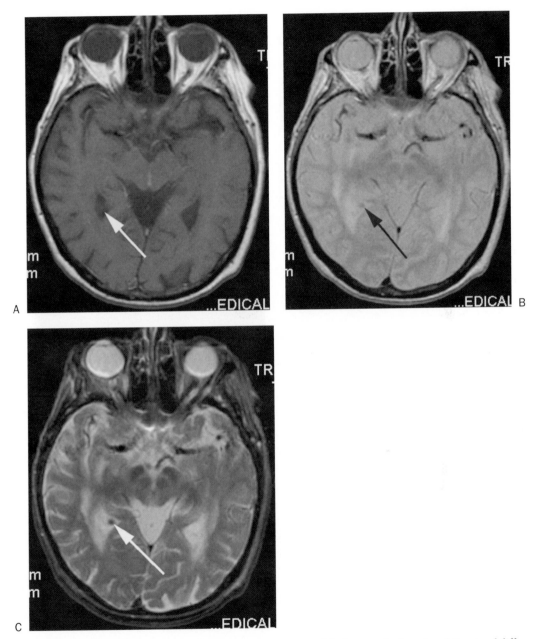

Figure 6-13. Axial T1 (**A**), proton density (**B**), and T2 (**C**) images of the brain again show the relative signal differences in normal structures between the three different sequences. The *arrow* points to a small intraventricular meningioma that has typical signal close to gray matter on all sequences.

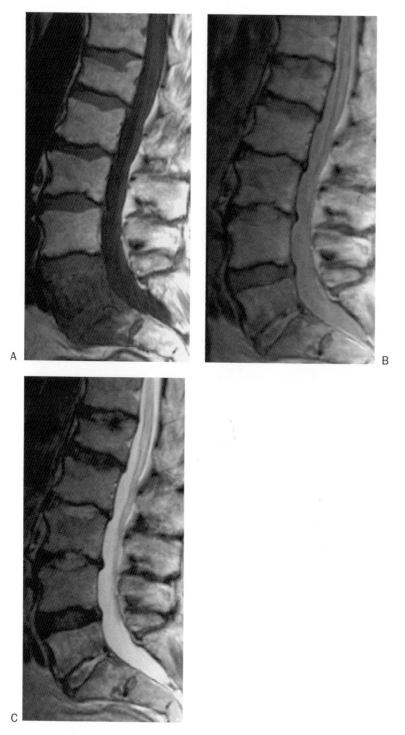

Figure 6-14. Sagittal T1 (**A**), proton density (**B**), and T2 (**C**) images of the lumbosacral spine show dark signal in the L5 and S1 vertebral bodies on the T1 sequence due to the longer T1 of edema compared with the shorter T1 of the fatty marrow at the other levels. The CSF and the intervertebral discs are normally dark on T1 due to fluid and/or dessication. The proton density and T2 images show the L5/S1 disc and a few others to be bright, as is the CSF. Note that the CSF is brightest on the T2. The combination of both abnormal bone marrow signal and the adjacent bright disc represent osteomyelitis and discitis, whereas bright discs at other levels with adjacent normal marrow represent hydrated discs.

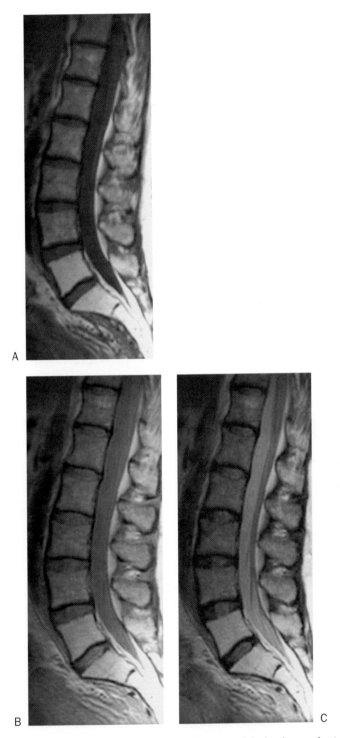

Figure 6-15. Sagittal T1 (**A**), proton density (**B**), and T2 (**C**) images of the lumbosacral spine show normally bright signal in all the vertebral bodies through L4; however, the L5 vertebral body and the sacrum have very bright signal on all sequences. The proton density and T2 images were acquired with a fast spin echo technique. This patient had radiation therapy for cervical cancer with subsequent complete fatty replacement of the marrow at L5 and the sacrum as opposed to the normal fatty-containing marrow at other levels.

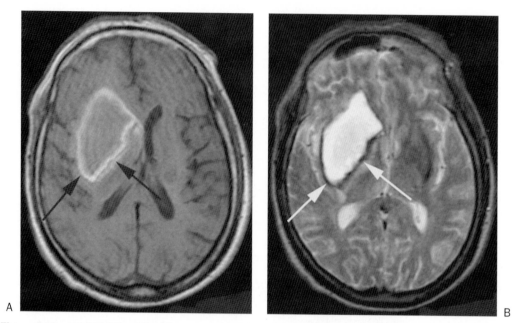

A

B

Figure 6-16. Axial T1 (**A**) and T2 (**B**) images demonstrate a large, right basal ganglia acute hypertensive hemorrhage (isointense on T1 and bright on T2—oxyhemoglobin). There is a rim of bright T1 and dark T2 signal (*arrows*) that represents a characteristic rim of the more temporally advanced intracellular methemoglobin.

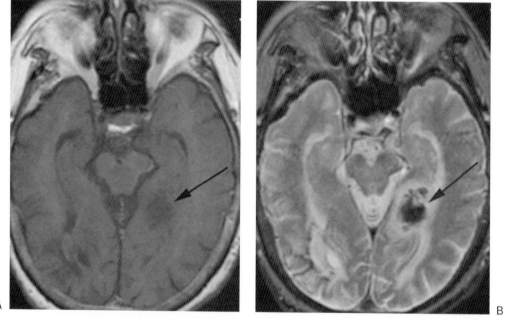

A

B

Figure 6-17. Axial T1 (**A**) and T2 (**B**) images demonstrate an acute (dark on T1 and T2—deoxyhemoglobin) left medial temporal intraparenchymal hematoma (*arrows*). Additional axial T1 (**C**) and T2 (**D**) images in the same patient at another level show a late subacute (bright on both T1 and T2—extracellular methemoglobin) right occipital hematoma (*arrows*) and acute (isointense on T1 and dark on T2) left medial temporal hematoma (*arrowhead*—best seen in image **D**). This patient had amyloid angiopathy.

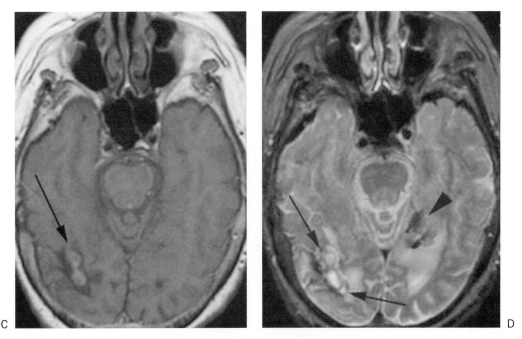

C

D

Figure 6-17. (*continued*)

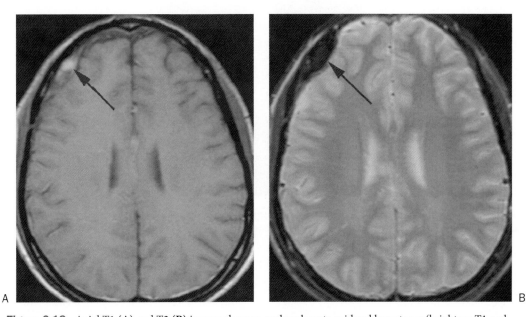

A

B

Figure 6-18. Axial T1 (**A**) and T2 (**B**) images show an early subacute epidural hematoma (bright on T1 and dark on T2—intracellular methemoglobin) along the right frontal lobe (*arrows*).

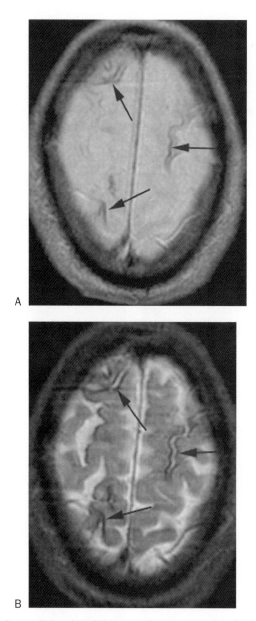

Figure 6.19. Axial proton density **(A)** and T2 **(B)** images demonstrate superficial gyriform dark signal from superficial siderosis (hemosiderin) in a patient with a history of subarachnoid hemorrhage (*arrows*).

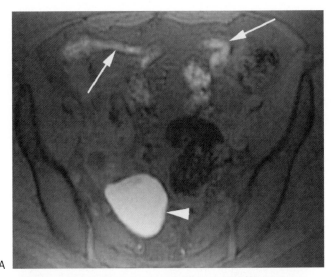

A

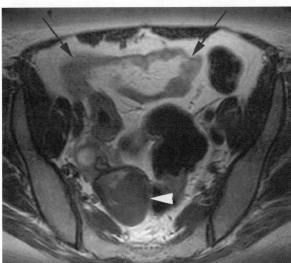

B

Figure 6-20. Axial T1 with fat saturation without gadolinium (**A**) and fast spin echo T2 (**B**) images show bright T1 and relatively dark T2 signal in the lumen of the small bowel consistent with proteinaceous solutions (*arrows*). Additionally, the patient has a right endometrioma (*arrowhead*) with predominantly bright T1 and dark T2 signal secondary to recurrent hemorrhage.

Questions

6-1 T/F Hydration layer water has a shorter T1 than bulk water.

6-2 Match (i) short T1 and T2; (ii) short T1, long T2; (iii) long T1, short T2; and (iv) long T1, long T2 with
  (a) air
  (b) fat
  (c) water
  (d) intracellular methemoglobin
  (e) extracellular methemoglobin

6-3 T/F The most efficient energy transfer occurs at the Larmor frequency.

6-4 Match the following: (i) short TR and TE; (ii) long TR and TE; (iii) short TR, long TE; (iv) long TR, short TE with
  (a) T1 weighted
  (b) T2 weighted
  (c) intermediate weighted

7

Pulse Sequences: Part I (Saturation, Partial Saturation, Inversion Recovery)

Introduction

A **pulse sequence** is a *sequence* of radio frequency (RF) *pulses* applied repeatedly during an MR study. Embedded in it are the TR and TE time parameters. It is related to a **timing diagram** or a **pulse sequence diagram** (PSD), which is discussed in Chapter 14. In this chapter, we discuss the concepts of **saturation** and consider pulse sequence partial saturation, saturation recovery, and inversion recovery (IR). In the next chapter, we'll talk about the important spin-echo pulse sequence. Figure 7-1 illustrates the notations used for three types of RF pulses throughout this book.

Saturation

Immediately after the longitudinal magnetization has been flipped into the x–y plane by a 90° pulse, the system is said to be **saturated.** Application of a second 90° pulse at this moment will elicit no signal (like beating a dead

horse). A few moments later, after some T1 recovery, the system is **partially saturated.** With complete T1 recovery to the plateau value, the system is **unsaturated** or fully *magnetized*. Should the longitudinal magnetization only be partially flipped into the x–y plane (i.e., flip angles less than 90°), then there is still a component of magnetization along the z-axis. The spins in this state are also **partially saturated.**

Partial Saturation Pulse Sequence. Start with a 90° pulse, wait for a short period TR, and then apply another 90° pulse. Keep repeating this sequence. The measurements are obtained immediately after the 90° RF pulse. Therefore, the signal received is a free induction decay (FID).

Let's see how this looks on the T1 recovery curve (Fig. 7-2). At time $t = 0$, flip the longitudinal magnetization 90° into the x–y plane. Right after that, the longitudinal magnetization begins to recover. Wait a time $t = TR$, and repeat the 90° pulse. Initially, at time $t = 0$, the longitudinal magnetization is at a maximum. As soon as we flip it, the longitudinal magnetization goes to zero and then immediately thereafter begins to grow. At time $t = TR$, the longitudinal magnetization has grown but has not recovered its plateau before it is flipped into the x–y plane again. (Note that the length of the longitudinal magnetization vector before the second 90° RF pulse is less than the original longitudinal magnetization vector.)

Now, with a third 90° RF pulse, we again flip the longitudinal magnetization into the x–y plane. Again, the longitudinal magnetization goes to zero and immediately begins to recover.

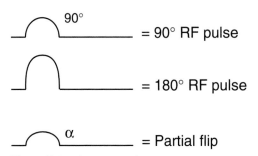

Figure 7-1. The notation for 90°, 180°, and partial flip pulses.

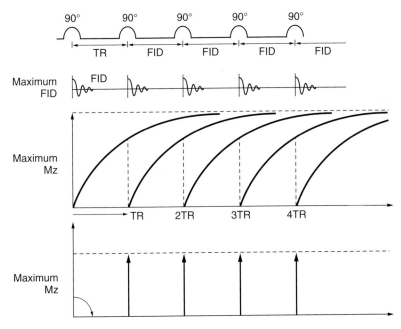

Figure 7-2. The recovery curves following the RF pulses in a partial saturation sequence.

Again, at time 2TR, it is less than maximum but is equal to the previous longitudinal magnetization (at time TR). Each subsequent recovery time TR after each subsequent 90° pulse will also be the same. Thus, the maximum FID occurs at time $t = 0$ after the first 90° RF pulse, and all subsequent FIDs will have less magnitude but will have the same value.

> *Question: Is there a residual transverse magnetization $\mathbf{M}_{xy}$ at time TR just before the next 90° RF pulse?*
>
> *Answer: No! Because T1 is several times larger than T2, after a time TR has elapsed, the magnetization in the x–y plane has fully decayed to zero.*

In partial saturation, TE is minimal. The signal is measured immediately after the 90° RF pulse.

> **Partial saturation: TR is short, TE is minimal.**

> *Question: With short TR and minimal TE, what kind of an image would we be getting?*
>
> *Answer: T1-weighted image.*

> **A partial saturation pulse sequence generates a T1-weighted image.**

Saturation Recovery Pulse Sequence

The previous sequence is called partial saturation because at the time of the second 90° RF pulse (at time TR), we haven't yet completely recovered the longitudinal magnetization. Therefore, only a portion of the original longitudinal magnetization ($\mathbf{M}_0$) is flipped at time TR (and subsequent TRs). Hence the name *partial saturation*.

In **saturation recovery,** we try to recover all the longitudinal magnetization before we apply another 90° RF pulse. We have to wait a long time before we apply a second RF pulse. Thus, TR will be long (Fig. 7-3).

After each 90° RF pulse, we measure it and an FID right away. Because we allow the longitudinal magnetization to recover completely before the next 90° pulse, the FID gives the maximum signal each time. In other words, we have recovered from the state of saturation.

> **In saturation recovery, TR is long and TE is minimal.**

> *Question: With long TR and minimal TE, what kind of image do we get?*
>
> *Answer: Proton density weighted (PDW).*

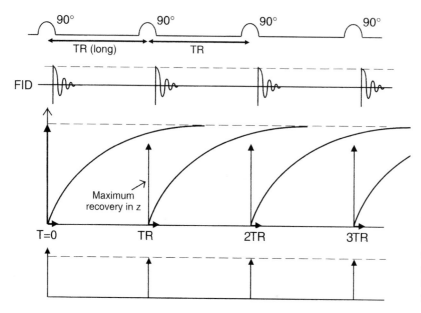

90°   90°   90°   90°

TR (long)   TR

FID

Maximum recovery in z

T=0   TR   2TR   3TR

Figure 7-3. In a saturation recovery sequence, TR is long and longitudinal magnetization vectors are near maximal.

> **The saturation recovery pulse sequence results in a proton density-weighted image.**

Neither of these sequences is really used any more, but they are so simple to understand that they are good springboards from which to learn about other, more complex pulse sequences. These pulse sequences are not used because it is very difficult to measure the FID without a delay period. Electronically we have to wait a certain period of time to make the measurements. Also, external magnetic inhomogeneity becomes a problem; that's why spin-echo sequences (which we will discuss in the next chapter) are used to eliminate this problem.

Inversion Recovery Pulse Sequence

In IR, we first apply a 180° RF pulse. Next, we wait a period of time (the inversion time TI) and apply a 90° RF pulse. Then we wait a period of time TR (from the initial 180° pulse) and apply another 180° RF pulse (Fig. 7-4), beginning the sequence all over again.

Before we apply the 180° pulse, the magnetization vector points along the z-axis. Immediately after we apply the 180° pulse, the magnetization vector is flipped 180°; it is now pointing south (−z), which is the opposite direction (Fig. 7-5).

We then allow the magnetization vector to recover along a T1 growth curve. As it recovers, it gets smaller and smaller in the −z direction until it goes to zero, and then starts growing in the +z direction, ultimately recovering to the original longitudinal magnetization.

After a time TI, we apply a 90° pulse. This then flips the longitudinal magnetization into the x–y plane. The amount of magnetization flipped into the x–y plane will, of course, depend on the amount of longitudinal magnetization that has recovered during time TI after the original 180° RF pulse. We measure this flipped magnetization. Therefore, at this point we get an FID proportional to the longitudinal magnetiza-

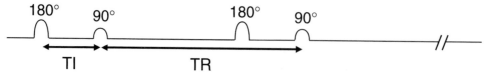

180°   90°   180°   90°

TI   TR

Figure 7-4. In inversion recovery, the time between the 180° pulse and the 90° pulse is denoted TI.

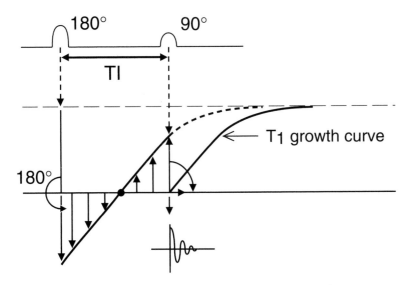

$$180° \qquad 90°$$

TI

T1 growth curve

180°

Figure 7-5. The recovery curves in inversion recovery. After the 180° pulse, the longitudinal magnetization vector is flipped 180° and starts to recover from a value that is the negative of its initial maximal value.

tion flipped into the x–y plane. Also, at this point, we begin the regrowth of the longitudinal magnetization. Recall that for a typical T1 recovery curve, the formula for the exponential growth of the curve is

$$1 - e^{-t/T1}$$

However, when the magnetization starts to recover from $-\mathbf{M}_0$ instead of zero (Fig. 7-6), the formula for recovery is

$$1 - 2e^{-t/T1}$$

Exercise

Verify the above formula mathematically.

At time $t = 0$,

$$\text{Signal intensity (SI)} = 1 - 2e^{-0/T1}$$
$$= 1 - 2(1) = -1$$

So at time $t = 0$,

Magnitude of signal intensity $= -1$.

At $t = \infty$ (infinity),

$$\text{Signal intensity} = 1 - 2e^{-\infty/T1}$$
$$= 1 - 2(0) = +1$$

So at time $t = \infty$, the signal is maximal. These values correspond to the graph in Figure 7-6.

Null Point. The point at which the signal crosses the zero line is called the **null point.** At this point, the signal intensity is zero. The time at this null point is denoted TI(null). We can

solve the equation mathematically for TI(null), at which point the signal intensity is zero:

$$\text{Signal intensity} = 0 = 1 - 2e^{-TI/T1}$$

The solution to this equation is (see Question 7-1 at the end):

$$\text{TI(null)} = (\log_e 2)\, T1 = (\ln 2)\, T1 \approx 0.693\, T1$$

Let's go back and re-examine the recovery curves. Actually, there are two different exponentially growing curves occurring sequentially (Fig. 7-7):

1. Recovery after the 180° RF pulse
2. Recovery after the 90° RF pulse

   1. The T1 recovery curve following the 180° pulse starts at $-\mathbf{M}_0$ and grows exponentially according to the formula:

$$\mathbf{M}_0 \,(1 - 2e^{-TI/T1})$$

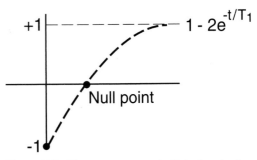

$$+1 \qquad\qquad 1 - 2e^{-t/T_1}$$

Null point

$$-1$$

Figure 7-6. The recovery curve in IR is given by the formula $1 - 2e^{-t/T1}$.

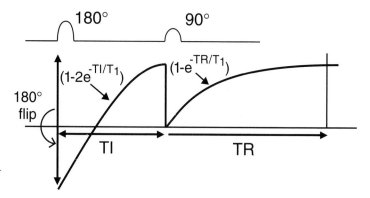

Figure 7-7. There are two recovery curves in one IR cycle.

2. The T1 recovery curve following the 90° RF pulse, after the longitudinal magnetization, flips into the x–y plane, starts at 0, and grows exponentially according to the formula:

$$\mathbf{M}_0 \, (1 - e^{-TR/T1})$$

If we combine both of these T1 recovery curves, we get a relationship that combines both T1 and TR together. The result is the product of the above two formulas:

$$SI \propto \mathbf{M}_0 \, (1 - 2e^{-TI/T1}) \, (1 - e^{-TR/T1})$$

Assuming that TI $\ll$ TR, the product of the terms within parentheses can be simplified to (see Question 7-2 at the end):

$$(1 - 2e^{-TI/T1}) + (e^{-TR/T1})$$

Clinical Applications of Inversion Recovery. In an IR pulse sequence, we start out with a 180° RF pulse followed, after a time interval TI, by a 90° RF pulse. Next, after a certain time interval TR, the sequence is repeated with another 180° pulse.

TI = inversion time, which represents the time interval between the 180° pulse and the 90° pulse

TR = time interval between successive 180° pulses (or successive 90° pulses)

Consider graphically what happens to two tissues: edema and white matter (Fig. 7-8). In IR, we first flip the longitudinal magnetization 180° with a 180° RF pulse. Subsequently, the magnetization vector still runs along the z-axis but points in the negative (south) direction. Next, the longi-

tudinal magnetization vectors begin to grow according to the T1 growth curves of edema and white matter. Edema has a greater proton density than white matter, so its maximum magnetization along the z-axis will be greater than the maximum for white matter. Likewise, after they have flipped 180°, the T1 recovery curve for edema begins lower, that is, it is more negative along the z-axis than is white matter.

From this initial position along the z-axis, the longitudinal magnetization for edema grows along its T1 recovery curve until it reaches its maximum. It starts decreasing in the negative z direction until it reaches zero (the null point), and then it continues increasing in the positive z direction until it reaches its maximum. The T1 growth curve for white matter, because of its lower proton density, starts closer to zero on the negative z-axis than edema after the 180° flip. Because of its shorter T1, it recovers more rapidly along its T1 curve than does edema to reach its maximum.

At time TI, a 90° excitation pulse is applied. Edema and white matter will have recovered their longitudinal magnetization at different rates depending on their individual T1s. When both longitudinal magnetization vectors are flipped into the x–y plane by the 90° pulse, they generate FID signals. Immediately after the 90° pulse, each longitudinal magnetization vector goes to zero but begins recovering according to its T1 recovery curve. Then, after a time interval TR, the process is repeated with another 180° inverting pulse.

We saw earlier that the T1 growth curve after the 180° pulse is given by the formula:

$$\mathbf{M}_0 \, (1 - e^{-TR/T1}) \, (1 - 2e^{-TI/T1})$$

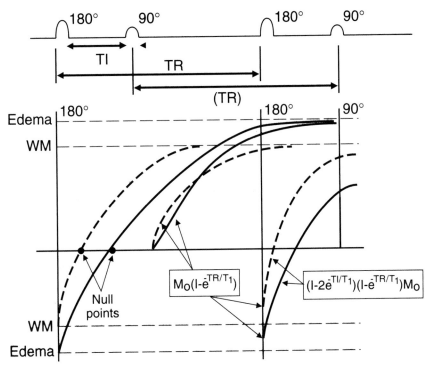

Figure 7-8. Recovery curves for WM and edema.

Magnitude Reconstruction. Magnitude reconstruction is another variable in IR. If we want to increase the signal-to-noise ratio by about 40% (more precisely, by a factor of $\sqrt{2}$), we can add the x and y channels of the coil together as the root mean square (rms), that is, $\sqrt{(S_x{}^2 + S_y{}^2)}$.

This gives us a **magnitude** image, which is always positive. It appears like the mirror image of the negative growth curves, flipped about the time axis (Fig. 7-9). The dashed lines going from the positive z-axis, down to the zero point, are actually the mirror image of the two T1 growth curves of edema and white matter, "flipped" so that we only register their *magnitude*, not their positive or negative phase. This new method of displaying the IR process is called **magnitude reconstruction.** Although it has $\sqrt{2}$ more signal to noise than the original **phase construction,** its dynamic range is less than the original, that is, 0 to $\mathbf{M}_0$ versus $-\mathbf{M}_0$ to $\mathbf{M}_0$. Thus, magnitude reconstruction is used whenever the signal-to-noise ratio is limited, and phase reconstruction is used when greater contrast is needed.

In IR, TR is always long. By picking a long TR, we reach a steady state with maximum value on the T1 growth curve of each tissue after the 90° pulse. What happens when TI is chosen to null white matter (Fig. 7-9)? If we consider just the *magnitude* of the signal, which is the distance of the T1 recovery curve above or below the time line, then edema has a greater *magnitude* than white matter. Because edema has a longer T2 than white matter, if we choose a long TE, then we will magnify the difference in intensity between the two tissues. In fact, the longer the TE, the greater the contrast difference will be between edema and white matter (Fig. 7-10).

Fat Suppression: STIR Imaging

STIR stands for short TI (or Tau) inversion recovery. Let's draw two T1 recovery curves, after the 180° RF pulse, for two tissues—fat and H_2O (Fig. 7-11). Pick the TI at the point where fat crosses the zero point. (The null point is equal to ln 2 [or 0.693] multiplied by the T1 of fat [see Question 7-1 at the end].)

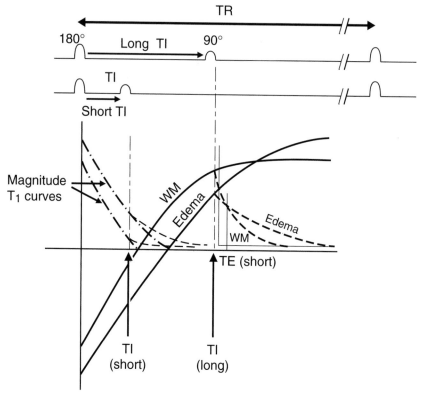

Figure 7-9. Recovery curves, magnitude recovery curves (mirror image curves to make everything positive), and associated decay curves for WM and edema.

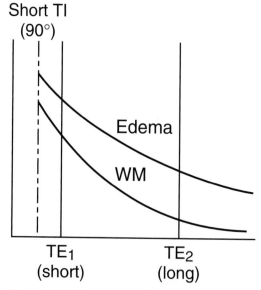

Figure 7-10. Tissue contrast for two different TEs.

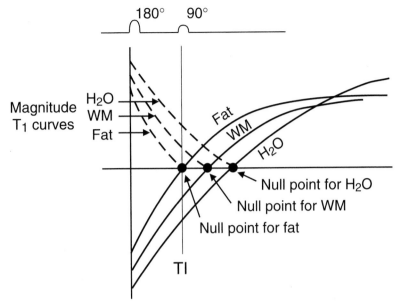

Figure 7-11. In the STIR fat suppression technique, TI is chosen so that the T1 recovery curve for fat crosses zero at the time of the 90° pulse.

At this null point for fat, if we draw the T2 decay curves, fat starts at zero and will stay at zero. There will be no transverse magnetization from fat in the x–y plane, and water will have its usual T2 decay curve. In effect, we have *suppressed* the fat signal. Therefore, after a 180° inverting pulse, we wait a time TI = 0.693 T1 (fat) and we give the 90° pulse. All other tissues will have longitudinal magnetization that will flip into the x–y plane and give off a signal according to their T2 curves. However, at its

null point, fat will not have any longitudinal magnetization to flip into the x–y plane and thus will not have any signal.

The term **STIR** is called *short TI inversion recovery* because fat has a very short T1; therefore, a very short TI must be chosen to null it (at high field [1.5 T] this TI is 140 msec, whereas at midfield [0.5 T] it is 100 msec). Fat will reach its null point before white matter, gray matter, H_2O, or edema (Fig. 7-11).

Key Points

We have discussed three types of pulse sequences: saturation recovery, partial saturation, and inversion recovery (IR). The latter is very important because it allows suppression of any tissue by selecting TI to be 0.693 times the T1 of that tissue:

$$TI(null) = 0.693 \times T1$$

This subject is further elaborated in Chapter 25 on tissue suppression techniques.

A partial saturation sequence results in T1 weighting (short TR and TE). A saturation recovery, however, results in PD weighting (long TR, short TE).

Questions

7-1 (a) Given an inversion recovery (IR) pulse sequence (Fig. 7-6), prove that TI that "nulls" or "suppresses" a certain tissue is equal to 0.693 × T1 (tissue), that is, TI(null) = 0.693 × T1

Hint: The IR curve is proportional to $SI \propto 1 - 2e^{-t/T1}$, where $t = TI$.

(b) Assuming a T1 = 180 msec for fat, what TI would "suppress" the fat?

7-2 Consider the inversion recovery (IR) pulse sequence shown in Figure 7-12. Prove that the signal measured after each 90° pulse (i.e., at A, A′) is given by $N(H)$ $(1 - 2e^{-TI/T1} + e^{-TR/T1})$ assuming that TI is much smaller than TR (i.e., $TI \ll TR$).

7-3 Match
(i) partial saturation
(ii) saturation recovery
with
(a) PD weighted
(b) T1 weighted

7-4 **T/F** In an IR sequence, a 180° pulse is followed TI millisecond later by a 90° pulse.

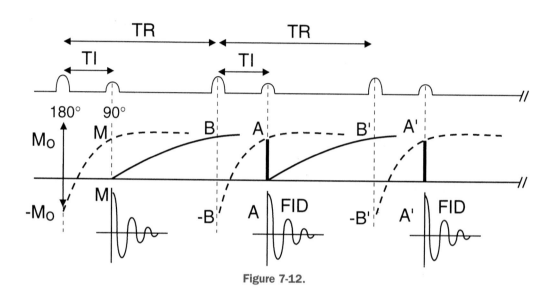

Figure 7-12.

Pulse Sequences
Part II (Spin Echo)

Introduction

This chapter focuses on the most frequently used pulse sequence—the spin echo (SE) pulse sequence. When the concept of **dephasing** was discussed in previous chapters, we brought up two main causes: (i) external magnetic inhomogeneity, and (ii) inherent spin–spin interactions. The SE pulse sequence eliminates the former by an additional **refocusing** or **rephasing** $180°$ radio frequency (RF) pulse. By using the SE pulse sequence, we can eliminate dephasing caused by fixed **external magnetic field inhomogeneities**. (We can't eliminate **spin–spin interactions** because they are not fixed, i.e., they fluctuate randomly.)

Spin-Echo Pulse Diagram

As a result of the $90°$ pulse, the magnetization vector $\mathbf{M}_z$ is flipped into the x–y plane. Consider the precession of three different magnetization vectors in the transverse plane, each in a slightly different magnetic environment (Fig. 8-1A). Initially, all these vectors are *in phase* and they are all precessing at frequency ω_0.

In Figure 8-1A, say one group of spins is exposed to the magnetic field $\mathbf{B}_0$, which causes them to precess at frequency ω_0. The adjacent group of spins sees a slightly higher field $\mathbf{B}_0^+$ and precesses at a slightly higher frequency ω_0^+, and another sees a slightly lower field $\mathbf{B}_0^-$ with a precessional frequency of ω_0^-. After the $90°$ pulse, the three spins will begin to get *out of phase* with each other (Fig. 8-1B). Eventually, the fast vector

and the slow vector become $180°$ out of phase and cancel each other out (Fig. 8-1C).

Analogy

Let's consider the analogy of three runners running around the track (Fig. 8-2). Initially, they start out at the same point. After they run for a time τ, they are no longer together—one is running faster and gets ahead of the others, and one is running slower, falling behind the others.

At this time, if we make the runners turn around and run the opposite way, each one will still be running at the same speed (precessing at the same frequency in the case of the spins). They have just changed direction and are running back to where they started. Each one will then run the same distance if they run the same amount of time τ. Therefore, at time 2τ, they will all come back at the starting point *at the same time* and will be back together in phase. The action of making the runners change direction is done with the use of a $180°$ refocusing pulse in the case of the spins.

Thus, at a certain time τ after the $90°$ pulse, when the spins have gotten out of phase, a $180°$ pulse is applied. Now all the spins flip $180°$ in the x–y plane and they continue precessing, but now in the opposite direction (Fig. 8-3). Let's look at the pulse sequence diagram (Fig. 8-4). We start off with a $90°$ RF pulse to flip the spins into the x–y plane. We wait a time τ and apply a $180°$ RF pulse. Then we wait a long time, TR, and repeat the process.

If we draw the free induction decay (FID) after the $90°$ pulse, we see that the FID dephases

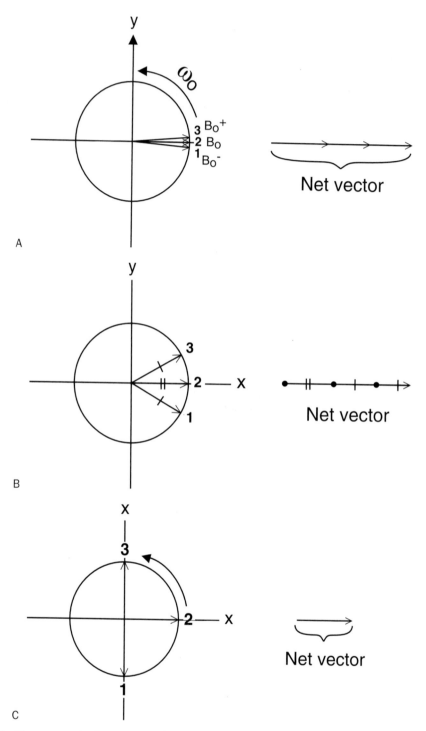

Figure 8-1. Three magnetization vectors in three slightly magnetic environments. In (**A**) they are in phase and their vector sum is three times each individual vector. In (**B**) they are slightly out of phase, yielding a smaller net vector. In (**C**) vector 1 and 3 cancel each other out because they are 180° out of phase, leaving only vector 2.

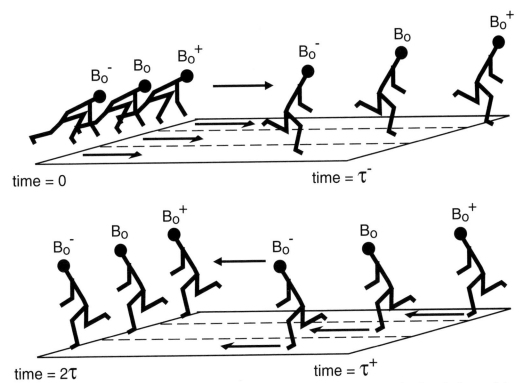

Figure 8-2. Analogy of three runners on a track. At time τ they are made to turn around and run back toward the starting point. Because the slowest runner is now in the lead, they will all reach the starting point at exactly the same time (at time 2τ).

very rapidly due to the T2* effect related to external magnetic field inhomogeneities and spin–spin interactions. The spins get out of phase. After time τ we apply the 180° refocusing pulse. After an equal time τ they will be completely in phase again, and the signal will reach a maximum.

1. Time τ is the time from the 90° RF pulse to the 180° RF pulse.
2. Time τ is also the time from the 180° RF pulse to the point of maximum rephasing, that is, the **echo.**
3. We call 2τ the **echo delay time (time to echo)—TE:** the time after the 90° pulse when we get maximum signal again.
4. The 180° pulse is, therefore, called a **refocusing** or **rephasing** pulse.

We can apply a second 180° pulse. Now, instead of one 180° pulse following the 90° pulse, we have two 180° pulses in sequence after a 90° pulse (Fig. 8-5). After the first echo, the spins

will begin to dephase again. A second 180° pulse applied at time τ_2 after the first echo will allow the spins to rephase again at time $2\tau_2$ after the first echo and a second echo is obtained. Each echo has its own TE.

1. The time from the 90° pulse to the first echo is TE_1.
2. The time from the 90° pulse to the second echo is TE_2.

Ideally, we would like to regain all the signal from the original FID. In practice, it can't happen. We are able to regain the signal lost due to fixed external magnetic field inhomogeneities by applying a refocusing 180° pulse, but dephasing caused by spin–spin interaction of the tissue cannot be regained. If we join the points of maximum signal due to rephasing as a result of the 180° pulses, we will get an *exponentially decaying curve* with a time constant given by T2. Therefore, the decay of the original FID and the decay of each subsequent echo is given by $e^{-t/T2^*}$, whereas the decay of the

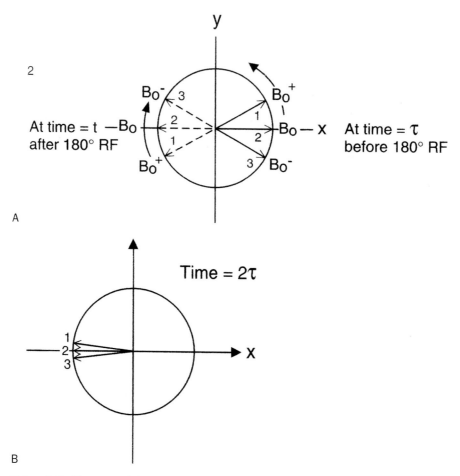

Figure 8-3. The vectors in Figure 8-1 are reversed 180° in direction at time τ (**A**), so that at time 2τ they'll get in phase again (**B**).

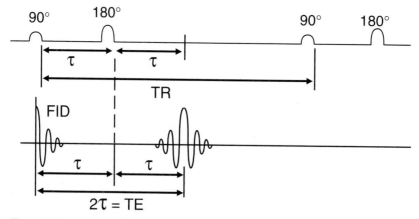

Figure 8-4. In a spin-echo pulse sequence, a 180° pulse is applied at time τ, causing the spins to get in phase at time 2τ. This leads to the formation of an echo from the FID.

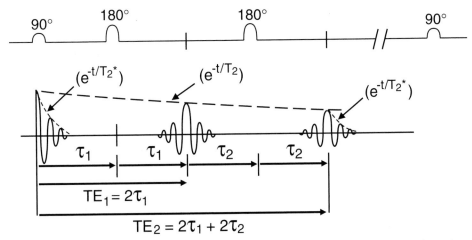

Figure 8-5. An example of a dual-echo, spin-echo pulse sequence in which two echoes are formed via application of two 180° pulses.

curve describing the maximum signal reached by each echo is given by $e^{-t/T2}$. This is the difference between T2* and T2.

Symmetric Echoes

In Figure 8-5, if $\tau_1 = \tau_2$, then we get **symmetric echoes.**

Example
Take TR = 2000, and TE = 40 and 80 msec.
Here, $\tau_1 = 20$, so that $TE_1 = 2\tau_1 = 40$, and $TE_2 = 80 = TE_1 + 2\tau_2 = 40 + 2\tau_2$; then $2\tau_2 = 40$ and $\tau_2 = 20$.
So $\tau_1 = \tau_2$ in symmetric echoes.

Asymmetric Echoes

If $\tau_1 \neq \tau_2$, then we get **asymmetric echoes.**

Example
Take TR = 2000, TE = 30 and 80 msec.
Here $TE_1 = 2(\tau_1) = 30$ msec, so $\tau_1 = 15$ msec. $TE_2 = 80$ msec $= TE_1 + 2(\tau_2) = 30$ msec $+ 2\tau_2 = 80$ msec.
Then $2\tau_2 = 50$ and $\tau_2 = 25$ msec.
So $\tau_1 \neq \tau_2$ in asymmetric echoes.

Question: *What does the 180° pulse do to the longitudinal magnetization?*

Answer: *It inverts it. However, at time TE/2 (on the order of 10 msec), the recovered longitudinal magnetization is negligible and its inversion*

does not cause any significant signal loss. In fact, at t = TE/2, we have

$$\mathbf{M}_z = \mathbf{M}_0 \left(1 - e^{-\text{TE}/2\text{TR}}\right) \cong 0$$

because TE/2 ≪ TR, so that $e^{-TE/2TR} \cong 1$.

Tissue Contrast

As discussed in Chapter 6, tissue contrast in SE depends primarily on TR and TE. There are three types of tissue contrast:

1. T1 weighted (T1W)
2. T2 weighted (T2W)
3. Proton density weighted (PDW; also called "balanced," "intermediate," and "spin density")

Let's see what TR and TE must be for these three imaging scenarios (Table 8-1):

1. For T1 weighting, we want to eliminate the T2 effect and enhance the T1 effect.
   (a) To eliminate (reduce) the T2 effect, we want a short TE.
   (b) To enhance the T1 effect, we want a short TR.
   (c) The signal is then proportional to $N(H) (1 - e^{-\text{TR}/\text{T1}})$.
2. For T2 weighting, we want to eliminate the T1 effect and enhance the T2 effect.
   (a) To eliminate (reduce) the T1 effect, we want a long TR.

Table 8-1

	TR	TE	Signal (Theoretical)
T1W	Short	Short	$N(H) (1 - e^{-TR/T1})$
T2W	Long	Long	$N(H) (e^{-TE/T2})$
PDW	Long	Short	$N(H)$

(b) To enhance the T2 effect, we want a long TE.

(c) The signal is, therefore, proportional to $N(H) (e^{-TE/T2})$.

3. For proton density weighting, we want to eliminate the T1 and T2 effects.

   (a) To eliminate (reduce) the T1 effect, we want a long TR.

   (b) To eliminate (reduce) the T2 effect, we want a short TE.

   (c) The signal is then proportional to $N(H)$.

Remember that in practice we never totally eliminate any of these factors. We would have to have an infinitely long TR to eliminate all T1 effects, and we would need a TE of 0 to eliminate all T2 effects. Therefore, all T1-weighted images in practice have some T2 influence (Fig. 8-6); all T2-weighted images have some T1 influence; and proton density-weighted images have some influence from both T1 and T2. This is why we use the terms *T1 weighting*, *T2 weighting*, and *proton density weighting*:

1. We put more *weight* on the differences in T1 by shortening the TE and the TR.

2. We put more *weight* on the differences in T2 by lengthening TR and the TE.

3. We put less *weight* on T1 and T2 by lengthening TR and shortening TE, thus giving more *weight* to proton density.

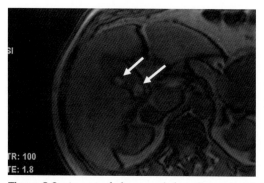 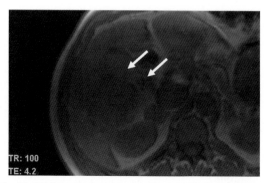

Figure 8-6. An out-of-phase spoiled gradient echo T1 (**A** with TE 1.8 msec) and an in-phase spoiled gradient echo T1 (**B** with TE 4.2 msec) demonstrate bright gallstones in (**A**), but dark gallstones in (**B**). This is due to the short T2* time of the gallstones with rapid signal loss between 1.8 and 4.2 msec. Also note the signal loss of the bile in the gallbladder on the out-of-phase image indicating a mixed amount of fat/cholesterol signal and water signal.

Key Points

1 The SE (spin echo) pulse sequence is composed of a 90° excitation pulse followed by one or more 180° rephasing pulses.

2 The purpose of the 180° pulse is to eliminate the dephasing effects caused by external magnetic field inhomogeneities by rephasing the spins at the time of echo (TE).

3 The resultant echo then depends on T2 decay rather than T2* decay, as seen with the FID (free induction decay).

4 Table 8-2 summarizes the tissue contrast in SE with respect to TR and TE.

<table>
<tr><td colspan="3">**Table 8-2**</td></tr>
<tr><td></td><td>**Short TE**</td><td>**Long TE**</td></tr>
<tr><td>Short TR</td><td>T1W</td><td>Mixed</td></tr>
<tr><td>Long TR</td><td>PDW</td><td>T2W</td></tr>
</table>

Questions

8-1 Consider a dual-echo SE sequence as in Figure 8-5:

(a) What are the received signals at the first echo and at the second echo?

(b) What would the signal at TE_1 be without a 180° refocusing pulse?

(c) Calculate the ratio of the signals at point A *without* a refocusing pulse to that with a refocusing pulse for $TE_1 = 25$, $TE_2 = 50$, $T2 = 50$, and $T2^* = 25$ msec.

8-2 Match
(i) T1W **(ii)** T2W **(iii)** PDW
with
(a) short TR and short TE
(b) long TR and short TE
(c) long TR and long TE

8-3 T/F The 180° pulses totally eliminate the dephasing of spins in the transverse plane.

9

Fourier Transform

Introduction

Fourier was an 18th century French mathematician. His picture, along with the Fourier transform of his picture, is shown in Figure 9-1. The Fourier transform (FT) is a mystery to most radiologists. Although the mathematics of FT is complex, its concept is easy to grasp. Basically, the FT provides a frequency spectrum of a signal. It is sometimes easier to work in the frequency domain and later convert back to the time domain.

Let's start by saying that we have a signal $g(t)$, with a certain waveform (Fig. 9-2). This signal is basically a *time* function, that is, a waveform that varies with time. Now, let's say we have a "black box" that converts the signal into its *frequency* components. The conversion that occurs in the "black box" is the **Fourier transform.** The FT converts the signal from the *time domain* to the *frequency domain* (Fig. 9-2). The FT of $g(t)$ is denoted $G(\omega)$. (The frequency can be angular [ω] or linear [f].)

The FT is a mathematical equation (you don't have to memorize it). It is shown here to demonstrate that a relationship exists between the signal in the time domain $g(t)$ and its Fourier transform $G(\omega)$ in the frequency domain:

$$G(\omega) = \int_{-\infty}^{+\infty} g(t)e^{-i\omega t}\,dt \quad \text{(Eqn. 9-1a)}$$

$$G(f) = \int_{-\infty}^{+\infty} g(t)e^{-i2\pi ft}\,dt \quad \text{(Eqn. 9-1b)}$$

where $\omega = 2\pi f$.

We are already familiar with the term ($e^{-i\omega t}$) from Chapter 1. This is the term for a vector spinning with angular frequency ω. The formula integrates the product of this periodic function and $g(t)$ with respect to time. It also provides another function, $G(\omega)$, in the frequency domain (Fig. 9-2).

One interesting thing about the Fourier transform is that the Fourier transform of the Fourier transform provides the original signal. If the Fourier transform of $g(t)$ is $G(\omega)$, then the Fourier transform of $G(\omega)$ is $g(t)$:

$$g(t) = 1/2\pi \int_{-\infty}^{+\infty} G(\omega)e^{+i\omega t}\,d\omega \quad \text{(Eqn. 9-2)}$$

FT provides the *range of frequencies* that are in the signal. Here are some examples of functions and their Fourier transforms:

Example 1

The cosine function: cos ($\omega_0 t$).

Obviously this signal (Fig. 9-3) has one single frequency. The frequency could be any number. The Fourier transform is a single spike representing the single frequency in the frequency domain (because of its symmetry, we also get a similar spike on the opposite side of zero[1]). The Fourier transform in this case tells us that there is only a single frequency because it shows only one frequency spike at ω_0 and is zero everywhere else on the line. We can, for simplicity, ignore the symmetric spike

---

[1] One can think of a negative frequency as oscillation in the opposite direction. For instance, if clockwise rotation is regarded as a positive frequency, then counterclockwise rotation would constitute a negative frequency. Also, see the discussion below regarding even and odd functions and their Fourier transforms.

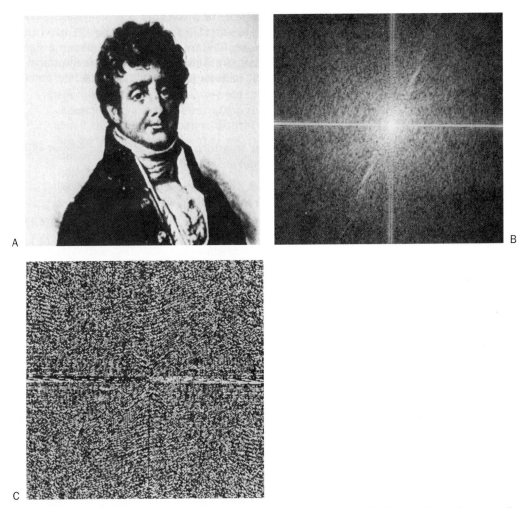

Figure 9-1. A: Picture of the French mathematician Fourier. **B:** The magnitude of Fourier's two-dimensional Fourier transform. **C:** The phase of his Fourier transform. (Reprinted with permission from Oppenheim AV. Signals and systems. Prentice Hall; 1983.)

on the negative side of zero and just consider the single spike on the positive side to tell us that there is a single frequency (ω_0). The spike represents frequency and amplitude of the cosine function.

Example 2

The sinc wave: $\text{sinc}(\omega_0 t) = \sin(\omega_0 t)/(\omega_0 t)$

The Fourier transform of this signal (Fig. 9-4) has a rectangular shape and shows that the signal

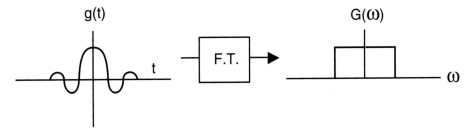

Figure 9-2. The FT of $g(t)$, designated $G(\omega)$.

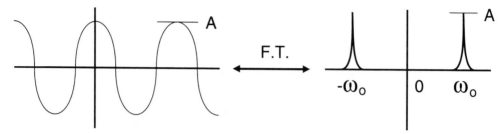

Figure 9-3. The FT of $\cos(\omega_0 t)$ consists of two spikes, one at ω_0 and one at $-\omega_0$.

contains, not just a single frequency, but a range of frequencies from $-\omega_0$ to $+\omega_0$.

The bandwidth of this range of frequencies is from $-\omega_0$ to $+\omega_0$.

$$\text{Bandwidth} = \pm\omega_0 = 2\omega_0$$

(We'll discuss bandwidth again later.) So the Fourier transform tells us the *range of frequencies* that there are in a signal, as well as the amplitude of the signals at those frequencies. What's nice about the Fourier transform is that if we have the range of frequencies and the amplitudes, we can reconstruct the original signal back.

Example 3

Let's consider two frequencies:

1. $\cos \omega t$ and
2. $\cos 2\omega t$ (which is twice as fast as $\cos \omega t$)

The signal $\cos(2\omega t)$ oscillates twice as fast as $\cos(\omega t)$ (Fig. 9-5). If we add them up, we get a complex signal (Fig. 9-6). If we were just given the signal in Figure 9-6, we would have no idea that it is the sum of two cosine waves.

Question: What is a good way to figure out the frequencies of which the signal is composed?

Answer: The Fourier transform of this complex signal (which we know is the sum of two cosine waves, one twice as fast as the other) contains two spikes, one twice as far from the origin as the other (Fig. 9-6). This FT, then, demonstrates the composition of the signal in terms of its frequencies.

Example 4

Let's now have a complex signal with two cosine waves, with the second cosine wave not only twice as fast, but with twice the amplitude as well. Again, by looking at the signal in Figure 9-7, we have no idea what it is composed of, but by looking at the frequency spectrum (the FT of the signal), we can tell the composition of the signal: in this case, two separate cosine waves with differing frequencies and differing amplitudes. The FT provides the frequency spectrum of a signal with its amplitudes.

Example 5

Let's consider the FT of a sine wave: $\sin \omega t$. The FT of a sine wave is different from the FT of a cosine wave:

1. FT of a cosine wave is symmetric with two symmetric spikes on either side of zero (Fig. 9-8a).

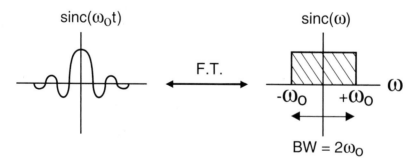

Figure 9-4. The FT of a sinc function (sinc $\omega_0 t = \sin \omega_0 t / \omega_0 t$) has a rectangular shape. The two ends of this rectangle are at ω_0 and $-\omega_0$ (where ω_0 is the frequency of the sinc function).

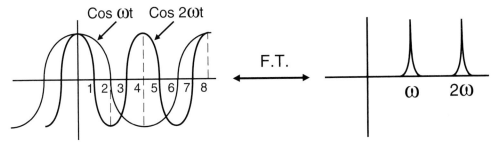

Figure 9-5. The FT of cos $2\omega t$ has two spikes: one at 2ω and one at -2ω. (Here, only the positive frequencies are shown.)

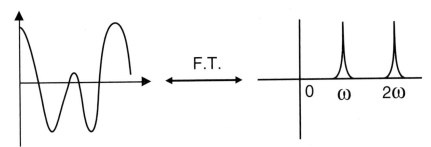

Figure 9-6. The FT of cos ωt + cos $2\omega t$ has two sets of spikes at $\pm\omega$ and $\pm 2\omega$. By looking at the FT signal, it is easy to figure out its composition in the time domain.

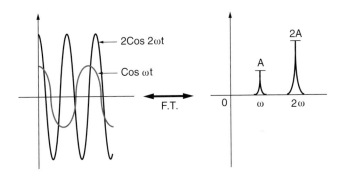

Figure 9-7. The signal cos ωt + 2cos $2\omega t$ and its FT. The FT has again two sets of spikes: one at $\pm\omega$ and one at $\pm 2\omega$ (but with twice the magnitude).

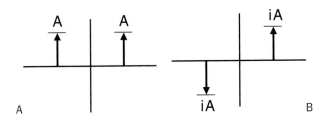

Figure 9-8. A: FT of cos ωt. **B:** FT of sin ωt. Here the spikes have opposite polarities and are also imaginary [iA in **(B)** as opposed to **(A)**].

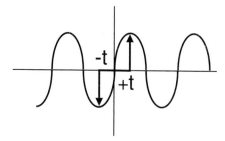

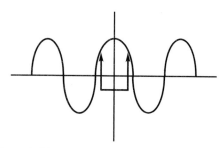

Figure 9-9. sin ωt is an example of an *odd* function where the value of the signal at −t is the negative of its value at +t.

Figure 9-10. cos ωt is an example of an *even* function where the values at the signal at ±t are the same.

2. FT of a sine wave is antisymmetric. It has a positive spike to the right of zero and a negative spike to the left of zero[2] (Fig. 9-8b).

The reason for this is that a *sine* function is an **odd** function. In other words, if we take a time interval of t to the right of zero, the *sine* value is positive, whereas, if we take a similar interval in the other direction, the *sine* value is negative (Fig. 9-9). The *cosine* function, however, is an **even** function. If we go a certain interval to the right or left of zero, the *cosine* value is the same (Fig. 9-10). The FT of an even function is **real,** whereas the FT of an odd function is **imaginary.** Thus, *cosine* functions have FTs that are real (Fig. 9-8a). *Sine* functions have FTs that are imaginary (Fig. 9-8b).

Fourier Transform Versus Fourier Series

There is a difference between a **Fourier transform** and a **Fourier series.** Admittedly this is confusing. Let's talk about the original function g(t). This function can be represented by an infinite number of sine and cosine waves:

$$g(t) = a_0 + a_1\cos(\omega_0 t) + a_2\cos(2\omega_0 t)$$
$$+ \cdots + b_1\sin(\omega_0 t) \qquad \text{(Eqn. 9-3)}$$
$$+ b_2\sin(2\omega_0 t) + \cdots$$

What does this mean? Let's say that we have the rectangular function (Fig. 9-11a). We said that

this is composed of an infinite number of *sine* and *cosine* waves:

1. If we start with a single *cosine* wave, the signal will be as in Figure 9-11b.
2. As we add *sine* and *cosine,* the signal will be as in Figure 9-11c.
3. As we continue to add *sine* and *cosine,* signal will be as in Figure 9-11d.
4. The more *cosine* and *sine* we add, the more the signal approximates a square wave (Fig. 9-11e).

It is impractical to go to infinity (∞). However, by eliminating the higher frequencies, we get a "ring-down" effect.

If we do an FT of the Fourier series of g(t) above, we get a series of spikes (Fig. 9-12). The **envelope** of this FT is the *sinc* wave.

The foregoing has emphasized temporal frequencies in cycles per second or hertz. This would apply to spectroscopy but not imaging. For imaging, we are interested in "spatial frequencies" with units of cycles per millimeter. If image data g(**r**) is distributed within a 3D volume, it is then possible to define the following *complementary* distribution G(**k**) using a Fourier transform:

$$G(\mathbf{k}) = \int_V g(\mathbf{r}) \exp[2\pi i(\mathbf{k} \cdot \mathbf{r})]\mathbf{dr}$$

Here **k** denotes a complex vector composed of three components and **dr** is a volume element integrated over the volume V described by the vector **r** = {x, y, z}. The vector **k** = {k_x, k_y, k_z} (the origin of the term "k-space") is complementary to the Euclidean **r**-space. The two distributions g(**r**) and G(**k**) carry exactly the same

---

[2]Actually, the negative spike has an imaginary rather than a real amplitude (in the form of iA, where i is the imaginary unit $\sqrt{-1}$ and A is the amplitude of the spike). This concept is rather important in understanding the symmetry that exists in k-space, discussed in Chapters 13 and 16.

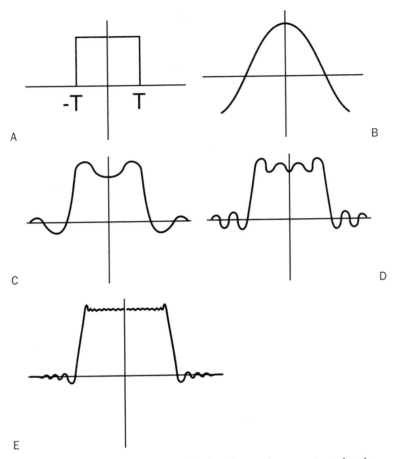

Figure 9-11. **A:** A square or rectangular function can be approximated as the sum of a finite number (N) of sine and cosine functions. **B:** $N = 1$. **C:** $N = 3$. **D:** $N = 7$. **E:** $N = 20$. The signal in (**E**) more closely approximates a rectangle, except for the presence of a ring-down effect.

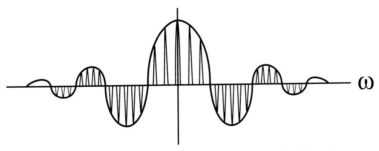

Figure 9-12. The FT of the signal in Equation 9-3 is a set of spikes whose envelope is a sinc function.

information. In fact, knowing $G(\mathbf{k})$, the function $g(\mathbf{r})$ can be computed from

$$g(\mathbf{r}) = \int G(\mathbf{k}) \exp[-2\pi i(\mathbf{k} \cdot \mathbf{r})] d\mathbf{k}$$

These are known as Fourier transforms and reverse Fourier transforms. Technically, acquiring an imaging in the presence of a gradient breaks the data down into its component frequencies (in k-space), which is the essence of a Fourier Transform. Turning the k-space data back into an image is technically a reverse Fourier transform.

In summary, the **Fourier series** tells us that a signal can be represented by a series of *sine* and *cosine* waves (in the time domain). The **Fourier transform,** however, gives the frequency spectrum of the function (in the frequency domain).

Key Points

The FT, as intimidating as it may appear, represents a simple concept. Every signal (in the time domain) is composed of a series of frequencies. The FT is a way of representing that signal in terms of its frequencies. The FT also allows mathematical manipulations performed in the frequency domain, which are sometimes easier than in the time domain. The one-to-one relationship between a signal and its FT allows reconstruction of the original signal from its FT.

In other words, the FT represents a function in the frequency domain whose amplitude varies with the frequencies present in the signal. The bandwidth (BW) is simply a measure of the range of frequencies present in the signal (in Hz or in radians/sec).

Questions

9-1 **T/F** The FT of an FT equals the original signal.

9-2 **T/F** **(a)** It is always easier to perform calculations in the frequency domain.

    (b) It is always easier to perform calculations in the time domain.

9-3 **T/F** The FT of a *cosine* function consists of two spikes, one on each side of the zero separated by the frequency of the *cosine.*

9-4 **T/F** The FT represents the frequency spectrum of a signal, whereas the Fourier series decomposes the signal into a series of sine and cosine waves.

10

Image Construction: Part I (Slice Selection)

Introduction

The signals received from a patient contain information about the entire part of the patient being imaged. They do not have any particular spatial information. That is, we cannot determine the specific origin point of each component of the signal. This is the function of the **gradients.** One gradient is required in each of the x, y, and z directions to obtain spatial information in that direction. Depending on their function, these gradients are called

1. The slice-select gradient
2. The readout or frequency-encoding gradient
3. The phase-encoding gradient

Depending on their orientation axis they are called G_x, G_y, and G_z. Depending on the slice orientation (axial, sagittal, or coronal), G_x, G_y, and G_z can be used for slice select, readout, or phase encode.

A gradient is simply a magnetic field that changes from point to point—usually in a *linear* fashion. We temporarily create magnetic field nonuniformity in a linear manner along all three axes to obtain information about position.

First, we'll consider the slice-select gradient, which is the easiest of all to understand. Once a slice has been selected, we worry about the problem of in-plane **spatial encoding,** that is, discriminating position within the slice. As we'll see shortly, the principles behind slice selection and spatial encoding in MRI are different from the principles used in computerized tomography (CT).

How to Select a Slice

Suppose that we have a patient on the table and we want to select a slice at a certain level and of a certain thickness (Fig. 10-1). Remember that the patient is lying in the external magnetic field $\mathbf{B}_0$, which is oriented along the z-axis. If we transmit a radio frequency (RF) pulse and get a free induction decay (FID) or an echo back, the received signal would be from the entire patient. There is no spatial discrimination. All we get is a

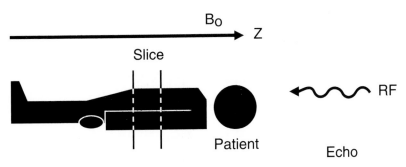

Figure 10-1. Selecting a slice of a certain thickness.

signal, and we have no idea yet from where exactly in the body the signal is coming.

The frequency of the RF pulse is given by the **Larmor frequency:**

$$\omega_0 = \gamma \mathbf{B}_0$$

If we transmit an RF pulse that does not match the Larmor frequency (the frequency of oscillation at magnetic field $\mathbf{B}_0$), we won't excite any of the protons in the patient.

However, if we make the magnetic field vary from point to point, then each position will have its own resonant frequency. We can make the magnetic field slightly weaker in strength at the feet and gradually increase in strength to a maximum at the head (Fig. 10-2). This effect is achieved by using a **gradient coil.**

Let's say the magnetic field strength is 1.5 T at the center, 1.4 T at the feet, and 1.6 T at the head. Then, the foot of the patient will experience a weaker magnetic field than the head. Therefore, a *gradient* in any direction (x, y, or z) is a variation in the field along that axis in some fashion (the most common form of which is *linearly* increasing or decreasing). If we now transmit an RF pulse of a single frequency into the patient, we will receive signals corresponding to a line in the patient at the level of the magnetic field corresponding to that frequency (according to the Larmor frequency), but it will be an infinitely thin line. What we need to do is transmit an RF pulse with a **range** of frequencies—a **bandwidth** of frequencies.

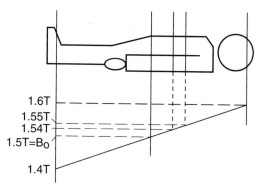

Figure 10-2. Slice thickness is determined by the slope of the gradient.

What will the RF pulse look like in the frequency domain? First, note that for a 1.5-T magnet, the Larmor frequency is 64 MHz for hydrogen protons:

64 MHz corresponds to $\mathbf{B}_0$ of a 1.5-T magnet.

To see how this is derived, recall that

$$\omega_0 = \gamma \mathbf{B}_0$$

where $\gamma \cong 42.6$ MHz/T and

$$\mathbf{B}_0 = 1.5 \text{ T}$$

This results in

$$\omega_0 = 42.6 \times 1.5 = 64 \text{ MHz}$$

The graph in Figure 10-3 shows the magnetic field strength and the corresponding Larmor

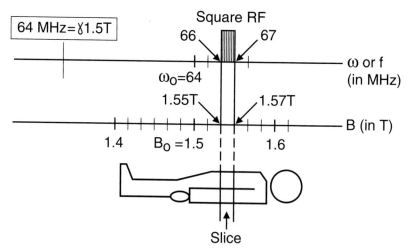

Figure 10-3. The relationship between field strength and Larmor frequency in determining slice thickness and position.

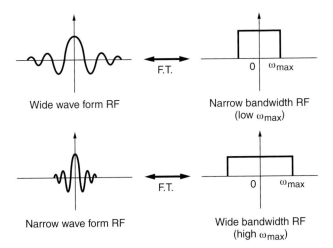

Figure 10-4. Comparison of wide and narrow waveforms and their FTs. The narrower the waveform in time domain, the wider its FT will be.

frequency range. We are concerned here about a magnetic field strength ranging from 1.4 to 1.6 T because, in our example, that is the magnetic field strength range to which we have exposed the patient. Let's excite one slice with an RF pulse. For example, let's excite a slice extending from 1.55 to 1.57 T. This corresponds to a frequency range from 66 to 67 MHz.

If the RF has a square shape in the frequency domain with a range of frequencies that correspond to a range of magnetic field strengths, then we will excite only the protons that are in the slice containing that range of magnetic field strengths. The other protons in the rest of the body are not going to get excited because the range of frequencies from which we are transmitting the RF pulse does not match the Larmor frequencies of the other protons. The range of frequencies in the RF pulse will only match the Larmor frequency of a single slice.

So, we transmit an RF pulse with a range of frequencies that we know will correspond to a range of magnetic field strengths in a particular slice. This range of frequencies determines the slice thickness and is referred to as the **bandwidth.**

> **Bandwidth = range of frequencies (determines the slice thickness)**

We can measure the bandwidth (range of frequencies) by looking at the Fourier transform of

the RF pulse. Let's now compare the RF signal with its Fourier transform. The RF pulse is generally a *sinc* wave and looks like Figure 10-4a with the Fourier transform that has a square shape.

If we have a narrower signal, we get a wider frequency bandwidth (Fig. 10-4b). The narrower signal reflects the fact that there are more oscillations in a given period of time so that the maximum frequency of the signal is greater. Because the Fourier transform depicts an infinite number of frequencies from zero to maximum, the bandwidth gets wider to depict a greater maximum frequency.

Let's apply this example to a *cosine* wave (Fig. 10-5a). The Fourier transform for this *cosine* wave contains two spikes, one on each side of zero (Fig. 10-5b). If we then take a *cosine* wave with twice the oscillation frequency and look at its Fourier transform, we see that the spikes are farther apart (Fig. 10-6). Thus, as the *cosine* wave goes two times faster, the Fourier transform shows that the maximum frequency (in this case, the only frequency) is two times farther away from the zero point. Furthermore, if we look at the diagram of the *cosine* waves, the faster *cosine* wave has a narrower oscillating waveform—the narrower the waveform, the faster the oscillation frequency. Again, the narrower the waveform of the RF signal, the wider its bandwidth (the greater the maximum frequency; Fig. 10-6).

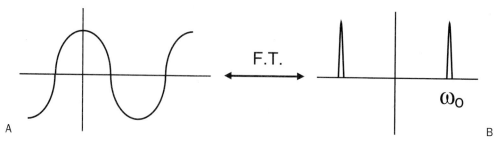

Figure 10-5. The FT (**B**) of (**A**) a cos signal (cos $\omega_0 t$) has two spikes at $\pm \omega_0$.

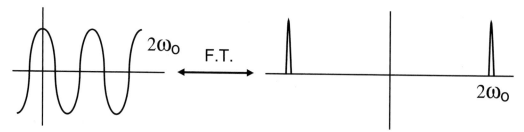

Figure 10-6. The FT of cos $2\omega_0 t$ has two spikes at $\pm 2\omega_0$.

Slice Thickness

Let's now talk about how we establish **slice thickness** (Fig. 10-7). The same principle would apply if we were to image from the base of the skull to the vertex rather than from the patient's head to toe. We establish a magnetic field strength **gradient** so that at the midpoint of the field of study (in this instance, the entire body), the field strength is 1.5 T; at the low end of the gradient (the foot), the field

strength will be 1.4 T; and at the high end of the gradient, the field strength will be maximum at 1.6 T. These magnetic field strengths also correspond to different frequencies. Using the Larmor equation, we can calculate that approximately:

$$1.6\ T \sim 68\ MHz$$
$$1.5\ T \sim 64\ MHz$$
$$1.4\ T \sim 60\ MHz$$

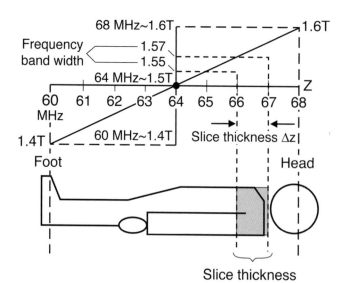

Figure 10-7. An example of the relationship between slice thickness and position, frequency, and field strength.

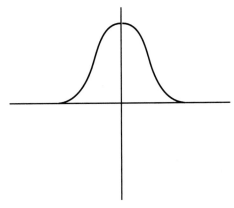

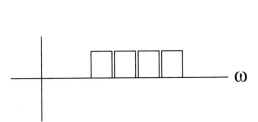

Figure 10-8. Ideal contiguous slices correspond to ideal rectangular-shaped FTs that are positioned side by side.

Figure 10-9. A more realistic FT has side lobes such as a Gaussian curve.

If we pick a frequency bandwidth of a certain range, we would then get a slice of a certain thickness. Therefore, we transmit an RF pulse with a specific frequency bandwidth and no frequencies outside of this range (ideally). The frequency bandwidth will match the Larmor frequencies of the protons only in a section of the patient of a certain thickness, which corresponds to the range of magnetic field strengths corresponding to the Larmor frequencies. The magnetic field strength everywhere outside this slice is going to be either more or less than the magnetic field strengths that correspond to the Larmor frequencies of the RF bandwidth.

Question: What happens if we put one slice right next to another?

Answer: Ideally, the contiguous slices are right next to each other and the Fourier transform has a rectangular shape (Fig. 10-8). In other words, we want to have frequency ranges that are discrete and next to each other, so that each range of frequencies excites a different slice, and we can obtain contiguous slices.

Cross-Talk. In reality, the frequency spectrum of the RF pulse does not have a rectangular shape. Instead, it may have a bell shape or "Gaussian" curve (Fig. 10-9). If we place these frequency spectrums close together, they will overlap; these areas of overlap cause "**cross-talk**" (Fig. 10-10).

Remember that cross-talk is best explained in the **frequency domain**. It is more difficult to comprehend this in the time domain. To avoid this cross-talk created by the overlap of adjacent frequency bandwidths, we create a **gap** between the consecutive bandwidths (in the frequency domain), thus creating a **gap** between consecutive slices in the actual image (Fig. 10-11). This will minimize or eliminate "cross-talk."

How to Change the Slice Thickness. There are two ways to change the slice thickness:

1. The first way to decrease the thickness is to use a *narrower bandwidth*. A narrower frequency bandwidth will excite protons in a narrower band of magnetic field strengths (Fig. 10-12a).

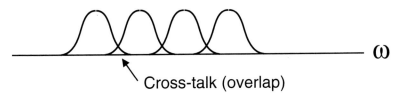

Figure 10-10. Cross-talk: in the absence of ideal rectangular-shaped FTs, the side lobes of the FTs may overlap.

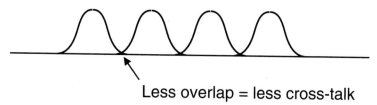

Less overlap = less cross-talk

Figure 10-11. To minimize cross-talk, the slices are set farther apart (by introducing gaps between successive slices).

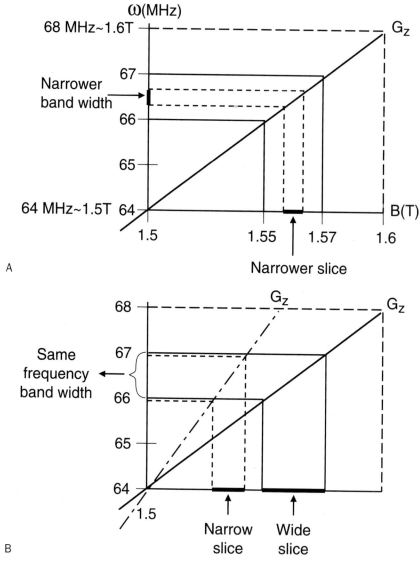

Figure 10-12. To decrease slice thickness, either a narrower BW (**A**) or a steeper gradient (**B**) is used.

2. The second way to decrease slice thickness is to *increase the slope of the magnetic field gradient* (Fig. 10-12b), that is, by increasing the gradient strength.

Slice-Select Gradient. The change in the magnetic field strength along the z-axis is called the **z gradient** (G_z). For an axial slice in a superconducting magnet, it is also called the **slice-select gradient.** If we increase the gradient and keep the frequency bandwidth the same, we get a thinner slice.

The slice thickness can be decreased by

1. **decreasing the bandwidth of the RF pulse, or**
2. **increasing the slice-select gradient.**

There is an electronic limitation as to how much we can decrease the bandwidth. There is also a machine limitation as to how much we can increase the gradient. These factors set an absolute limit on how *thin* a slice can be.

By the foregoing procedure, we select a slice with a certain thickness. The slice is selected with a frequency range in the RF pulse that corresponds to the slice location and its thickness. The echo signal that we get back from the slice is from the entire slice. We have no way yet of discriminating points within the slice. This is where the **frequency-encoding** and the **phase-encoding** steps come into play.

Review

RF Pulses. There are two types of RF pulses:

1. Nonselective
2. Selective

By **selective**, we mean an RF pulse that is slice selective—an RF pulse whose frequency bandwidth corresponds to a specific band of magnetic field strengths along a magnetic field gradient. Ideally, this RF pulse will select only a certain slice of the body that we are imaging (used in two-dimensional [2D] imaging).

A **nonselective** RF pulse excites every part of the body that is in the coil (used in three-dimensional [3D] imaging).

Sinc RF Pulse

Earlier, we talked about one type of RF pulse in which we had a *sinc* wave in the time domain. The *sinc* function is mathematically expressed as

$$\text{sinc } (t) = \sin(t)/t$$

This simply means that the oscillating function sin t is divided by t. Therefore, because t goes into an oscillating function (sin t), the result will be an oscillating function. As t goes from a large value to a small value, the result of (sin t/t) will get larger and will reach maximum when t approaches zero. The rectangular transform in the frequency domain has a positive maximum frequency (f_{max}) and a negative maximum frequency ($-f_{max}$), as shown in Figure 10-13. The bandwidth is thus 2 × (maximum frequency), that is,

$$\text{BW} = 2f_{max}$$

This is only one type of selective RF pulse. There are other types of selective RF pulses.

Gaussian RF Pulse

The first generation of MR machines used an RF pulse that had a **Gaussian** shape (Fig. 10-14a).

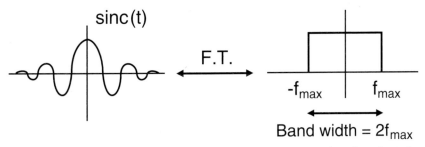

Figure 10-13. The sinc function and its FT. The bandwidth (BW) is $2f_{max}$ where f_{max} is the frequency of the sinc function.

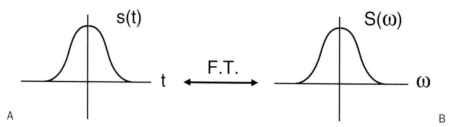

Figure 10-14. The FT (**B**) of a Gaussian signal (**A**) is itself Gaussian.

The Gaussian RF pulse has a bell shape in the time domain.

> **The Fourier transform of a Gaussian function is also a Gaussian curve (Fig. 10-14).**

If we take another Gaussian curve in the narrower time domain, its Fourier transform will be wider (Fig. 10-15). An inverse relationship exists between the range of frequencies and the duration of the RF pulse, as we have discussed before.

A short pulse results in a wider bandwidth. The MR machine uses different types of RF pulses for different purposes, but for the sake of discussion, let's assume that we are dealing with an ideal *sinc* wave RF pulse that has an ideal square Fourier transform.

Remember that the RF pulse is an electromagnetic wave generated by an electric current through a coil. If we use the body coil to generate the RF pulse, we generate the RF throughout the body. If we use a transmit/receive coil, then the coil transmits the RF pulse and also

receives the signal from the body resulting in less RF energy in the body and more signal. Most coils are receive only which do not change the RF energy placed in the body, but increase the signal.

Going back to the *sinc* wave, in reality we can't go all the way to infinity in time when transmitting a signal. We have to **truncate** the signal and deal with a certain finite time domain (Fig. 10-16). The Fourier transform of this truncated signal gives the "**ripples**" effect on the square wave as we have seen in Chapter 9. The more we truncate the signal, the more "ripples" we get. Ripples are also called "overshoot" and "undershoot" artifacts.

Bandwidth. Bandwidth is a measure of the range of frequencies. We know that for a 1.5-T magnet, the Larmor frequency is about 64 MHz. The RF pulse that we generate is in the RF range, but its bandwidth is in the **audible** frequency range.

This is analogous to a radio. When we tune into the FM station KSON 97.3 FM in San Diego, are we really getting 97.3 MHz of sound waves? If the signal you receive on your radio

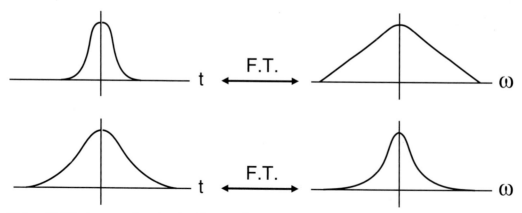

Figure 10-15. A narrow Gaussian signal has a wide Gaussian FT, and vice versa.

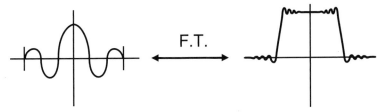

Figure 10-16. The FT of a truncated sinc function has a rectangular-like profile containing rings or ripple effects.

has this high a frequency, you can't hear it (we can't hear a MHz frequency signal [maybe dolphins can, but humans can't!]). However, the frequency that we receive is actually in the **audible** range. Each station has a certain frequency range that they deal with, and the bandwidth that they use is nearly the same for all radio stations in the audible frequency range; it is about 1 to 2 kHz (Fig. 10-17).

Now, the bandwidth of 1 kHz is 100,000 times smaller than the 97.3 MHz frequency. The audible frequency range gets **modulated** to the **center frequency** (e.g., FM 97.3 MHz). The modulated frequency is then transmitted. The antenna receives this modulated signal. The signal then goes into the radio and is **demodulated** (Fig. 10-18). Depending on which station we tune into (e.g., KSON FM at 97.3 MHz), we get that range of frequencies demodulated back to zero frequency.

Thus, the bandwidth of a signal transmitted by a radio station always stays at about 1 kHz, but it is transmitted as a 1-kHz bandwidth *modulated* to, say, 97.3 MHz. Then, in the radio, it is demodulated back to zero center frequency, still with a bandwidth of about 1 kHz. What we send and what we receive are in the same frequency range. In between, the frequency gets modulated from 0 to 97.3 MHz. We are just changing *the center frequency*. Everything else stays the same.

The reason radio transmission does this is that each radio station is only allowed a narrow bandwidth (in the kHz range) for transmission. However, we cannot transmit a kHz frequency. It just doesn't travel very far, and radio transmissions have to travel for miles. Besides, the signals from different stations will get all mixed up if they all work in a small frequency range in the order of a few kilohertz. Therefore, the kHz frequency bandwidth is modulated to the MHz range, still maintaining the same kHz bandwidth. Now with the MHz frequency as a **carrier,** the narrow 1-kHz bandwidth can be transmitted over long distances.

In MRI, the **center frequency** is the Larmor frequency. Thus, the RF pulse that we transmit into the patient is *centered* at the Larmor frequency of 64 MHz at 1.5 T (Fig. 10-19). However, the bandwidth of frequencies in the RF pulse is *very narrow*. Again, for simplicity, we will assume that the bandwidth of the RF pulse has been demodulated to a center frequency of zero.

Slice-Select Gradient. Let's go back to the slice-select gradient. We purposely create a linear magnetic nonuniformity, so the foot will experience a weaker magnetic field than the head. The slope of magnetic field versus distance is called the **gradient.** A gradient is a measure of change of magnetic field with distance. We can have a **linear** gradient or a **nonlinear** gradient. The gradients that we use in MRI are usually linear. (In fact, nonlinearities may be present in the gradients that cause **geometric distortion artifacts** [see Chapter 18].)

By creating this gradient, different magnetic fields are experienced from the foot to the head

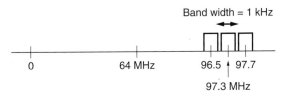

Figure 10-17. An example of frequencies of FM radio stations.

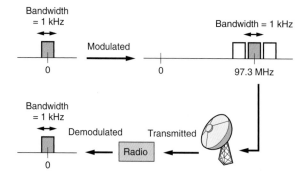

Figure 10-18. Each radio station has a limited audible BW. To transmit this to the listeners, this BW is "modulated" via a carrier frequency (which is several orders of magnitude higher). In the radio, this frequency is demodulated back to the audible range.

in an increasing order. The protons in the body will also experience a gradient in terms of their precessional frequency in that the protons in the foot are going to precess slower than the protons in the head.

We then transmit an RF pulse that matches the proton precessional frequency in a certain section of the body. Then, only the protons in this section will **resonate**; none of the other protons in any other portion of the body will resonate (i.e., flip into the transverse plane).

If we want to select a specific slice, then we transmit an RF pulse with a bandwidth that has the appropriate *center frequency*. This gradient is turned on only when we transmit the RF pulses. This makes sense because we only want

the RF pulse to excite a thin slice of the body. When we transmit the 180° pulse for the same slice, we activate the same gradient.

When we study another slice, the gradient stays the same. We just alter the *center frequency* of the RF pulse. In this manner, we can excite different slices in any order desired.

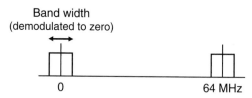

Figure 10-19. The process of demodulation in MRI.

Key Points

We have seen how one goes about selecting a slice in the body. This is done via a slice-select gradient. To vary the slice *thickness*, we can either vary the bandwidth of the transmitted RF pulse or the slope of the gradient. Thus, we can decrease the slice thickness by

1 decreasing the bandwidth of the RF pulse, or

2 increasing the slice-select gradient.

Because the RF profiles are not ideal and may have side lobes or tails, if you try to have contiguous slices, you'll run into a problem called *cross-talk*. Basically, the transmitted signals in the frequency domain (i.e., their Fourier transforms)

will overlap and "cross-talk." To avoid this, you must introduce *gaps* between the slices. This is done by excluding a certain range of frequencies (i.e., bandwidths) in the transmitted RF pulses. The larger the gaps, the less cross-talk you get, but the chance of missing a lesion within the gaps is greater.

The center frequency for each transmitted bandwidth is like a *carrier* frequency around which the desired bandwidth is centered, much like what goes on in radio-communication. Once a slice is selected, the question arises as to how to determine the pixels within that slice. This is the topic of the next chapter.

Questions

10-1 (a) The range of frequencies included in an RF pulse is referred to as its bandwidth (BW). Suppose that an RF pulse has frequencies ranging from -500 to 500 Hz (i.e., BW $= 1,000$ Hz $= 1$ kHz). Now, to achieve a slice thickness of 5 mm, determine the amplitude of the slice-selection gradient.

(b) What is the minimum achievable slice thickness given a minimum RF BW $= 426$ Hz and a maximum gradient $G_z = 10$ mT/m?

Hint: $\omega = \gamma \mathbf{B}$ so $\Delta\omega =$ BW $= \gamma \Delta \mathbf{B}$. Now, $\mathbf{B} = G_z z$ so that $\Delta \mathbf{B} = G_z \Delta z$. Thus BW $= \gamma \Delta \mathbf{B} = \gamma G_z \Delta z$ or $\Delta z =$ BW$/(\gamma G_z)$, where $\Delta z =$ slice thickness and $\gamma = 42.6$ MHz/T.

10-2 Thinner slices can be achieved by
(a) decreasing the transmit (RF) BW
(b) decreasing the receive (signal) BW
(c) increasing the slice-select gradient strength
(d) all of the above
(e) only (a) and (b)
(f) only (a) and (c)

10-3 T/F The FT of a *sinc* function is rectangular.

10-4 T/F The FT of a bell-shaped Gaussian function is also bell-shaped.

11

Image Construction: Part II (Spatial Encoding)

Introduction

In the last chapter, we learned how to select a slice and how to adjust its thickness. However, we did not address the question of from where within a particular slice each component of the signal comes. In other words, we still don't have spatial information regarding each slice. To create an image of a slice, we need to know how much signal comes from each **pixel** (picture element) or, more accurately, each **voxel** (volume element). This is the topic of spatial encoding, of which there are two parts: (i) frequency encoding and (ii) phase encoding.

Frequency Encoding

After selecting a slice, how can we get information about individual pixels within that slice? As an example, consider a slice with three columns and three rows, for a total of 9 pixels. This slice is selected using a selective 90° pulse (Fig. 11-1). We turn the G_z (slice-select gradient) on during the 90° pulse and turn it off after the 90° pulse.

We also send a selective 180° RF refocusing pulse, and we again turn the G_z gradient on during the 180° pulse. The **echo** is received after a time TE. The echo is a signal from the *entire* slice. To get spatial information in the x direction of the slice, we apply another gradient G_x called the **frequency-encoding gradient** (also called the **readout gradient**) in the x direction (Fig. 11-2). With this gradient in the x direction, the center of this 3×3 matrix (the center volume) is not going to experience the gradient, that is, it's not going to experience any change in magnetic field from that prior to turning on the G_x gradient. The column of pixels to the right of midline will experience a higher net magnetic field. The column of pixels on the left will have a lower net magnetic field.

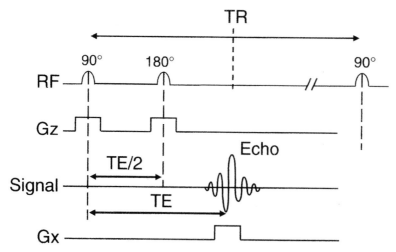

Figure 11-1. Spin-echo pulse sequence diagram.

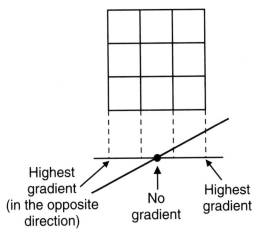

Figure 11-2. Frequency-encoding gradient along the x-axis.

0	1	1
1	2	0
-2	0	1

Figure 11-3. In the previous example of a 3 × 3 matrix, each pixel is assigned a value (magnitude).

> **The G_x gradient is applied during the time the echo is received, that is, during readout.**

Let's now assign some magnitude numbers to the pixels in the matrix (Fig. 11-3).

The numbers in each pixel and their specific location is what we ultimately want to discover because this corresponds to an image. We want to *recreate* this image using MRI.

Initially, all the protons in this section experience the same frequency of precession. Let's call that frequency ω_0. Now let's assign each pixel its frequency at a specific point in time before turning on the G_x gradient, while they all still have the same frequency, and combine it with the magnitude we've assigned to each pixel (Fig. 11-4). For simplicity, we'll use a *cosine* wave as the received signal. In reality, the received signal is a more complicated one, such as a *sinc* wave.

Each pixel has a designated magnitude (amplitude), and they all have the same precessional frequency ω_0 (except those pixels that have zero signal amplitude). Without any gradient in the x direction, this is the signal we're going to get. The signal will be the *sum* of all the signals from each pixel.

The sum of the amplitudes

$$= (0) + (1) + (-2) + (1) + (2) + (0) + (1) + (0) + (1) = 4$$

The frequency is the same for each pixel (i.e., ω_0), as is the shape of the signal (i.e., cos $\omega_0 t$). So the sum of the pixels

$$= \text{signal from whole slice} = 4 \cos \omega_0 t$$

We know that, in reality, the signal is more complex. For example, the signal is a decaying signal with time such as a *sinc* wave, but, for simplicity, let's accept that we are dealing with

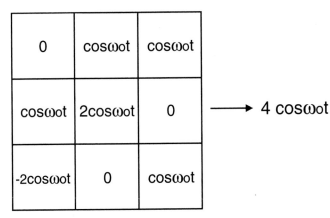

0	cosωot	cosωot
cosωot	2cosωot	0
-2cosωot	0	cosωot

→ 4 cosωot

Figure 11-4. Each pixel is also assigned a frequency ω_0 and is represented as $A \cos \omega_0 t$, where A is the magnitude.

a simple *cosine* wave as our signal with an amplitude of 4.

In summary, when we transmit an RF pulse with frequencies appropriate for a particular slice, all the protons in that slice will start to precess in phase at the Larmor frequency (ω_0). Each pixel contains a different number of protons designated by a number. For purposes of illustration, the number we have assigned to each pixel is proportional to the number of protons in each pixel. This number corresponds to the **amplitude** of the signal. The signal is designated as a *cosine* wave because it oscillates as a result of the precessing protons. However, we still do not have any spatial information; all we have at this point is a signal coming from the *entire slice* without spatial discrimination. What we want to be able to do is to separate the summed signal into its components and to tell, pixel by pixel, where each component of the received signal originated.

Let's now apply the frequency-encoding gradient in the x direction and see what happens to the pixels (Fig. 11-5). Let's look at the three columns in the matrix:

1. The pixels in the center column will not feel the gradient. Thus, they will remain with the same frequency (ω_0). (And, of course, the amplitude of each pixel is constant because the number of protons doesn't change.)
2. The column of pixels to the right of midline is going to have slightly higher frequency. We'll call this (ω_0^+). This is because at a higher magnetic field strength, the protons in this column will oscillate at a higher frequency.
3. The column of pixels to the left of midline will experience a slightly lower field strength and thus have a precessional frequency a little lower than the other columns. We'll call this (ω_0^-).

The signal that we get now is still the sum of all the individual signals; however, now each column of pixels has a different frequency, so we can *algebraically* only add up the ones that have the same frequency, as follows:

Column #1: $0 + (\cos \omega_0^- t) + (-2 \cos \omega_0^- t)$
$$= -\cos \omega_0^- t$$

Column #2: $(\cos \omega_0 t) + (2 \cos \omega_0 t) + 0$
$$= 3 \cos \omega_0 t$$

Column #3: $(\cos \omega_0^+ t) + 0 + (\cos \omega_0^+ t)$
$$= 2 \cos \omega_0^+ t$$

> **Sum of signals = $(-\cos \omega_0^- t) + (3 \cos \omega_0 t)$**
> **$+ (2 \cos \omega_0^+ t)$**

Let's look at the Fourier transform of the signal *before* the G_x gradient is applied (Fig. 11-6A) and look at it again *after* the G_x gradient is applied (Fig. 11-6B). For a *cosine* wave, the Fourier transform is a symmetric pair of spikes at the *cosine* frequency, with an amplitude equal to the magnitude of the signal. (Remember that this is simplified. Usually, we deal with a band of frequencies, i.e., the *bandwidth*, as opposed to a single frequency. However, right now, for simplicity, we leave it as a single frequency, with its Fourier transform as a single spike.)

Now the computer can look at the Fourier transform and see that we are now dealing with three different frequencies:

1. The center frequency comes from the central column, and the amplitude of the frequency spike represents the sum of the amplitudes of the pixels in that column, that is, ($3 \cos \omega_0 t$).
2. The higher frequency comes from the column to the right, and the amplitude of that frequency spike represents the sum of the amplitude of the pixels in that column, that is, ($2 \cos \omega_0^+ t$).
3. The lower frequency comes from the column to the left, and the amplitude of that frequency spike represents the sum of the amplitude of the pixels in that column, that is, ($-\cos \omega_0^- t$).

The way frequency encoding works is that frequency and position have a one-to-one relationship:

> **frequency ↔ position**

So far we have done some spatial encoding and have extracted some information from the slice.

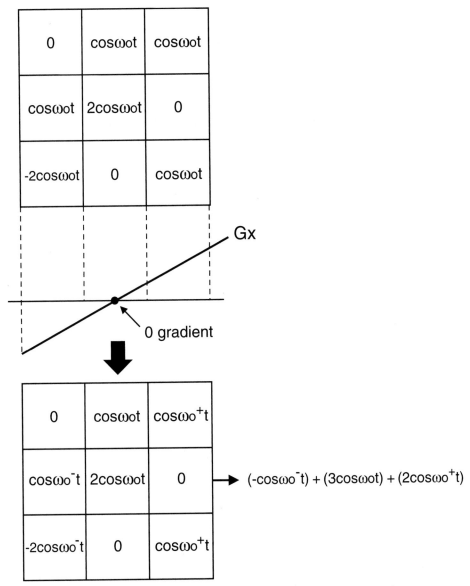

Figure 11-5. When the matrix is exposed to the frequency gradient, different frequencies result in each column: ω_0, ω_0^+, and ω_0^-.

We are now able to decompose the slice matrix into three different columns (Fig. 11-7). That is, we have three different shades of gray corresponding to the three columns.

So, now we've done our job in the x direction. The next thing we want to do is to decompose the individual columns into their three individual pixels (i.e., work in the y direction). The two ways of doing this are as follows:

1. Back projection
2. Two-dimensional Fourier transform (2DFT)

Back Projection. If we think in terms of CT imaging and apply gradients, we start out with an area we want to image and apply a gradient (Fig. 11-8A). Then we can rotate the gradient by an angle θ and reapply the gradient (Fig. 11-8B). We can continue this to complete 360°, and

Received Signal s(t) = (4cosωot)

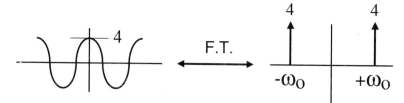

A

Received Signal s(t) = (-cosωo⁻t) + (3cosωot) + (2cosωo⁺t)

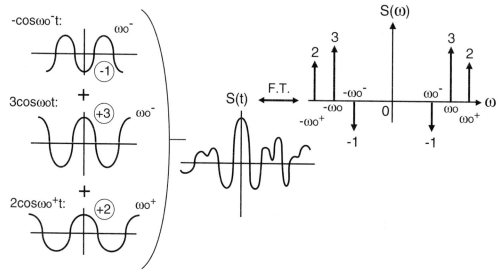

B

Figure 11-6. **A:** The signal and its Fourier transform (FT) prior to the application of the gradient. The signal has a single frequency ω_0. **B:** After application of the frequency gradient G_x, the resulting composite signal will be composed of three frequencies with a more complicated waveform and FT.

each time we do this we get different numbers. At the end, we end up with a set of equations, which can be solved for values of the pixels in the matrix. This is the **back projection** approach performed by rotating the frequency gradient.

Figure 11-7. The sum of the signals in each column. Since the signals belonging to the same column have the same frequency, they are additive.

Advantage

1. It is possible to pick a small field of view (FOV).

Disadvantages

1. This technique is very dependent on external magnetic field inhomogeneities (i.e., it is sensitive to $\Delta \mathbf{B}_0$).
2. This technique is also very sensitive to the magnetic field gradients. If the gradient is *not* perfect, you get artifacts.

Because of these disadvantages, this technique was given up.

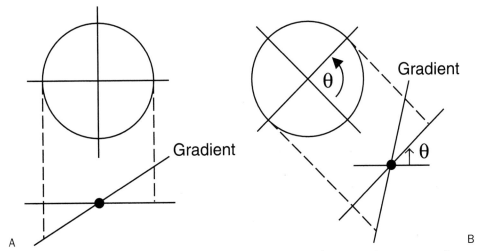

Figure 11-8. Back projection. By gradually rotating the gradient (from **A** to **B**), we get a set of equations the solution to which gives the pixel values.

2DFT: Two-dimensional Digital. Fourier transform (2DFT) is the method currently used and is the topic of the remainder of this chapter.

Advantages

1. Lack of sensitivity to external magnetic field inhomogeneities
2. Lack of sensitivity to gradient field inhomogeneities

Phase Encoding

In the 2DFT technique, in addition to using the G_z gradient for slice selection and the G_x gradient for encoding in the x direction, we add another gradient G_y in the y direction. This is called the **phase-encoding gradient** (Fig. 11-9).

We turn on the G_y gradient before we turn on the G_x (readout) gradient. It is usually applied right after the RF pulse or just before the G_x gradient or anywhere in between.

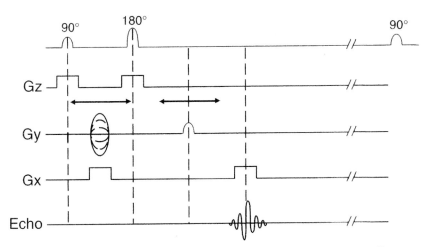

Figure 11-9. The phase-encode gradient G_y is applied along the y-axis. It is usually applied between the 90° and the 180° pulse or between the 180° pulse and the echo. The first G_x gradient is used for offsetting any phase shift induced during frequency readout (further discussion in Chapter 14).

G_y is usually applied between the 90° and the 180° RF pulses or between the 180° pulse and the echo.

So now let's again look at the slice with its 9 pixels before either the G_x (frequency-encoding) gradient or the G_y (phase-encoding) gradient is applied (Fig. 11-10A). The designation of the pixels on the right in Figure 11-10A is a way of denoting phase and frequency. The arrow represents the hand of a clock and denotes the position of precession (i.e., the phase) at a given point in time. After the 90°

RF pulse, all the protons in the selected slice precess at the same frequency (ω_0). At any point in time *before* being exposed to a magnetic field gradient, the protons in all the pixels will all be pointing in the same direction (e.g., north) without any phase difference among them.

This is precisely what the clock diagram shows: Prior to being exposed to a magnetic field gradient, all the protons in each pixel are in phase with each other, oscillating at the same frequency. (Note that we have eliminated magnitude from the clock diagram. All we are concerned about for

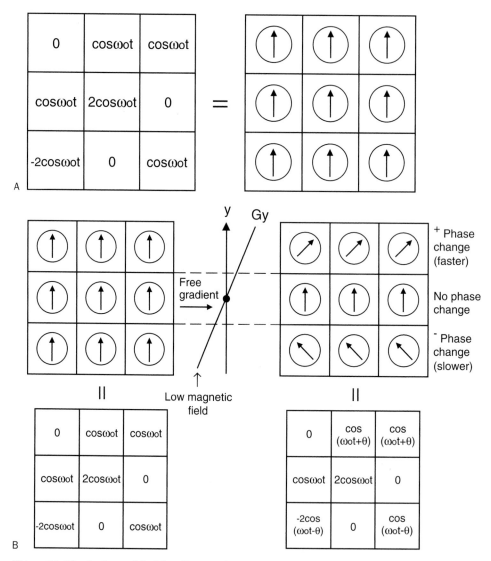

Figure 11-10. Analogy of clock handle. **A:** Before application of G_x or G_y, the handles point north. **B:** After application of G_y (*right*), the handles in different rows get out of phase. (*Continued on next page.*)

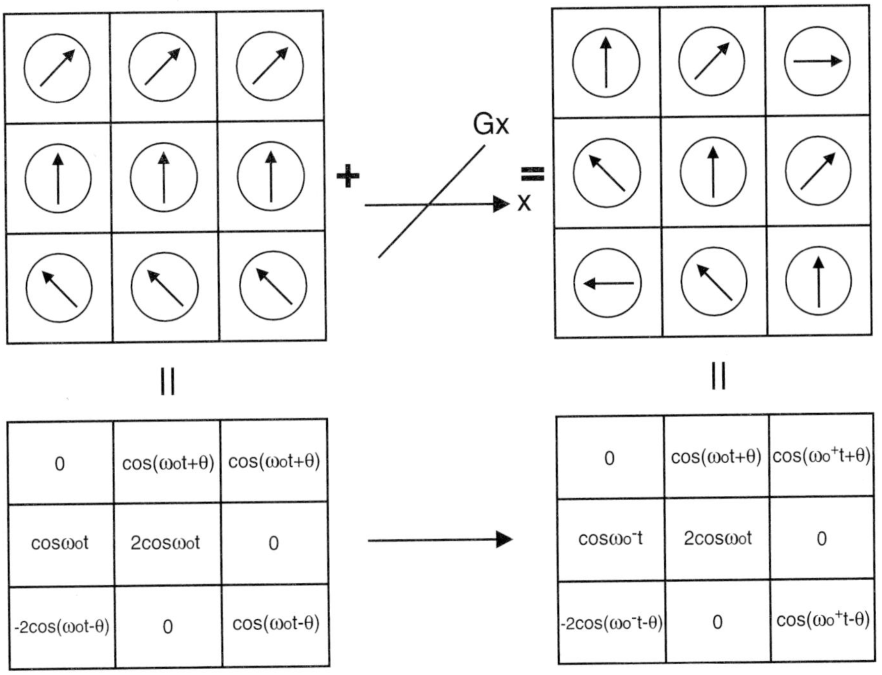

C

Figure 11-10. (*continued*) C: After application of G_x (*right*) and G_y (*left*), each pixel has a different frequency and phase (i.e., the handles rotate at different speeds and with different phase, keeping in mind that the speed is the same for all the elements belonging to the same column).

now is the phase and frequency of the direction of the spins at a particular point in time.)

Now let's expose the slice to a G_y gradient—a magnetic field gradient in the y direction (Fig. 11-10B). With the gradient now applied in the y direction, the pixels in the upper row will experience a higher net magnetic field, the pixels in the middle row will experience no change in the magnetic field, and the pixels in the lower row will experience a lower net magnetic field.

Consequently, the pixels in the middle row, because they experience no change in the magnetic field, will have no phase change after the gradient is turned on. They will continue to point in the same direction as they did before activation of the gradient.

Protons in the pixels on the top row will all start precessing faster because they are now experiencing a stronger magnetic field. Therefore, they will all remain in phase with one another but will be out of phase with the protons in the middle row.

The pixels in the bottom row will all start precessing more slowly because they are now experiencing a weaker magnetic field. They will all be in phase with one another but will be out of phase with the protons in the middle and upper rows.

Once the G_y gradient is turned off, all the protons will now be at the same magnetic field strength once again, so they will all again precess at the same frequency.

However, look at what has happened. A permanent **phase shift** has occurred in the protons of each row. True, they are now all spinning at the same frequency; however, those that were previously exposed to the higher magnetic field and were out of phase with the protons in the middle row will continue to be out of phase now that all protons are spinning at the same frequency again. Likewise, those protons previously exposed to the lower magnetic field that went out of phase with the protons in the middle now will continue to be out of phase now that all protons are spinning at the same frequency again.

Now we have caused a difference in the rows of pixels based on phase (designated by θ in Fig. 11-10B). Differences in spatial position up and down are reflected in that phase value. Hence the term **phase encoding.**

Remember that the G_y gradient is turned on before reading out the signal. So when we read the signal, we turn on the G_x gradient, which, as we learned from our earlier discussion, allows us to frequency encode in the G_x direction (Fig. 11-10C). With the G_x gradient on, the middle column protons won't experience any change in their precessional frequency, so their frequency is unchanged. However, as you can see, each pixel in the middle column already has a distinct *phase shift,* which had occurred when the G_y gradient was on, and this phase shift persists.

With the G_x gradient turned on, the protons in the columns to the right of midline will experience a greater magnetic field so that all the protons in this column will have a faster precessional frequency. However, we notice that each pixel in this column was already out of phase with the other pixels in the column due to the phase shift that had occurred when the G_y gradient was on. Therefore, protons in each pixel of the right column shift the same amount (because they all have the same increased frequency). However, because they shift from a unique position, they will then each move to a phase shift that is different for each pixel.

Likewise, the protons in the column to the left of midline will experience a lower preces-sional frequency with the G_x gradient on, but, again, we notice that each pixel in this column is already out of phase with the other pixels in the column due to the phase shift that had occurred when the G_y gradient was on. So, again, after the G_x gradient is turned on, each pixel will move to a specific phase shift distinct for each pixel. In summary, x position is represented by a unique *frequency* and y position by a unique *phase.*

The protons in each pixel have a distinct frequency and a distinct phase, which are unique and encode for the x and y coordinates for that pixel.

Question: How does one determine the phase shift between adjacent rows?

Answer: First, to figure out the phase shift, we divide 360° by the number of rows:

$$\Delta\theta = 360/\text{Number of rows}$$

Because we have three rows, the phase shift between rows is (Fig. 11-11): $\Delta\theta = 360/3 = 120°$ (or $2\pi/3$).

Therefore, in the middle row, there will be no phase shift. In the upper row, the phase shift will be 120°. In the lower rows, the phase shift will be $+240°$ (which is the same as $-120°$).

0	$\cos(\omega ot+120°)$	$\cos(\omega o^+t+120°)$
$\cos(\omega o^-t)$	$2\cos(\omega ot)$	0
$-2\cos(\omega o^-t-120°)$	0	$\cos(\omega o^+t-120°)$

Figure 11-11. The received signal after application of both G_x and G_y for the 3 × 3 matrix used in previous examples.

Each *row* has its own *unique phase shift* caused by the G_y gradient:

Row 1: phase shift of $+120°$

Row 2: no phase shift

Row 3: phase shift of $-120°$

Also, each *column* has its own *unique frequency* caused by the G_x gradient.

Column 1: frequency of ω_0^-

Column 2: frequency of ω_0

Column 3: frequency of ω_0^+

When combined, as it is during the readout of the signal, we see that each pixel has its own unique phase shift and frequency.

Question: Why does it take time to do phase encoding?

Answer: It takes time because we need to do a separate phase encode for each row of pixels that we need to discriminate in the slice. In this case, we have three rows of pixels, so we would do three phase-encoding steps. Each time we do a separate phase encode, it is a new spin echo taking time TR after a new 90° RF pulse. With each new phase-encoding step (taking time TR), we change the magnetic gradient Gy.

TR#1: no gradient—no phase shift between rows

TR#2: gradient with 120° phase shift between rows

TR#3: gradient with 240° (or −120°) phase shift between rows

We wouldn't need another TR because 240° + 120° = 360° phase shift, and this would give us the same information as a 0° phase shift. What would happen to the signals with the three different phase-encoding steps (Fig. 11-12)?

During TR#1, where we don't apply a gradient G_y in the y direction, we get no phase shift between the rows. Then, when we apply the frequency-encoding gradient G_x in the x direction, we get the frequency difference between the columns.

During TR#2, we apply a G_y gradient so that there is a 120° phase shift between the rows. Then, when we apply the frequency-encoding

gradient G_x in the x direction, we get the frequency difference in the columns on top of the 120° phase shift between the rows.

During TR#3, we apply a steeper G_y gradient so that now there is a 240° (or −120°) phase shift between the rows. Then, when we apply the frequency-encoding gradient in the x direction, we get the frequency difference in the columns on top of the 240° phase shift between the rows.

Notice that in each case the middle row never experiences any phase shift, and the middle column never experiences any frequency change. Therefore, the center pixel never experiences any frequency or phase shift. Also notice that we need a separate TR for each phase-encoding step. That is why phase encoding takes time. We need one TR time period to perform each phase-encoding step. Hence, part of the formula describing the acquisition time for a sequence includes TR and the number of phase-encoding steps (as well as the number of excitations).

As an example, if we need to discriminate 256 rows, then we need to perform 256 phase-encoding steps, each with a different gradient G_y, taking time 256 × TR. The difference in the phase shift between the rows in this case would be 360°/256 phase-encoding step ≈ 1.40°.

1. TR#1 = no gradient, ∴ no phase shift
2. TR#2 = gradient to allow a phase shift = 1.40° between rows
3. TR#3 = steeper gradient to allow a phase shift = 2 × (1.40°) between rows
4. TR#4 = steeper gradient to allow a phase shift = 3 × (1.40°) between rows
5. TR#256 = the steepest gradient to allow a phase shift = 255 × (1.40°) between rows

If we do these steps once more, we get the same information as the first phase-encoding step, which is redundant. Each time we do a phase-encoding step followed by frequency encoding, we get a *signal*. The first signal we get is without any phase shift (TR#1). Then we activate the phase-encode gradient, add some phase shift, and get another signal (TR#2), and so on. Each signal is different because it has a different phase shift.

Data Space. Each of these signals fills one line in a set of rows referred to as the **data space** (Fig. 11-13). **k-space** can be thought of as a digitized version of the data space (more on this in Chapter 13). Let's see how this is done within each TR period:

1. With TR#1, we have no phase shift. After the frequency-encoding step, a signal is

received and placed into one row of the data space. In the previous example, we happened to put it into the center row of the data space (this is arbitrary, though).

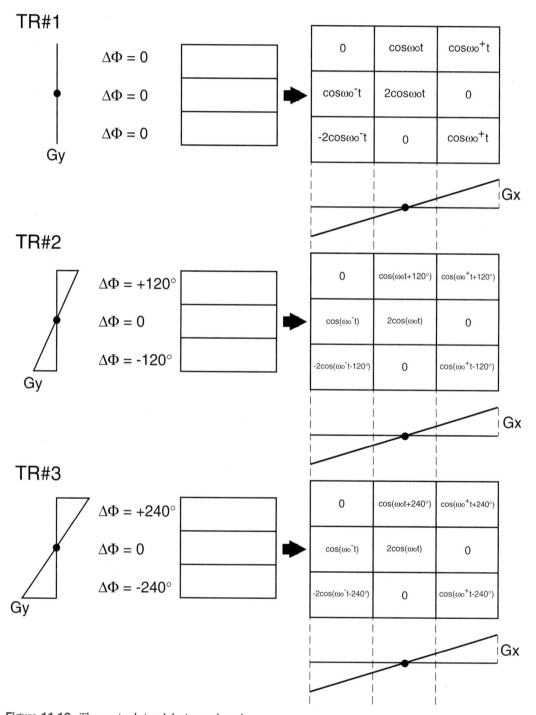

Figure 11-12. The received signal during each cycle.

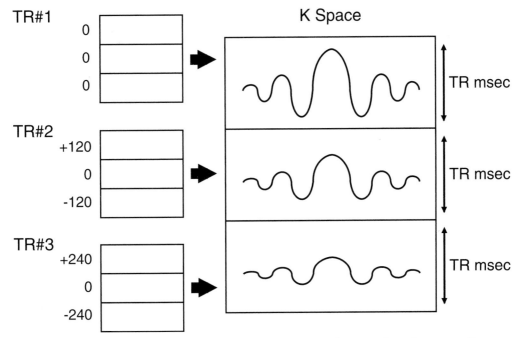

Figure 11-13. Each row in the data space (analog k-space) contains the received signal corresponding to a particular phase-encode gradient.

2. With TR#2, we add a phase shift, and, after the frequency-encoding step, a signal (which will be different from the signal from the first TR) is received and put into another row in the data space. In the previous example, we put it into the top row of the data space (again, this is arbitrary).

3. With TR#3, we add more phase shift. After the frequency-encoding step, a third signal (which is different from the other two signals because of the increased phase shift) is received and put into another row of the data space. In the previous example, we put it into the bottom row of the data space.

The interval between the rows in the data space is given by TR msec, going through a cycle from one 90° pulse to the next 90° pulse.

Summary

TR#1: place the signal into the center of the data space

TR#2: place it one above the center of the data space

TR#3: place it one below the center of the data space

If we had a TR#4, we would place it two above the center, and if we had a TR#5, we would place it two below the center. We could continue along filling the data space in this manner.

Remember that in our example, we start in the center of the data space with TR#1, which has no phase shift. In each subsequent row (as we go farther out in the data space) there is progressively greater and greater phase shift in each phase-encoding step. Also remember that each phase-encoding step has a different magnetic field gradient; thus, its phase shift will be different from each preceding and each subsequent phase-encoding step.

However, also note that the selection of phase-encoding steps, that is, the order in which we perform them, is *arbitrary*. We can start with no phase shift and go progressively to maximum phase shift, or we can start with maximum phase shift and go down to no phase shift. Likewise, the position to which they are assigned in the data space is also *arbitrary*.

When we discuss fast spin echo in later chapters, we will see the arbitrariness of this

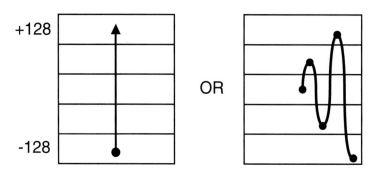

Figure 11-14. Various k (or data) space trajectories.

phase-encoding assignment. Even in conventional spin-echo imaging, the placement of signals into the data space can vary. For example, two different patterns of the data space filling with 256 phase-encoding steps are shown in Figure 11-14. We can put the first signal in the bottom of the data space and work up with successive phase-encoding steps. Or, as in our example, we can start in the center and go alternately up and down. Usually, the center row of the data space corresponds to no phase gradient.

Note, however, that the center of the data space does not represent the center of your picture. Each signal has information in it about the entire picture. Remember that each signal that goes into each row of the data space is the *sum* of all the signals from individual pixels in the slice.

The information in the data space is in the **time domain** (so it is not as scary as it looks). In fact, it is in the time domain in both directions: the received signal is displayed over a period of time (*t*), and signals in two successive rows are obtained at every TR (Fig. 11-15).

The information in this data space has not yet been digitized. In fact, a digitized version of this information is the true **k-space.** We will see in a later chapter (Chapter 16) that the "digitized" k-space is in a **spatial frequency domain.** But let's not get confused now! Let's see how we can digitize this information in the data. This is accomplished via sampling.

Sampling

The signal that goes into the data space has been phase encoded and frequency encoded, but it has not yet been **sampled** (more on this in the next chapter).

When we describe a matrix of, say, 256 × 192, what do we mean by it? If we only have 192 phase-encoding steps, why do we have 256 (instead of 192) frequency encodes if we only need one frequency encode for every encoding step?

Actually, the 256 number refers to the different number of frequencies we have for each phase-encoding step. These two steps are thus independent from one another. For example, let's look at a 4 × 5 matrix. This means that we do five different frequencies for each phase-encoding step, with the center column having no change in frequency and two different frequencies for the columns on either side; there will be

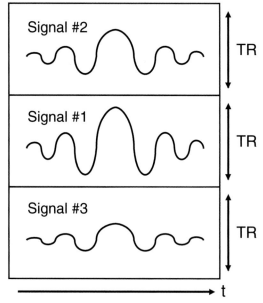

Figure 11-15. The data space is in the time domain.

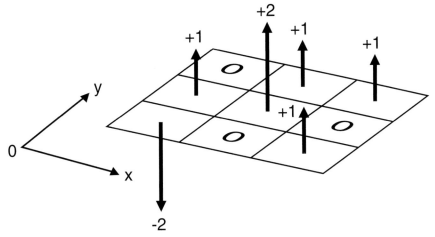

Figure 11-16. The Fourier transform of the data space (Fig. 11-5) is the desired image, shown here in three dimensions.

four different phase-encoding steps. Therefore, the result will be **asymmetric** pixels. Let's go back to our original 3 × 3 matrix, with its data space as in Figure 11-15.

How do we go from the data space to the desired image? The answer is via **Fourier trans-formation.** The Fourier transform of the signals in Figure 11-15 is a set of spikes, which in a three-dimensional space looks like Figure 11-16. More on this in chapters to come.

Key Points

In the previous chapter, we learned how to select a slice using a slice-select gradient G_z. In this chapter, we saw how to determine the pixel values in a slice using two gradients: (i) a frequency-encoding (or readout) gradient G_x and (ii) a phase-encoding gradient G_y.

The G_x gradient is the same strength for each echo, and since it is applied during the readout (i.e., during reception of the echo), it alters the Larmor frequency along the x-axis. This provides specific information along the x-axis. Each TR interval contains one readout (G_x) per slice.

The G_y gradient, however, is applied in increments between the 90° RF pulse and each echo. Since this gradient is applied at a time apart from the echo, it does not change the echo frequency, but merely induces a phase shift. Thus, for every slice, each TR interval contains one phase-encoding step (i.e., one unique value of G_y). This process completes one line in k-space corresponding to the selected G_y. This process is repeated N_y times to fill all of k-space.

We have not yet discussed the mechanism of performing frequency- and phase-encoding operations. This is the topic of the next chapter.

Questions

11-1 Match
(i) G_x (ii) G_y (iii) G_z
with
(a) applied during the echo

(b) applied during the RF transmission
(c) applied between the RF and the readout

11-2 **T/F** The purpose of the gradients is to determine the position of the originating signals from the patient (i.e., spatial encoding).

11-3 What is the phase increment for 128 phase-encode steps (i.e., $N_y = 128$)?

11-4 Match
  (i) position along x-axis
  (ii) position along y-axis
  with

(a) phase-encode gradient G_y
(b) frequency-encode gradient G_x
(c) absolute phase ϕ_y
(d) absolute frequency f_x

11-5 **T/F** In conventional spin-echo imaging, during each cycle (one TR period), only a *single* value of the phase-encode gradient strength G_y is applied.

12

Introduction

Signal processing refers to analog and/or digital manipulation of a signal. The signal could be an electric current or voltage, as is the case in magnetic resonance imaging (MRI). **Image processing** is a form of signal processing in which the manipulations are performed on a digitized image. **Analog-to-digital conversion** (**ADC**) is a process by which a time-varying (analog) signal is converted to a digitized form (i.e., a series of 0s and 1s) that can be recognized by a computer. An understanding of signal processing requires a basic understanding of the concept of frequency domain and Fourier transform (FT) because most of the "processing" of a signal is accomplished in the frequency domain and, at the end, the results are converted back into the time domain.

One of the key concepts in signal processing, as we shall see shortly, is the **Nyquist sampling** theorem. An understanding of the sampling procedure allows one to appreciate the relationship between the samples of a signal (in the time domain) and its bandwidth (in the frequency domain). Once this concept is grasped, the issue of **aliasing (wraparound)** artifact can be explained very easily. A knowledge of signal processing will also help the reader understand the more complicated, newer fast scanning pulse sequences presented in later chapters.

Sequence of Events

First, let's summarize what has been discussed so far. Figure 12-1 illustrates a summary of a spin-echo pulse sequence. The following is a summary of the sequence of events:

1. We have 90° and 180° pulses separated by a time of TE/2 msec.
2. After a time of TE millisecond after each 90° radio frequency (RF) pulse, we get an **echo.**
3. We turn on the slice-selective gradient (G_z) during the two RF transmissions. This causes a linear gradient of magnetic field along the z-axis. By choosing an RF pulse with an appropriate frequency and bandwidth, we can select a slice at a particular position with a particular thickness.

As an aside, consider Figure 12-2. Plotting field strength versus position (Fig. 12-2), the gradient is represented as a sloped line. The slope of the line is a constant that we call G. The value y along this line with slope G at point x is $y = G_x$. This is a simple linear equation. Figure 12-2B plots gradient strength versus time. Figures 12-2A and 12-2B are used interchangeably to illustrate a *linear* gradient with strength G.

4. Right before we receive the echo, we apply a phase-encoding gradient (G_y). The symbol for the phase-encoding gradent is in Figure 12-3. This symbol denotes the *multiple* phase-encoding steps that are necessary as we cycle through the acquisition. Remember that one of the phase-encode steps may be performed without any gradient.

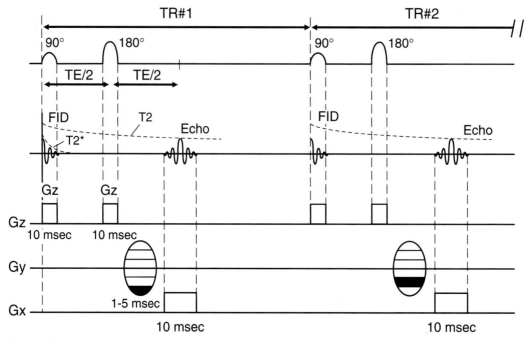

Figure 12-1. Spin-echo pulse sequence diagram.

5. The frequency-encoding gradient (G_x) is turned on during the time period during which the echo is received.

6. Time requirements

    (a) The frequency-encoding step takes about 10 msec (4–8 msec at high field; 16–30 msec at lower fields).

    (b) The phase-encoding step takes 1–5 msec.

    (c) Each RF pulse (with a G_z gradient) takes 2–10 msec.

Then we repeat the whole sequence of events after time TR. The time spent from the center of the 90° pulse to the end of the echo readout is

TE + 1/2 (sampling time) = (TE + Ts/2)

The **sampling time** T_s is the time it takes to sample the echo, which is the time that the G_x gradient (readout or frequency-encode gradient) is on. The G_x gradient is on throughout the echo readout—from beginning to end (Fig. 12-4). The time from the beginning of the 90° pulse to the midpoint of the echo is TE. Because half of the sampling time continues past the midpoint of the echo, we need to add half the sampling time to TE to account for the entire "active time" from the beginning of the RF pulse to the end of the sampling time:

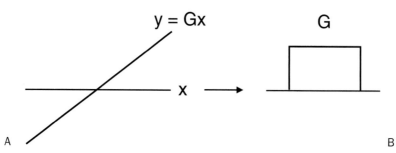

Figure 12-2. A linear G represents a linear function G_x, which can be represented either as a linear line with slope G (**A**) or as a rectangle with height G (**B**).

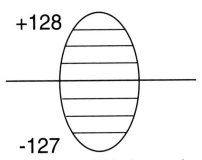

Figure 12-3. The symbol for phase-encode gradient.

Active time = TE + $T_s/2$

There may also be time taken up by other events that occur before the RF pulse (such as presaturation pulses) that we include as **overhead time** (T_o). Thus,

---

Active time = TE + $T_s/2$ + T_o

Let's assume a TE of 40 msec, a sampling time T_s = 10 msec, and an overhead time T_o = 5 msec. Then,

$$\text{Active time} = 40 \text{ msec} + 10 \text{ msec}/2 + 5 \text{ msec}$$
$$= 50 \text{ msec}$$

Therefore, it takes 50 msec to read out the signal from one echo. We then place this signal into the data space (Fig. 12-5). We have designated 256 rows in the data space (from -127 to $+128$), and in this instance we've placed the first signal at position -127.

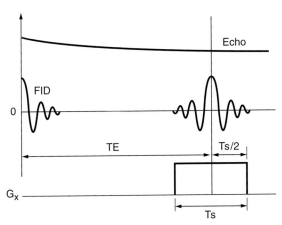

Figure 12-4. The frequency gradient is turned on during readout (i.e., during the echo).

7. In the next TR cycle, we do exactly the same thing, except this time, the phase-encoding step will be done with a slightly weaker magnetic gradient and will be one step higher in k (data) space.

Question: Why does the magnitude of the signal differ with each phase-encoding step? For example, in Figure 12-5, the signal from the echo of TR#2 seems to have higher maximum amplitude than the signal from the echo of TR#1.

Answer: The strength of the phase-encoding gradient affects the magnitude of the signal.

When the phase-encode gradient is at a maximum (when we have the largest magnetic field gradient), we have the maximum dephasing of proton spins. Recall that we are dealing with proton spins that have been flipped into the transverse plane by a 90° pulse, and the signal is maximum as long as these proton spins stay *in phase*. By using a magnetic field gradient, we are introducing an artificial external means of dephasing. Also, remember that when we flip the protons into the transverse plane, they are initially in phase and then rapidly go out of phase due to external magnetic inhomogeneities and spin–spin interactions (Fig. 12-6A). Next, the protons are flipped with a 180° pulse and, after a period of time = TE/2, they go back in phase (Fig. 12-6B).

On top of this, we introduce a magnetic inhomogeneity by way of a linear gradient in which the inhomogeneity increases linearly, causing *additional dephasing* of proton spins. We realize that we have to accept this additional dephasing because this is the way we obtain *spatial* information along the axis of this gradient. This process is called **phase encoding.**

However, this explains why, when we use the magnetic field gradient for phase encoding, the additional dephasing caused by the gradient will necessarily decrease the overall signal we receive during that phase-encoding step. It then allows us to conclude as follows:

(a) The largest magnetic gradient we use for maximum phase encoding will give us the lowest magnitude signal.

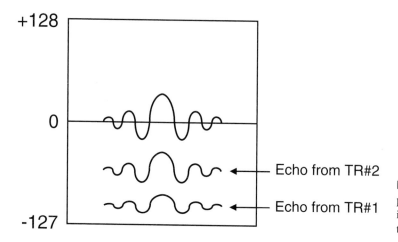

+128

0

-127

Echo from TR#2

Echo from TR#1

Figure 12-5. For each phase-encoding step, a signal is obtained that is placed in the data space.

(b) When the magnetic gradient in the phase-encode direction is zero, we will not introduce any additional dephasing, and we will get the largest magnitude signal.

Therefore, if we go back and examine the signal from TR#1 and TR#2, we see that

(a) TR#1 at position −127 in the data space has a lower amplitude signal than TR#2

at position −126. This is because during TR#1 a larger phase-encoding gradient is used than during TR#2. (Keep in mind, however, that assignments of gradients to different TR intervals in the data space are *arbitrary*.)

k-space, as we mentioned in the last chapter (with more to come in Chapters 13 and 16), can

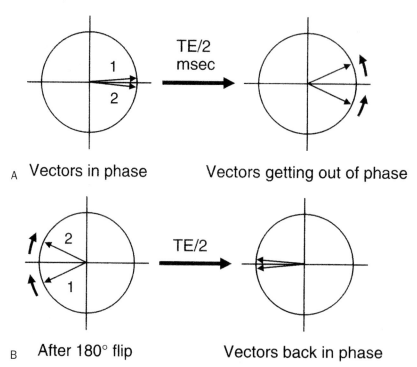

TE/2 msec

A Vectors in phase   Vectors getting out of phase

TE/2

B After 180° flip   Vectors back in phase

Figure 12-6. The spins are initially in phase (**A**) and then get out of phase at time TE/2. At this point, a 180° pulse is applied, reversing the vectors (**B**) so that they come back in phase after another period TE/2 (i.e., at time TE).

be thought of as a digitized version of the data space. The signal in the center of k-space (at position 0) has the maximum amplitude. This is because this signal is obtained at a phase-encoding step at which no magnetic field gradient is used (i.e., no phase gradient and hence no extra dephasing due to phase encoding). In fact, the center line of k-space will always be occupied by the phase-encoding step that uses no gradient.

> **The center line of k-space will always contain the phase-encoding step with the weakest gradient and thus with the most signal.**

The most peripheral lines of k-space will be occupied by the phase-encoding steps that use the strongest gradients.

> **The periphery of k-space will contain the phase-encoding steps with the largest gradients and thus with the least signal.**

8. Multislice technique

Remember that TR is much longer than the *active time* needed to perform all the functions necessary to select a slice, phase encode, and frequency encode. The TR might be, say, 1000 msec. The *active time* in our example was 50 msec. There is a lot of **"dead time"** in between the 50 msec of active time and the next 90° pulse. We can take advantage of this "dead time" in order to get information regarding other slices.

As an example, in Figure 12-7 we will have time for two additional slices to be studied during the dead time within one TR period. After we obtain the signal from slice number 1, we can apply another 90° pulse of a different center frequency ω, but with an identical transmit bandwidth to specify the next slice (Fig. 12-8). Here we are talking about the transmitted bandwidth (of the RF pulse) that determines slice thickness, not to be confused with the receiver bandwidth (of the echo) that determines noise. More on this later.

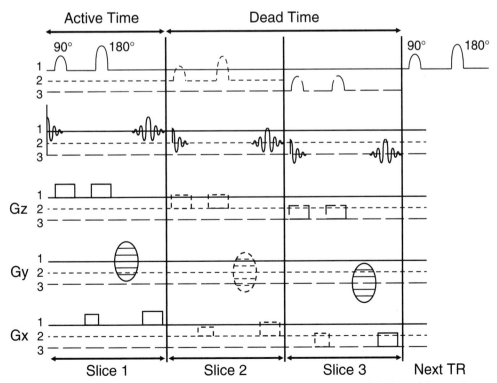

Figure 12-7. Multislice acquisition. During each TR cycle, there is a certain "dead time" that can be used to acquire other slices.

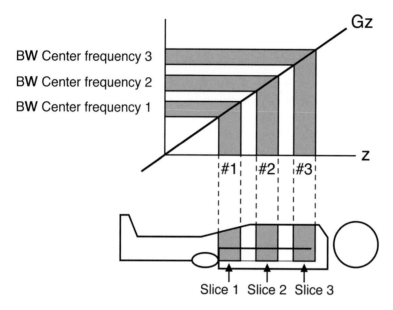

Figure 12-8. During each TR period, several RF pulses with different frequencies (and BWs) corresponding to different slices are transmitted.

To choose the next slice, we keep the same magnetic gradient G_z, but we choose a bandwidth at a higher or lower *center* (or Larmor) frequency to flip the protons 90° in a different slice. The *bandwidth is the same* as the first slice, but the *center frequency is different.*

We choose the same phase-encoding gradient G_y so we get the same amount of dephasing in this next slice. We sample the echo with the same frequency-encoding gradient as we did with the first slice. Because we still have time during the dead time to acquire a third slice, we repeat everything and again choose a 90° RF pulse of a different Larmor frequency so we can flip the protons of a different slice into the transverse plane. The signal from each slice will be placed in a different k-space.

Each slice has its own k-space.

Slice selection can be performed in several different ways. We can have *contiguous slices; sequential slices* with a *gap* between slices; and *interleaved slices,* where we do odd-numbered slices (i.e., 1, 3, 5) and then go back and do even-numbered slices (i.e., 2, 4, 6).

9. Number of slices (coverage)
    The number of slices we can do within any TR is limited by the *dead time* after

$(TE + T_s/2 + T_o)$. Furthermore, if we choose to have two echoes per TR (as in a dual-echo, spin-echo sequence), the number of slices we could have would be cut back more. The formula for the maximum number of slices one can obtain is

$$\text{Number of slices} < \frac{TR}{TE + T_s/2 + T_o}$$
$$= \frac{TR}{\text{active time}}$$

If we do multiple echoes (or just one long echo), the formula is governed by the *longest* TE.

Examples
1. TR = 1000, TE = 35 msec, T_s = 10 msec, T_o = 10 msec (short TE)

$$\text{Maximum number of slices} = \frac{TR}{TE + T_s/2 + T_o}$$
$$= \frac{1000}{35 + 5 + 10}$$
$$= 1000/50 = 20 \text{ slices}$$

2. TR = 1000, TE = 75, T_s = 10 msec, T_o = 10 msec (long TE)

$$\text{Maximum number of slices} = \frac{1000}{75 + 5 + 10}$$
$$= 1000/90 \cong 11 \text{ slices}$$

We usually don't know what the sampling time (T_s) or overhead time (T_o) is; therefore, a rough approximation is

Maximum number of slices < TR/TE.

It is said that in a double-echo sequence, the first echo is "free." This means that the number of slices in a double-echo sequence is determined only by the TE of the second echo

$$TR = 1000, TE_1 = 30, TE_2 = 80$$

Maximum number of slices

$$= \frac{TR}{TE \text{ (second echo)} + T_s/2 + T_o}$$
$$= 1000/(80 + 15) = 1000/95$$
$$\cong 10.5$$

In fact, the maximum number of slices is determined by TR, and the time it takes to get one line in the data space as follows:

Maximum number of slices < TR/time to get one line of signal into the data space

$$= TR/(TE + T_s/2 + T_o)$$

Also remember that each slice has its own data space (and, thus, its own k-space), and if we are doing a double-echo sequence, *each echo has its own data space (k-space)*. The signal obtained from each slice during the same TR will be obtained with the same phase-encoding step. Thus, the equivalent line in each data space of the slices for a given TR will be subject to the same dephasing effects of the phase-encoding gradient (Fig. 12-9).

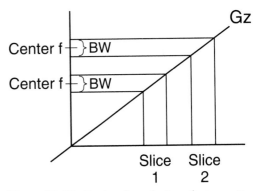

Figure 12-10. During slice selection, the transmit BW of RF pulses remains the same but their center frequencies vary.

10.   Center frequency

A few more words about the *center frequency* and *transmit bandwidth*. As we go from slice to slice, the RF center frequency (i.e., the Larmor frequency) changes, but the bandwidth remains the same. In Figure 12-10, the bandwidth (the range of frequencies) remains the same. The *center frequency* of the bandwidth changes: it increases as we go higher on the magnetic field gradient and it decreases as we go lower on the magnetic gradient.

The bandwidth (range of frequencies) should be constant because we want each slice to be of the same thickness. At the low end of the magnetic gradient the frequencies are lower, and at the top end of the gradient the frequencies are higher. Thus, as we go up the gradient, we approach higher center frequencies for the RF pulse; however, the bandwidth won't change.

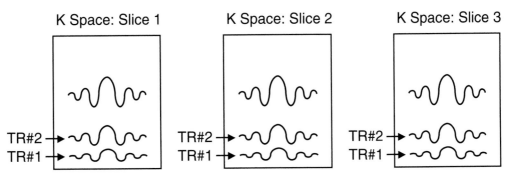

Figure 12-9. Each slice has its own k (data) space.

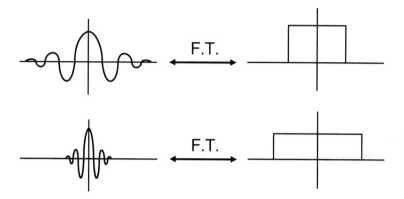

Figure 12-11. An inverse relationship exists between the duration of a pulse and its BW.

If the duration of the RF pulse is short, then its bandwidth will be wide and vice versa (Fig. 12-11). In our pulse sequence, we use the same RF bandwidth (i.e., the same RF duration) each time, but the center frequency is changed. Think of the center frequency as a **carrier** frequency. We are sending the same signal, but we are carrying it at a different center frequency, and the bandwidth around it is the original signal (Fig. 12-12).

If we use a *wider* bandwidth with the same center frequency, then we get a *thicker* slice; a *narrower* RF pulse whose FT has a wider bandwidth gives us a thicker slice. A *carrier* is a signal that determines the center frequency. For more details, refer to the discussion on bandwidth in Chapter 10.

Figure 12-13A displays a typical signal from the echo. After the signal is received at the receiver coil, it is digitized (through signal sampling) because the computer analyzing the signal can only work with digitized numbers. The vertical bars in Figure 12-13A demonstrate the sampling procedure. Instead of having a continuum of signal amplitudes, **samples** of the signal at certain time intervals (usually equidistant intervals) are taken.

The computer now only has these **discrete** (as opposed to analog) values. Each value is represented in the computer as a **binary number** (0s and 1s) so the computer doesn't deal with the whole signal—just discrete samples of the signal. A computer **bit** is either a 0 or a 1. A **byte** consists of 8 bits and represents the basic building block of computer characters. Each sample of an analog signal is encoded into a series of bytes, which is recognized by every computer. This process is the basis for **ADC.**

> The idea behind ADC is to just use the samples of a signal and be able to reconstruct the original signal from its samples.

Let's consider a *sinc* signal with frequency ω. As we have seen in previous chapters, this signal has a rectangle-shaped FT (Fig. 12-13B). The time between successive sampling points is called the sampling interval ΔT_s (or dwell time).

$$\Delta T_s = \text{sampling interval}$$

After it is sampled, the aforementioned signal will look like Figure 12-14A. The **envelope** of this function is a curve connecting the sample points (which resembles the original *sinc* function). The FT of this sampled signal is given in

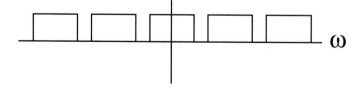

Figure 12-12. The FT of RF pulses—the BWs are the same, but the center frequencies are different.

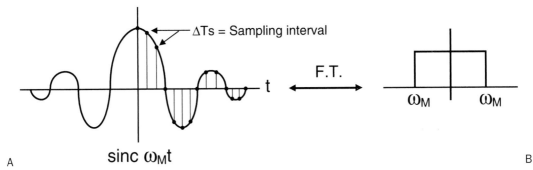

A   sinc $\omega_M t$ B

Figure 12-13. The FT of a sinc function (**A**) contains a single rectangle (**B**).

Figure 12-14B. This FT looks like a *periodic* version of the original FT (Fig. 12-13B) because the FT of a discrete and periodic function is also periodic (see later text). If ΔT_s is the sampling interval, the first center frequency is given by the following formula (Fig. 12-14B):

$$\text{Center frequency} = 1/\Delta T_s$$

If we make the sampling interval very short, we will spread out the square waves in the FT, that is, if we take several samples per cycle, the square waves spread out (Fig. 12-15). If we make the sampling interval very wide, the square waves of the FT are going to get closer, that is, if we take few samples per cycle, the square waves get closer (Fig. 12-16).

Aliasing

We don't want to take too few samples per cycle, that is, we don't want the sampling interval to be too wide because then the square waves will **overlap** and **aliasing** will result (Fig. 12-17).

Why is the FT of a continuous *sinc* function a single wave, whereas that of its sampled version

shows repetitive square waves (Fig. 12-18)? The reason for this is *mathematical*. We will try to give an explanation that doesn't involve the complicated mathematics behind it.

To sample the signal, we have to multiply the signal by a sequence of spikes (each spike is called a delta function). Each spike is separated from the next by the sampling interval (ΔT_s) (Fig. 12-19).

Because the value of the series of spikes is zero everywhere between the spikes and is positive where the spikes are located, then multiplying the signal by the spikes will result in a value of 0 throughout the signal except where the spikes are located (Fig. 12-20).

Now, the FTs of a series of spikes are also a series of spikes (Fig. 12-21). Whereas the spikes are separated by ΔT_s, the FTs of the spikes are in the frequency domain and are separated by $1/\Delta T_s$ (Fig. 12-21). The FT of the signal multiplied by the spikes is the FT of the signal **convolved** with the Fourier transfer of the spikes. (This has to do with a mathematical operation called **convolution.**) Convolution basically means that we take the FT of the signal and center it around each spike (Fig. 12-22).

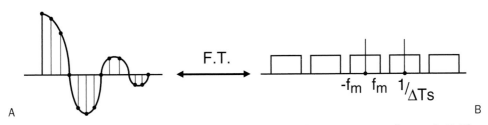

A   B

Figure 12-14. The FT of a sampled (discrete) sinc function (**A**) contains a series of rectangle. **B:** The midpoint of each rectangle is a multiple of $1/\Delta T_s$.

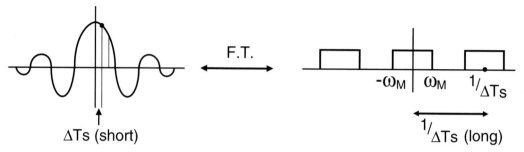

Figure 12-15. A short sampling interval ΔT_s (i.e., taking more samples) causes the rectangles to spread out.

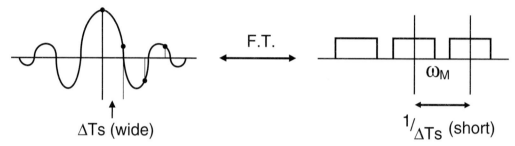

Figure 12-16. A longer sampling interval (i.e., taking fewer samples) causes the rectangles to move closer to one another.

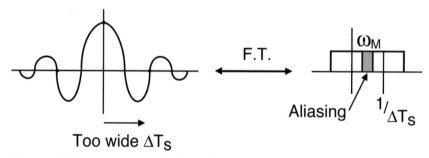

Figure 12-17. When the sampling interval is too long (i.e., not enough samples are taken), the rectangles may overlap (causing aliasing).

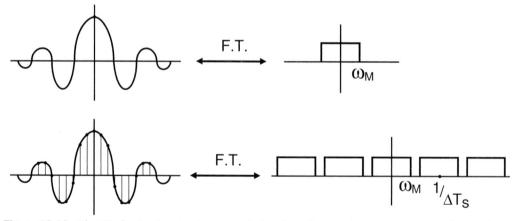

Figure 12-18. The FT of a sinc function is a rectangle, but that of its sample variant is a series of rectangles.

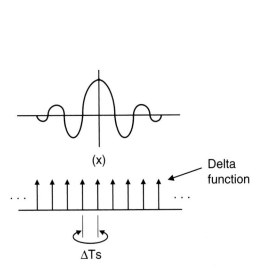

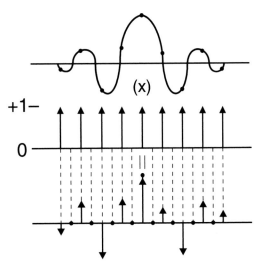

Figure 12-19. To sample a continuous, analog signal, a series of spikes (called delta functions) is multiplied by the signal.

Figure 12-20. After multiplying the signal by a series of spikes, the result is zero except at the points of the spikes. The value of each resulting spike is equal to the value of the signal at that point.

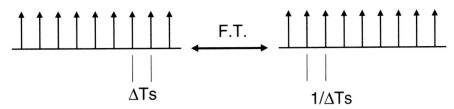

Figure 12-21. The FT of a series of spikes (separated by ΔT_s) is also a series of spikes (separated by $1/\Delta T_s$).

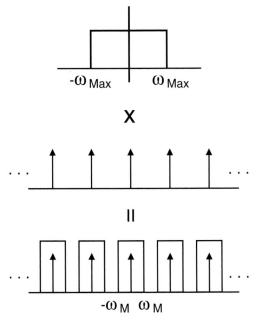

Figure 12-22. The FT of the product of a signal and a series of spikes is the FT of that signal (e.g., a rectangle) "convolved" with a series of spikes. The result is the FT of that signal replicated an infinite number of times.

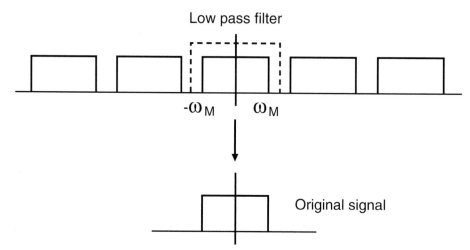

Figure 12-23. When the previous FT is passed through a low-pass filter, the result is the desired FT.

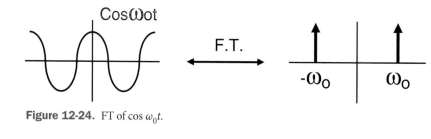

Figure 12-24. FT of cos $\omega_0 t$.

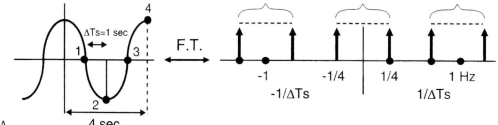

Figure 12-25. **A, B:** The FT of a sampled cosine signal.

Eventually, we want to get back our original signal. If we take these repetitive FTs and pass them through a **low-pass filter** (LPF), we will ultimately retrieve our original signal (Fig. 12-23). But remember, we really don't need to know the above mathematics to understand the principles of sampling.

Let's consider an easier signal: a *cosine* function cos $\omega_0 t$ and its FT (Fig. 12-24). The sampled version of this signal (with four samples per interval) is shown in Figure 12-25A with its FT in Figure 12-25B. Notice how the FT of this digitized cosine function has multiple replicas. Briefly,

1. The cycle is 4-sec long.
2. ΔT_s is 1 sec.
3. Frequency = number of cycles/sec = 1/4 cycle/sec = 1/4 Hz.
4. $1/\Delta T_s = 1/1$ sec = 1 Hz.

On the FT (Fig. 12-25A), we have the center frequency 1/4 Hz, corresponding to one replica, and the center frequency $1/\Delta T_s$ (= 1 Hz), corresponding to the second replica. If we now pass this FT through an *LPF* as in Figure 12-26 to eliminate all the high frequencies, we will recover our original pair of frequency

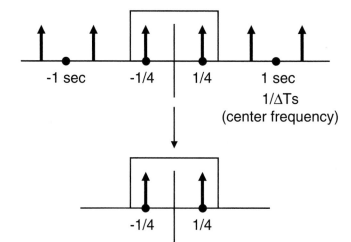

-1 sec   -1/4 | 1/4   1 sec
1/ΔTs
(center frequency)

-1/4 | 1/4

Figure 12-26. The previous FT passed through an LPF gives the FT of the original cosine function.

spikes, which is the FT of the original *cosine* wave.

Visually, if we had the four sampling points in Figure 12-25A, we could still see quite easily what the original signal should look like (Fig. 12-27) by connecting the dots. It would be easier if we had more samples because the more samples we use, the easier it is to see the shape of the original signal (Fig. 12-27B).

Let's now take another example in which we have fewer than four samples. Let's try two samples per cycle (Fig. 12-28A). In this case,

1. The period is still 4 sec.
2. ΔT_s = sampling interval is 2 sec.
3. $1/\Delta T_s = 1/2 = 0.5$ Hz.

Let's see the FT of this example (Fig. 12-28B). Frequency is still 1/4. The sampling interval is

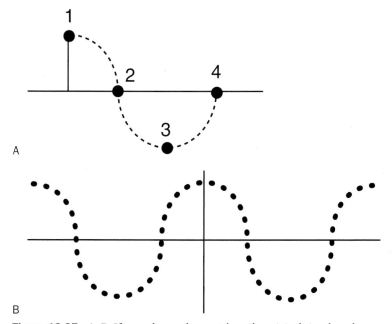

Figure 12-27. A, B: If enough samples are taken, the original signal can be visually reconstructed by connecting the dots. The more samples taken, the easier it is to visualize the original signal.

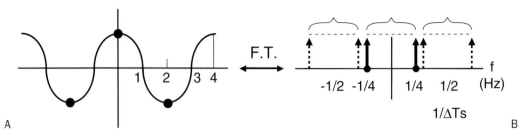

A

B

Figure 12-28. A, B: If exactly two samples are taken per cycle of a cosine function, the spikes will overlap exactly and the original signal is still decipherable.

now 2 sec, so $1/\Delta T_s = 1/2$ Hz. We show two spikes on either side of 1/2 Hz, which is the frequency range around the center frequency of 1/2 Hz.

We see now that the pair of spikes centered at 1/2 Hz come right next to the original pair of spikes of 1/4 Hz. They practically overlap. If we pass this FT through an LPF to eliminate the higher frequencies, we still recover the two frequency spikes, which are the FTs of the original *cosine* signal; however, they will be increased in amplitude because of the overlap (Fig. 12-29).

Now let's see what happens if we take even fewer samples (Fig. 12-30A). Here,

1. The period is still 4 sec.
2. But $\Delta T_s = 3$ sec.
3. $1/\Delta T_s = 1/3$ Hz.
4. The frequency is still 1/4 cycles/sec.

So, let's look at the FT (Fig. 12-30B). If we put this FT through an *LPF*, the spikes associated with the center frequency $(1/\Delta T_s)$ will *interfere* with the original signal (Fig. 12-31). We will not only have the original spikes but also have two extra spikes that are closer to the center. Now we have the *sum of two cosine waves* rather than the spikes of the single original *cosine* wave. We have the spikes of another *cosine* wave, which are closer together, meaning that its transform is a *cosine* wave of *lower frequency*. This is called **aliasing.**

What we wanted to approximate by sampling was the original signal, having a frequency of 1/4 Hz. But as a result of undersampling, we also obtain an undesired signal with a much lower frequency (Fig. 12-32).

Aliasing: An Analogy. As an analogy, let's consider a stage-coach wheel in a Western movie. Sometimes, it appears as if the wheel is

turning in the reverse direction. Let's see how this happens. When we take a motion picture, we are actually taking *samples* in time. Let's take one point on the wheel and take a sample at time $t = 0$ (Fig. 12-33). At a later time (t_1), we take another frame. The point rotates a certain distance forward as the wheel turns. When we watch this in a motion picture we see this point rotating in a *clockwise* direction.

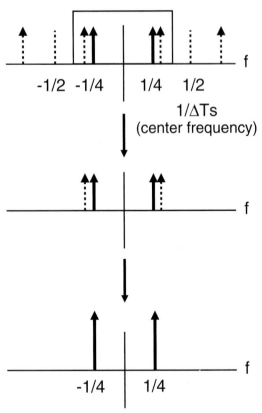

Figure 12-29. An LPF applied to the previous FT allows recreation of the original signal (although the height of the spikes is doubled).

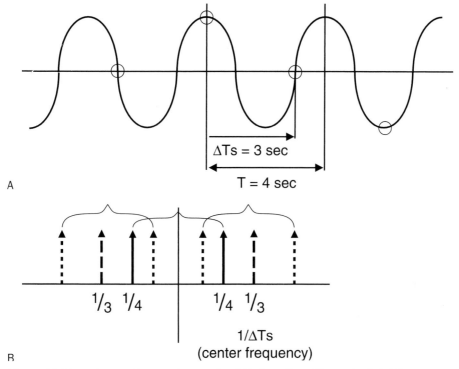

Figure 12-30. When too few samples are taken (**A**), the spikes will get mixed up (**B**).

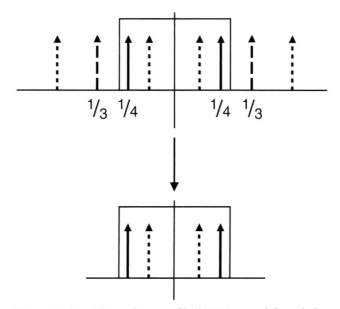

Figure 12-31. When a (low-pass filter) LPF is passed through the previous example, two sets, instead of one set, of spikes are produced, which would yield a different signal than the original cosine function. This is called aliasing.

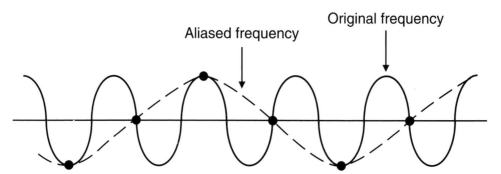

Figure 12-32. When too few samples are taken, the perceived (aliased) frequency is different from the actual (original) frequency.

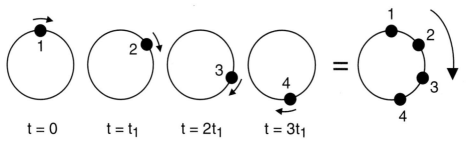

Figure 12-33. Analogy of aliasing. If the motion picture frames of a stage-coach wheel are taken fast enough, the wheel appears to rotate correctly in the clockwise direction.

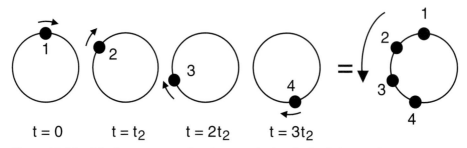

Figure 12-34. If the frames are not taken fast enough, the wheel will deceptively appear to be rotating in the counterclockwise direction.

Now let's see what happens when we **undersample** (Fig. 12-34). Let's say the first frame starts at the same point as before at $t = 0$. But on the next frame, we wait longer (t_2) to sample and don't sample until the point almost comes around to its original spot. We wait a similar time for the next sample and the point again comes around almost to the spot on the second frame. If we take a motion picture of this, the wheel will appear as if it's turning *counterclockwise*. This is because we are *undersampling*. This is an example of *aliasing*. The wheel is actually turning in a forward direction, but because of undersampling, it *appears* to be doing something else.

Undersampling causes aliasing.

Aliasing comes from the term **alias:** a *fake name*. We have a real frequency, but because of undersampling, we appear to have a *fake* frequency. In the previous example in which the *cosine* wave was undersampled, the real signal was a *cosine* wave with a frequency of 1/4 Hz,

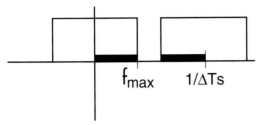

Figure 12-35. Nyquist law: To avoid aliasing, the maximum frequency in the signal (f_{max}) should be less than half the sampling frequency ($1/\Delta T_s$). In other words, the sampling interval (ΔT_s) should be at least twice the minimum period ($1/f_{max}$). That is, at least two samples per cycle (corresponding to the highest frequency in the signal) are required to avoid aliasing.

but the "alias" *cosine* wave had a *lower frequency* (Fig. 12-31). In the example of the wagon wheel, the real rotation was in a clockwise direction, but the alias was in a counterclockwise direction, probably with a slower rotation.

Sampling Theorem (Nyquist Law)

Consider Figure 12-35. The sampling theorem states:

> Nyquist law: If ω_{max} is the maximum frequency in the signal, then the sampling rate must be at least twice the maximum signal frequency to avoid aliasing, that is, $\omega_{sampling} = 1/\Delta T_s \geq 2\omega_{max}$.

This is easy to see in the diagram (Fig. 12-35). We want the sampling rate to be at least equal to the sum of the maximum frequencies of adjacent boxes (to keep the boxes from overlapping).

In other words, the sampling rate should be at least twice ω_{max}. In terms of sampling interval (ΔT_s), it should be less than half of the period of the signal (remember that $\Delta T_s = 1/\omega_{max}$):

$$\Delta T_s < 1/2 \text{ (period)}$$

This is the **Nyquist theorem.** Basically, it means that if we want to recover a signal from its samples, we need to take *at least two samples per cycle*. We can take as many samples as we like, but sampling takes time, so we want to *take the minimum number of samples necessary* to recover the signal accurately from its FT. We saw diagrammatically how, with a minimum of two samples per cycle, we could accurately approximate the original *cosine* signal (Fig. 12-36).

Nyquist Theorem The maximum frequency we can recover is one-half of the sampling rate.

$$\text{Max frequency} = 1/2(\Delta T_s)^{-1}$$

or

$$1/\Delta T_s = 2(\text{Nyquist frequency})$$

Question: What is the difference between sampling interval and sampling time?

Answer: Sampling interval (ΔT_s) is the time between sampling points (Fig. 12-37). When we sample a signal, we can't possibly take an infinite number of samples. So we take (N) samples and then we stop. This gives the sampling time (T_s) the time it takes to sample the entire signal.

$$T_s = N \times (\Delta T_s)$$

The sampling time (T_s) is the sampling interval (ΔT_s) multiplied by the number of samples taken (N). The MR machine samples at a certain inter-

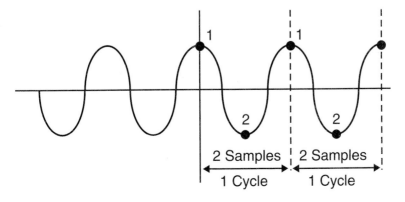

Figure 12-36. The original signal can be reconstructed with a minimum of two samples per cycle.

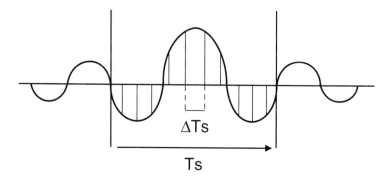

Figure 12-37. The sampling interval ΔT_s is the time interval between two successive samples. The sampling time is the product of ΔT_s and the number of samples N_x, that is, $T_s = N_x \cdot \Delta T_s$.

val (say, about $\Delta T_s = 50 \ \mu sec$). Let's say we have 256 frequency-encoding steps ($N = 256$). Then, sampling time = $256 \times 50 \ \mu sec \cong 13$ msec.

Let's prove the following:

Bandwidth = 1/sampling interval

Bandwidth = $1/\Delta T_s$

If the samples are close together, we get a higher bandwidth. If the samples are further apart, we get a lower bandwidth. Earlier, we were dealing with the bandwidth of an RF pulse. Now we are talking about the bandwidth of the received signal, that is, the bandwidth of the echo. The Nyquist theorem says that we should do a minimum of two samples per cycle to reconstruct the original signal. Is there any benefit in doing more samples per cycle?

The RF bandwidth is the **"transmission" bandwidth.** However, the bandwidth associated with the sampled signal is the **"receiver" bandwidth.** To prove the above relationship between bandwidth and ΔT_s, recall that frequency (which is number of cycles per second) is the reciprocal of time (1/time).

ΔT_s is the sampling interval (in the time domain), $1/\Delta T_s$ = frequency, and if we're operating at the Nyquist frequency,

$1/\Delta Ts$ = receiver bandwidth (Fig. 12.38)

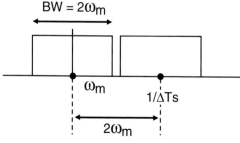

Figure 12-38. At Nyquist frequency, $1/\Delta T_s = \omega_{max}$ or $\Delta T_s = 1/(2\omega_{max})$.

From the diagram, we see that if we operate at the Nyquist frequency, then the bandwidth is equal to 2 × (maximum frequency ω_{max}). Thus,

$$\text{Bandwidth} = 2(\omega_{max}) = 1/\Delta T_s$$

We generally do not want to take more than the minimum number of samples to recreate the signal because more samples require more time. We want to operate as efficiently as possible, that is, take as few samples as possible, without causing *aliasing*.

We can, under certain circumstances, take more samples than two samples per cycle. For example, when we activate the feature on the scanner to avoid wraparound along the frequency-encode direction, the scanner automatically performs **oversampling** to prevent aliasing. This is done to play it safe by doubling the number of samples taken.

Digitized k-Space

We've already shown how we fill lines of the data space with our signal, with each line performed using a different phase-encoding step. What we actually put into each line of the data space are the *sampled* data from each signal. Once we put these samples into each line of data space, we complete the data space.

All MRI machines operate under the same principle when it comes to sampling the signal. A minimum of two samples per cycle is taken and put into the data space (Fig. 12-39A). If more than two samples per cycle are taken, then the bandwidth is wider, but it won't give us a better approximation of the signal (Fig. 12-39B). If we take less than two samples per cycle, the adjacent bandwidths may overlap and cause aliasing (Fig. 12-39C).

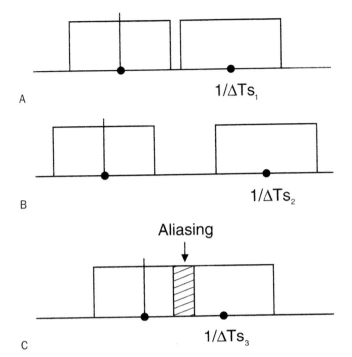

A

$1/\Delta Ts_1$

B

$1/\Delta Ts_2$

Aliasing

C

$1/\Delta Ts_3$

Figure 12-39. A: Operating at Nyquist frequency. **B:** When more samples are taken, the BW will be increased. **C:** When too few samples are taken, aliasing may occur $(T_{s3} > T_{s1} > T_{s2})$.

Signal-to-Noise Ratio

When the bandwidth is narrowed, the signal-to-noise ratio (SNR or S/N) is increased. (This topic is discussed at length in a later chapter.) SNR is inversely proportional to the square root of the bandwidth. SNR is also proportional to the volume of the pixel and to the square root of the number of phase-encoding steps (N_y), the number of frequency-encoding steps (N_x), and the number of excitations (NEX):

$$SNR \propto (\text{pixel volume}) \sqrt{\frac{N_y \cdot NEX \cdot N_x}{BW}}$$

Therefore, when we activate the feature on the scanner to lower the bandwidth (BW) on the second echo of a dual-echo T2-weighted spin-echo image, we increase the SNR on the second echo. Remember that when we decrease the bandwidth, we are increasing the sampling interval (ΔT_s). By increasing the sampling interval, we necessarily increase the sampling time (T_s) because $T_s = N(\Delta T_s)$. We do this only on the second echo because the magnitude of the signal is always weaker on the second echo, so we want to increase the SNR on the second echo. However, as we decrease the bandwidth to improve SNR, we

are necessarily decreasing the number of samples per cycle; thus, we are increasing the possibility of aliasing. This is the reason why there is a limit on how much the bandwidth can be decreased. If we sample too fast, the bandwidth is wider and SNR goes down. If we sample too slowly, the bandwidth is narrow and we may get aliasing.

If we increase the sampling time (T_s), we then decrease the number of slices we can take per TR because of the following formula:

$$\text{Number of slices} = \frac{TR}{TE + T_s/2 + T_o}$$

$\downarrow BW \rightarrow \uparrow \Delta T_s$ and $\uparrow \Delta T_s \rightarrow \uparrow T_s$
since $T_s = N(\Delta T_s)$.
Also $\downarrow BW \rightarrow \downarrow$ number of slices
since $\uparrow T_s \rightarrow \downarrow$ number of slices.

Sampling of Composite Signals

Let's discuss the sampling theorem in the case of a more complicated signal such as in Figure 12-40. When we have a *composite* signal (i.e., a signal composed of two or more frequencies), we need

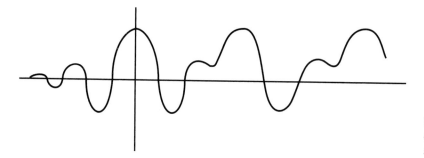

Figure 12-40. An example of a composite signal.

to take a minimum of two samples per cycle of the highest frequency present in the signal.

Presume that the complex signal above is a combination of three different *cosine* waves, each of a different frequency (Fig. 12-41). We have three different signals that are added up to give us a certain signal. The sampling theorem refers to the component of the signal that has the highest frequency. Therefore, we want to take two samples per cycle of the highest frequency component of the signal; this obviously means more than two samples per cycle for the other lower frequencies of the signal.

We are taking samples of the composite signal. Therefore, even though we take a minimum of two samples per cycle of the highest frequency component of the signal, we will necessarily be taking more than two samples per cycle of all the lower frequency components of the signal.

> **Nyquist sampling theorem: A minimum of two samples per cycle (corresponding to the highest frequency present in the signal) are required to reconstruct the original signal accurately from its samples.**

Example 1

(a) At 1.5 Tesla, it typically takes 8 msec to perform one readout: $T_s = 8$ msec.
(b) We have a matrix of, say, 256 × 256 pixels.

By convention, the first number refers to the number of frequency-encoding steps. The second number refers to the number of phase-encoding steps. What is the bandwidth? We know that

$$BW = 1/\Delta T_s$$

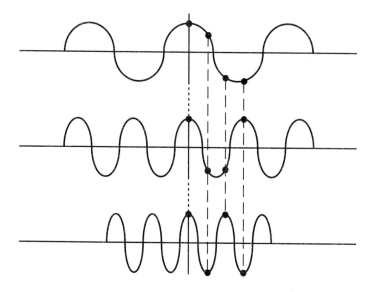

Figure 12-41. In a composite signal, two samples per cycle of the highest frequency component are required to avoid aliasing.

What is ΔT_s?

$$\Delta T_s = \text{sampling time/number of samples}$$
we test
$$= 8 \text{ msec/256 samples}$$
$$\text{BW} = 1/\Delta T_s = 1/(8 \text{ msec/256})$$
$$= 256/8 \text{ msec} = 256/0.008 \text{ sec}$$
$$= 32{,}000 \text{ Hz} = 32 \text{ kHz} = \pm 16 \text{ kHz}$$

This is a typical bandwidth for a typical readout with 256 frequency-encoding steps and a sampling time of 8 msec. Therefore, a frequency bandwidth of 32 kHz (± 16 kHz) is a fairly typical frequency bandwidth that we deal with in routine imaging. This means that the bandwidth extends to $+16$ kHz on the right and -16 kHz on the left side of the center frequency.

Example 2
What would happen if we go to a 512×512 matrix, that is, with 512 frequency-encoding steps?

(a) We could either have a larger frequency bandwidth:

$$\text{BW} = \frac{1}{\Delta T_s} = \frac{1}{T_s/N}$$
$$= \frac{1}{.008 \text{ sec}/512}$$
$$= 512/.008 \text{ sec} = 64 \text{ kHz} = \pm 32 \text{ kHz}$$

(b) Or, we could double the sampling time and keep the sampling interval (and the bandwidth) the same.

(We'll get into the relationship between the field of view and bandwidth later.)

Key Points

In this chapter, we have presented the basic concepts of signal processing, of which image processing is a subset. As mentioned in the introduction, the understanding of these concepts is crucial in understanding the intricacies of image optimization, which is one of the goals of every imager. Again, memorizing the formulas is not as important as understanding the concepts behind them.

Let's summarize:

1 ADC (analog-to-digital conversion) is the process in which an analog (time-varying) signal is *encoded* to a digital signal (containing a series of binary numbers 0s and 1s) represented as *bytes* (8 *bits*) in the computer.

2 This is done by *sampling* the signal.

3 To be able to reconstruct the original signal from its discrete samples, the *Nyquist law* must be satisfied. Otherwise, *aliasing* will occur.

4 The Nyquist theorem states that the sampling frequency must be at least twice the highest frequency present in the signal.

5 Stated differently, if you take the waveform of the component signal with highest frequency (remember that each signal is a *composite* of many different signals with varying frequencies), then at least *two samples per cycle* are required to avoid aliasing.

6 Therefore, aliasing occurs because of *undersampling*. To ensure that aliasing will not happen, MR scanners may automatically perform *oversampling*.

7 The bandwidth (BW) is defined as the range of frequencies in the signal.

8 $\text{BW} = 1/\Delta T_s$, where ΔT_s is the sampling interval (interval between two samples).

9 At Nyquist frequency, $\text{BW} = 2\omega_{max}$, where ω_{max} is the highest frequency in the signal, so that $\Delta T_s = 1/\text{BW} = 1/(2\omega_{max})$.

10 Sampling time $T_s = N_x \cdot \Delta T_s$, where N_x is the number of frequency encodes.

11 SNR is given by

$$\text{SNR} \propto \text{voxel volume } \sqrt{(N_y \cdot N_x \cdot \text{NEX})/\text{BW}}$$

12 So,

$$\text{SNR is } \uparrow \text{ if BW } \downarrow$$

13 A narrower BW is used when a higher SNR is desired (e.g., on the second echo of a dual-echo SE image).

14 BW is $\downarrow$ if ΔT_s is $\uparrow$ (i.e., less samples are taken), which may cause aliasing!

15 Now, if ΔT_s is $\uparrow$ then $T_s = N_x \cdot \Delta T_s$ is $\uparrow$, which causes TE to $\uparrow$. Because

$$\text{Number of slices} \cong \text{TR/TE}$$

then a narrower BW will reduce the *coverage*.

Questions

12-1 According to the Nyquist theorem, to avoid aliasing:
- **(a)** At most, two samples per cycle corresponding to the highest frequency are required.
- **(b)** At least two samples per cycle corresponding to the highest frequency are required.
- **(c)** At most, two samples per cycle corresponding to the lowest frequency are required.
- **(d)** At least two samples per cycle corresponding to the lowest frequency are required.

12-2 According to the Nyquist theorem, to avoid aliasing:
- **(a)** The sampling frequency must be at least half the highest frequency in the signal.
- **(b)** The sampling frequency must be at least twice the lowest frequency in the signal.
- **(c)** The sampling frequency must be at least twice the highest frequency in the signal.
- **(d)** The sampling frequency must be at least half the lowest frequency in the signal.

12-3 **T/F** The bandwidth (BW) is the inverse of the sampling interval (ΔT_s).

12-4 **T/F** SNR is directly proportional to 1/BW.

12-5 A narrower BW (all other things remaining unchanged) will result in
- **(a)** more SNR
- **(b)** less coverage
- **(c)** longer sampling time
- **(d)** all of the above
- **(e)** only (a) and (b)

12-6 **T/F** Aliasing occurs because of oversampling.

13

Introduction

Before we can understand k-space, we need to discuss the data space, which is a matrix of the processed image data. To most radiologists, k-space is in the twilight zone! We have already seen some of the basic concepts of the data space and k-space in the previous chapters. In this chapter, we will learn some of the properties of k-space in greater detail. The understanding of k-space is crucial to the understanding of some of the newer MRI fast scanning techniques such as fast spin-echo (FSE) and echo planar imaging (EPI).

Where Does k-Space Come From?

k-Space is derived from the data space, so it's really not as intimidating as it initially appears. Figure 13-1 demonstrates a typical representation of the data space with a 256 × 256 matrix.

1. Figure 13-1 is an **"analog"** version of k-space. The true k-space, as we'll see later, is a **digitized** version of this figure, with axes referred to as **spatial frequencies.**
2. In Figure 13-1, we have 256 phase-encoding steps. We keep the zero-step (i.e., no

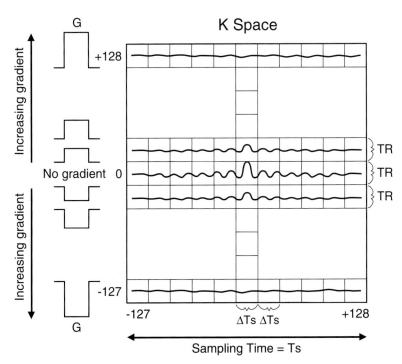

Figure 13-1. The data space (with both axes as time variables) is an "analog" version of k-space.

phase encoding) in the middle of k-space, so we go from -127 phase encode to $+128$ phase encode (bottom to top).

3. We also have 256 frequencies.
4. The y-axis, then, is the phase-encoding direction.
5. In the center, we put the signal acquired with no phase-encoding gradient.
6. As one advances on the y-axis, each set has signal acquired with an increasing phase-encoding gradient with maximum gradient at $+128$ phase-encoding step. Likewise, as one goes down from zero gradient in the y-axis, each step has signal acquired with an increasing phase-encoding gradient in the opposite direction with maximum gradient at -127 phase-encoding step.

Let's now go back and review the spin-echo pulse sequence (Fig. 13-2).

1. We apply the 90° pulse using an appropriate slice-select gradient, G_z.
2. Next, we apply a 180° pulse and, after a time, TE receives an echo.
3. During this time, we apply the readout gradient, G_x.
4. Then we place a *sampled version* of this echo in one of the rows in k-space. Let's say that this echo was obtained without using a phase-encoding gradient in the y direction. We *sample* the signal and then put it into the zero line in the data space.
5. With, say, a 256 × 256 matrix, we take 256 samples. Each of the 256 points in a row of the data space is a *sample* of the echo.

(It's hard to draw discrete samples, so we'll draw continuous signals in the data space rows, realizing that each point in a row is a **digitized sample** of the signal.)

6. For the second row in the data space, we do the exact same thing, except in this step the signal is obtained using a largar phase-encoding gradient in the y-axis.

Remember that the phase-encoding gradient causes **dephasing** of the signal. Therefore, the signal for the second line of the data space will be similar in shape to the first signal (because both are signals from the same slice of tissue, just obtained at a different time) but smaller in **magnitude** than the first signal (because it undergoes additional dephasing due to the phase-encoding gradient). Thus, when we draw this signal into the second line in the data space, we see that it is similar in shape to the first signal, but slightly *weaker*—because it's been *dephased*.

The signal that goes into the last line of the data space ($+128$) will be almost flat because it has undergone maximum dephasing; likewise, as we alternate to the signals placed below the zero line (i.e., $-1, -2, \cdots, -127$), a certain symmetry results. For instance, line (-1) is similar in strength to line $(+1)$ in that, whereas line $(+1)$ experiences mild dephasing due to a slight increase in magnetic field strength, line (-1) experiences similar mild dephasing due to a slight decrease in magnetic field strength. Likewise, the signal that goes into the first line in the data space (-127) will be almost flat due to maximum dephasing in the opposite direction of line $(+128)$.

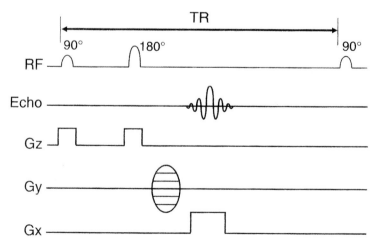

Figure 13-2. A spin-echo pulse sequence diagram.

Remember that each line in the data space contains the signal obtained from the entire image slice during a single TR. Each TR is obtained using a different phase-encoding step in the y-axis.

Question 1: How long does it take to go from one row in the data space to another?

Answer: It takes the time of one TR.

Question 2: How long does it take to go from one point (sample) in a row to the next point (sample) in the same row of the data space?

Answer: It takes the time spent between samples, that is, the sampling interval (ΔT_s).

Question 3: How long does it take to fill one row of the data space?

Answer: Let's say that $\Delta T_s \cong 31\ \mu sec$ and that there are 256 (N) samples along the readout axis. The sampling time is

$$\begin{aligned} T_s &= (\Delta T_s)(N) \\ &= (31\,\mu sec)\,(256) \\ &= 7.9\ msec \end{aligned}$$

Therefore, it takes about 8 msec to fill one line of the data space. In general, it takes

$$T_s = N_x \cdot \Delta T_s$$

to fill one line of the data space.

Question 4: How long does it take to fill one column of the data space?

Answer: It is the acquisition time $N_p \times$ TR, where N_p is the number of phase-encoding steps.

Let's say TR = 3000 msec and N_p = 256.

$$\begin{aligned} \text{Acquisition time} &= (3000\ msec)\,(256) \\ &= 12.8\ min \end{aligned}$$

If TR = 500 msec, then

$$\text{Acquisition time} = (500)\,(256) \cong 2\ min$$

> **It takes several milliseconds to fill one row of the data space. But it takes several minutes to fill the columns of the data space.**

Motion Artifacts

The preceding concept is one of the reasons why motion artifacts manifest themselves mainly in the phase-encoding direction. In other words, it takes much longer to gather the signal in the phase-encoding direction than in the frequency-encoding direction, leaving more time for motion to affect the image in the phase direction. Another reason, as we shall see later, is that motion in any direction results in a phase change; thus, motion artifact propagates along the phase-encoding direction.

Properties of k-Space

Center of k-Space. The center of the data space contains maximum signal. This finding is caused by two factors:

1. Each of the signals has its maximum signal amplitude in the center column (Fig. 13-3). Recall that when we apply the 180° refocusing pulse, the dephased signal begins to rephase and reaches maximum amplitude when the protons are completely rephased. It then decreases in amplitude as the protons dephase once more.

   The middle column in the data space corresponds to the center of each individual echo, and the more peripheral columns refer to the more peripheral segments of the echoes: columns to the left of center depict rephasing of the echoes toward maximal amplitude in the data space; columns to the right of center depict dephasing of the echoes away from maximal amplitude in the data space.

   Therefore, as we go further out to the more peripheral columns, the signal weakens. The most peripheral points in the signal to the left are the weakest point of the signal as the signal just begins to rephase (Fig. 13-3). Likewise, the most peripheral point in the signal to the right is the weakest point after the signal has been refocused and then has regained maximum dephasing.

2. The maximum amplitude occurs in the center row because this line is obtained without additional dephasing due to phase-encoding gradients; subsequent rows with progressively larger phase-encoding gradients have weaker signal amplitude.

Therefore, because the middle row has the strongest of all echoes and the middle column contains all the peaks of the echoes, the center

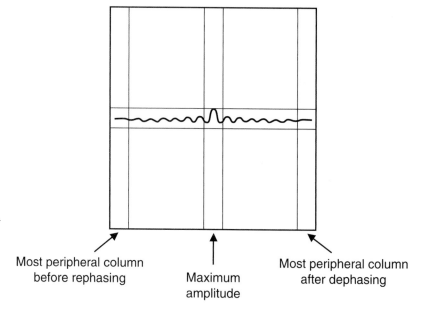

Figure 13-3. The peripheral points in the signal have the weakest amplitude; the center point has the maximal amplitude.

Most peripheral column before rephasing

Maximum amplitude

Most peripheral column after dephasing

point of the data space contains maximum amplitude, that is, maximum signal-to-noise ratio (SNR) (Fig. 13-4).

As we go farther out to the periphery in both directions, the signal weakens:

1. In the y direction because of progressively larger phase-encoding steps
2. In the x direction because the echo signal has either not yet reached maximum

amplitude or is losing maximum amplitude due to dephasing

Image of k-Space. Because of the *oscillating* nature of the signals, the image of the data space (and, thus, k-space) will appear as a series of concentric rings of signal intensity with alternating bands of high and low intensity as the signal oscillates from maximum to minimum, but an

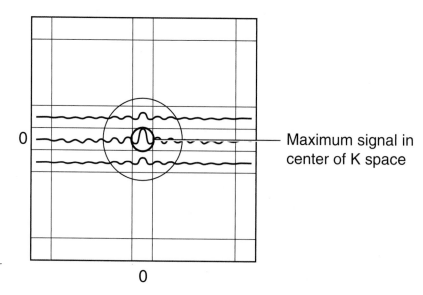

0

Maximum signal in center of K space

Figure 13-4. The center of k-space always contains maximum signal.

0

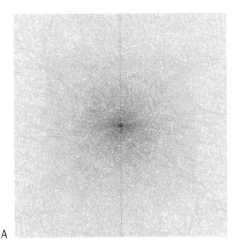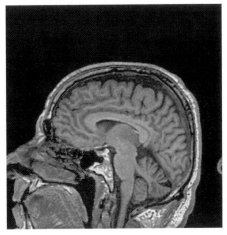

A   B

Figure 13-5. A: The original raw data (k-space) of **(B)** the original image (midline sagittal T1-weighted image of the brain).

overall decrease in intensity as one goes from the center to periphery (Fig. 13-5A). So, the white and dark rings in k-space correspond to the peaks and valleys of the echoes, respectively. The original raw data (k-space) and the original image are shown in Figure 13-5.

Edges of k-Space. You might be thinking that if the center of k-space contains the maximum signal, why not eliminate the periphery of the signal and just make an image from the central high signal intensity data (Figs. 13-4 and 13-6A)? We can actually make an image with this data, but

the edges of the structures imaged will be very coarse (Fig. 13-6B). The periphery of k-space contributes to the *fine detail* of the image. Let's see how this happens.

Question: What type of information is available in the periphery of k-space?

Answer: The periphery of k-space provides information regarding "fineness" of the image and clarity at sharp interfaces.

Recall the following Fourier transforms of a *sinc* wave and its truncated version from an earlier chapter (Fig. 13-7). As you can see, by truncating

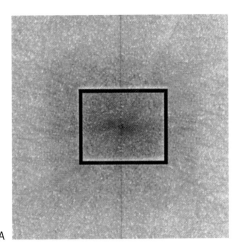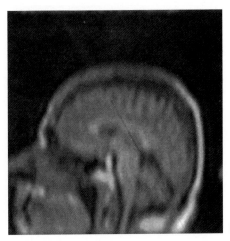

A   B

Figure 13-6. A: k-Space. **B:** The image constructed from only the center of k-space. The details are reduced due to exclusion of peripheral points in k-space.

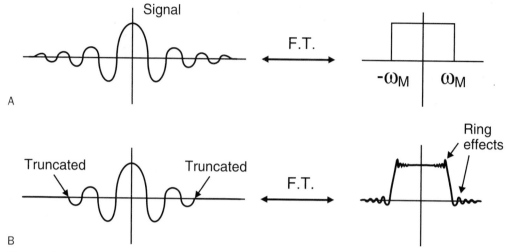

Figure 13-7. **A:** The FT of an ideal sinc function is a rectangle. **B:** The FT of a truncated sinc function has ring down effects.

the signal (echo), ring artifacts are introduced in the Fourier transform. Therefore, by eliminating the samples in the periphery of the data space, the sharp interfaces in the image are degraded and the image gets coarser. In other words, the *fine detail* of the image is compromised when the edges of k-space are excluded. Figure 13-8B is the image corresponding to the periphery of k-space (Fig. 13-8A).

Image Construction. We can take a single line in k-space and make a whole image. It wouldn't be a very pretty image, but it would still

contain all the information necessary to construct an image of the slice.

> There is absolutely no direct relationship between the center of k-space and the center of the image. Likewise, there is no direct relationship between the edges of k-space and the edges of the image.

A point at the very edge of k-space contributes to the entire image. It doesn't contribute as much to the image in terms of the SNR as does a point

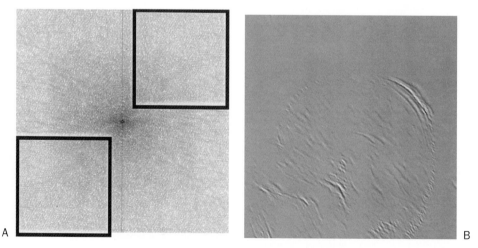

Figure 13-8. **A:** k-Space. **B:** The image constructed from only the periphery of k-space. This image has minimal signal but contains details about the interfaces in the original image.

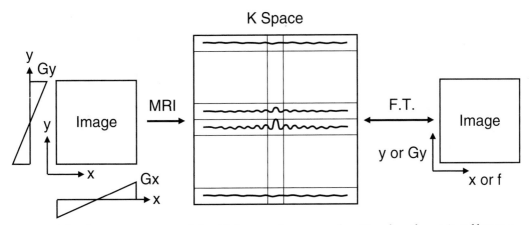

Figure 13-9. There is a one-to-one relationship between frequency and position along the x-axis and between phase-encoding gradient increment and position along the y direction.

in the center of k-space because the center of k-space has maximum signal, but the peripheral points still contribute to the clarity and fineness of the image.

Once we have all the data in k-space, we take the Fourier transform of k-space to get the image.

Question 1: Why is the Fourier transform of k-space the desired image?

Answer: Because there is a one-to-one relationship between frequency and position in the x direction and between phase-encoding gradient strength[1] and position in the y direction.

Question 2: Why is there a one-to-one relationship between frequency and position?

Answer: Because, in our method of spatial encoding, we picked a linear gradient in the x direction that correlated sequential frequency increments with position; likewise, we picked a linear gradient in the y direction that correlated sequential phase gradient increments with position in the y direction (Fig. 13-9).

Thus, the center of the field of view of the image experiences no frequency gradient and no phase gradient, and the points in the periphery of the image experience the highest frequency and phase gradients. In other words, there is a 1:1 relationship between frequency and position in the image.

In summary, the frequency- and phase-encoding gradients provide the position of a signal in space. They tell us which pixels each component of the signal goes into in the slice under study.

Question: How are the shades of gray determined?

Answer: The shades of gray are determined by the **magnitude** or **amplitude** of the signal (actually its Fourier transform) at each pixel.

Recall that the image of k-space looks like a series of concentric circles of alternating intensity on a two-dimensional surface. If we now incorporate *amplitude* as a third dimension, we would have the areas of greater amplitude coming off the surface of k-space toward us like a "warped" image (Fig. 13-10).

k-Space Symmetry. One step needs to be completed after receiving the signal and before placing it in k-space that we have so far ignored. This step is called **phase-sensitive detection.** We want to take the echo signal, which is on a **carrier frequency,** shift it to zero frequency, and divide the signal into its real (*cosine*) and imaginary (*sine*) components.

First, we start off with the signal that is being frequency- and phase-shifted around a carrier frequency of 64 MHz for a 1.5-T magnet. However, it's hard to tell whether a signal has been frequency- or phase-shifted unless we "ground" the signal back to "zero."

---

[1]The one to oneness in the y direction is related to the phase-encoding gradient strength—and not just the phase. This is because the rows in data space are differentiated by different phase-encoding gradient strengths G_y.

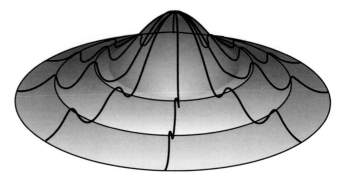

Figure 13-10. A three-dimensional line drawing of k-space.

Therefore, we first subtract the carrier frequency of 64 MHz from the signal (Fig. 13-11). We first take the signal and subtract a *cosine* wave of center frequency ω_0 from the signal. Then we take the signal and, in a separate computation, subtract the *sine* wave of center frequency ω_0 from the signal.

If we subtract ω_0 from the signal, we center the signal at zero (in the frequency domain). We then have a resultant signal whose center frequency is 0. Perform this step twice to separate the signal into its real component (*cosine*) and its imaginary component (*sine*).

Each data space has two components:

1. The data space with "real" (*cosine*) data: the signal that has (cos $\omega_0 t$) subtracted from it and brought back to 0 frequency.

2. The data space with "imaginary" (*sine*) data: the signal that has (sin $\omega_0 t$) subtracted from it and brought back to 0 frequency.

We now have two data spaces (Fig. 13-12): one with *cosine* data (real); one with *sine* data (imaginary). Both have data centered at 0 frequency. In the data space with *cosine* data, we know that a great deal of symmetry exists. A cosine function is an example of an **even** function. If we look at a *cosine* function, we see that there is symmetry to the right and left of zero. In addition, there is symmetry above and below zero. Thus, if we put a pixel in a line of the data space to the right of the 0 column, and above the 0 line (point *a*), the symmetry of the *cosine* function would make us unable to discriminate between the other (*a*) positions. The computer

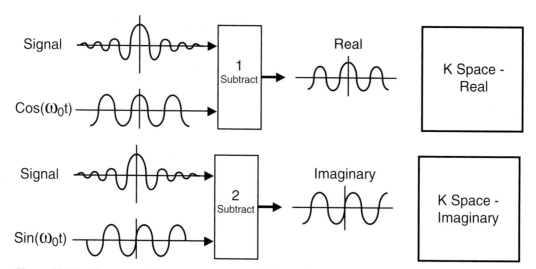

Figure 13-11. The process of image construction includes a preliminary decomposition of signal into its real and imaginary components. This in turn yields a real and an imaginary k-space, that is, a real and an imaginary image.

K space - Real (cos)   K space - Imaginary (sin)

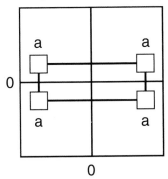
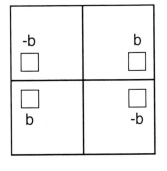

A   0

B

Figure 13-12. A, B: Spatial direction in k-space. The imaginary k-space provides a series of left–right or up–down directions.

couldn't tell the difference between any of the four pixel positions. This is why we use the *sine* version of the data space.

Now look at the data space with the *sine* data (Fig. 13-12B). Again, the pixel is in the same place as the *cosine* data space; it is in a line of the data space above the 0 line and to the right of the 0 column. However (unlike the *cosine* data space), here we can distinguish it from the pixel below the 0 line ($-b$). We can also differentiate it from the pixel to the left of the 0 column ($-b$).

Why are these pixels different in the *sine* data space? Let's review the *sine* function ($sin\ \omega_0 t$) of the two pixels to the right of the 0 frequency (Fig. 13-13A). The *sine* function is an example of an **odd** function because of its inherent antisymmetry. The *sine* function changes polarity above and below the 0 line. This allows us to differentiate the two pixels.

Now, let's examine the *sine* function ($sin\ \omega_0 t$) above the zero line of the data space (Fig. 13-13B). Again, because of inherent antisymmetry of the *sine* function on either side of the 0 frequency, the pixels will have opposite polarity.

Complex Numbers

We said in Chapter 1 that a complex number can be divided into its real (*cosine*) and imaginary (*sine*) parts. If we consider the *cosine* function as the real component and the *sine* function as the imaginary component, then we can add the *sine* and *cosine* together to get the **magnitude** of the signal as well as its **direction.**

So now let's add up the data of the 4 pixels (Fig. 13-14). Because of the changing polarity of the *sine* function, when we add the *sine* function to the *cosine* function, we can distinguish the *direction* of the four pixels (whereas with *cosine* function alone, we couldn't tell the direction).

In the lines above 0 phase encoding:

Pixel $a - ib$ is to the left of the 0 frequency.

Pixel $a + ib$ is to the right of the 0 frequency.

In the lines below 0 phase encoding:

Pixel $a + ib$ is to the left of the 0 frequency.

Pixel $a - ib$ is to the right of the 0 frequency.

Conjugate (Hermitian) Symmetry. The **conjugate** of a complex number $a + ib$ is the complex number $a - ib$ (i.e., with the same real component but a negative imaginary component). From this and from Figure 13-14, it is clear that **k-space possesses conjugate symmetry,** also known as **Hermitian symmetry.**

Half NEX (½ NEX). In a "½ NEX"[2] technique (half-Fourier in phase), we acquire the data from the upper half of k-space and construct the lower part mathematically (Fig. 13-15), thus reducing the scan time. The trade-off is a reduced SNR by a factor of $\sqrt{2}$, to be exact (see Chapter 17). Due to the presence of phase errors in the data, the symmetry previously discussed may not be perfect. This is why when employing such techniques, a few extra rows in the center of k-space—which contains maximum signal—are always added to

---

[2] ½ NEX is a misnomer because we are really halving the number of phase-encoding steps, not the NEX.

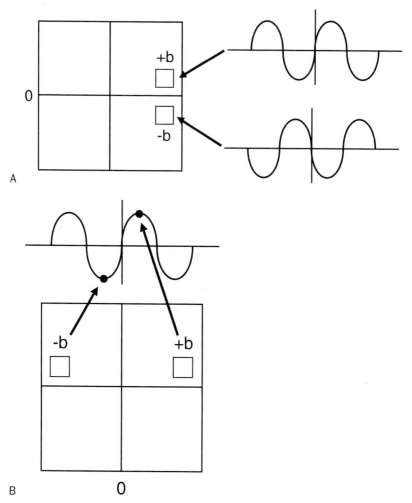

Figure 13-13. **A:** Because the phase gradients corresponding to the top and bottom half of k-space generally have opposite polarities, the values in the corresponding imaginary k-space also will have opposite polarities. **B:** Because the sine function is an odd function, the left half of the signal is the reverse of the right half; thus the corresponding points in the imaginary k-space will also have opposite signs.

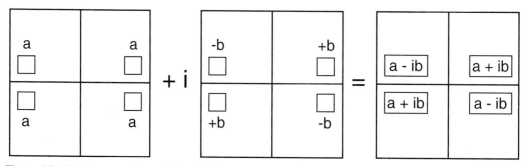

Figure 13-14. k-Space conjugate (Hermitian) symmetry can be seen by adding the real and imaginary components of four corresponding data points. Notice the conjugate symmetry between left and right and between top and bottom.

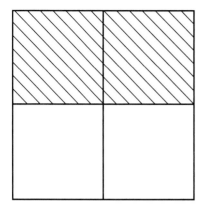

Figure 13-15. In half (or fractional) NEX, only half (or a fraction of) of the rows in k-space (plus a few extra central rows) are used, and the rest is constructed by symmetry.

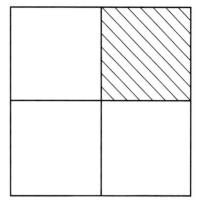

Figure 13-17. Due to conjugate symmetry of k-space, *theoretically* you should be able to reconstruct the entire k-space from just one of its quadrants. In reality, however, this may create excessive phase errors due to actual imperfections in data symmetry.

allow for such phase corrections. That is, slightly more than 50% of k-space must be sampled to maintain phase information.

Fractional Echo. In **fractional echo,** only the right half of the echo is sampled, and the left half is constructed based on the right half (Fig. 13-16). (This allows TE to be shorter for fast scanning techniques like turbo FLASH and Fast SPGR—see Chapter 21.)

¼ NEX. Because of the *conjugate symmetry* discussed previously, *theoretically* you should be able to create an image using only one *quadrant* of the combined real and imaginary data spaces (Fig. 13-17). That is, you should be able to construct the entire k-space data from only one

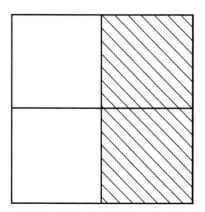

Figure 13-16. In fractional echo, only a fraction of the echo is sampled.

quadrant. In reality, however, due to the presence of data acquisition errors, perfect symmetry does not exist and doing so may lead to phase errors and image distortion, which is probably why this technique is not being used.

Real and Imaginary Images. We discussed two components of the data space, namely, the real and imaginary components. Their respective Fourier transforms provide the real and imaginary components of the image (Fig. 13-18).

Magnitude (Modulus) and Phase Image. Recall that given a complex number $c = a + ib$, with a being the real and b the imaginary component, the phase (angle) is given by $\tan \theta = b/a$ and the magnitude by $\sqrt{(a^2 + b^2)}$.

This concept can be applied to the real and imaginary components of the image (Fig. 13-18) to generate the **magnitude and phase images** (Fig. 13-18).

The **magnitude image (modulus)** is what we deal with most of the time in MRI. The **phase image** is used in cases in which the *direction* is important. An example is phase contrast MR angiography, in which the phase indicates the direction of flow, i.e., up versus down, anterior versus posterior, or left versus right. In summary, tangent (phase angle) = (imaginary/real), or phase angle = arctan (imaginary/real), and

$$modulus = \sqrt{(real)^2 + (imaginary)^2}$$

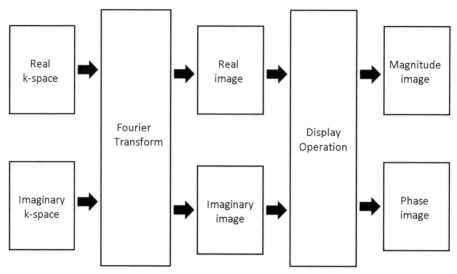

Figure 13-18. The FTs of the real and imaginary k-spaces provide the real and imaginary images, respectively. The real and imaginary images are used to create magnitude and phase images.

In actuality, when we do ½ NEX, we sample half of the phase-encoding steps plus a few lines above or below the 0 line. We can then compensate for phase errors and determine the actual phase. This is referred to as **overscanning.**

Ideally, we want to have a *real* image with the *imaginary* part being *zero,* and thus a zero phase. In reality, however, we have all sorts of motion artifacts and gradient errors that create phase artifacts. Therefore, in reality, phase is never zero. Sometimes, when service engineers try to debug a system, they will sometimes look at the phase image to figure out the problem.

We too can look at the phase image. In flow imaging, the phase image is a *velocity image* and indicates magnitude and direction. For example, in imaging the cerebrospinal fluid (CSF) flow through the aqueduct, flow in the *ante-grade* direction could be *black,* and flow in the *retrograde* direction could be *white* on the phase images. Thus, phase images in phase-contrast studies display the *direction* of flow (Fig. 13-19).

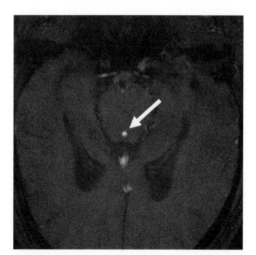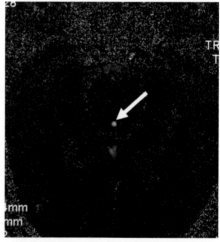

Figure 13-19. Magnitude image (**A**) and phase image (**B**) from a CSF flow study in a patient with normal pressure hydrocephalus. Notice the bright signal in the aqueduct of Sylvius (*arrows*) with image **B** reflective of flow direction in this instance superior to inferior flow.

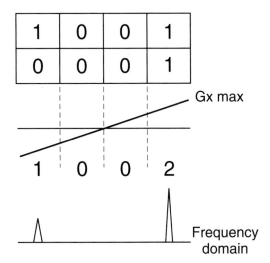

Figure 13-20. An example of a 2 × 4 matrix exposed to a frequency gradient and no phase gradient.

Because the phase is never zero, we can combine the "real" image and the "imaginary" image to get a composite image, which is the image that we look at when we read an MR study. The **modulus** is the image we look at; it combines the data corresponding to the Fourier transform of the real and imaginary data spaces:

image = modulus

$$= \sqrt{(\text{real image})^2 + (\text{imaginary image})^2}$$

k-Space: An Example. The following is an example of a 2 × 4 matrix:

1	0	0	1
0	0	0	1

The number of frequency-encoding steps = $N_x = 4$.

The number of phase-encoding steps = $N_y = 2$.

We will give magnitudes of either 1 or 0 to each pixel, so that:

A pixel with a magnitude = 1 will be white.

A pixel with a magnitude = 0 will be black.

In the first phase-encoding step, with no gradient in the y direction, we apply a frequency-encoding gradient in the x direction, which allows us to distinguish the columns. What we get then is a sum of pixels in each column, without knowing from which row the components of the sum originated (Fig. 13-20).

Remember that the Fourier transform can differentiate between different columns because each column has a different frequency. The Fourier transform of the signal will have two frequency spikes, with column 1 having an amplitude of 1 + 0 = 1, and column 4 having an amplitude of 1 + 1 = 2. Thus, applying the readout gradient allows us to differentiate between different columns. However, we still haven't differentiated between different rows. For instance, the amplitude = 2 in column 4 could be

1 + 1 or 0 + 2 or 2 + 0

With the single phase-encoding step, we have no idea how the sum of the amplitudes is decomposed to provide the amplitude of individual elements in each column. Remember that this first set of data was obtained with no gradient in the phase-encoding (y) direction.

The first phase-encoding step was at zero value of the phase-encoding gradient. For the next phase-encoding step, let's apply a gradient. The gradient will be 360° divided by 2, or 180°. This means that the first row will experience no gradient, and the second row will experience a gradient such that the spins will be 180° out of phase with

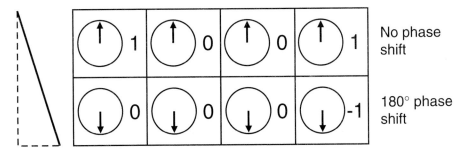

Figure 13-21. The same example exposed to phase encoding. The first row has no phase shift. The second row has a 180° phase shift (thus changing the sign of the pixel values).

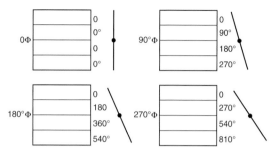

Figure 13-22. An example of a 4 × 4 matrix. The phase increments here are 0°, 90°, 180°, and 270°. (In general, the phase increment is $360°/N_y$, where N_y is the number of phase-encoding steps.)

the first row. This will result in no change in the numbers of the first row. But the numbers in the second row will be 180° phase shifted (i.e., they will be the negative of the original numbers).

1	0	0	1
0	0	0	−1

If we use the clock analogy to evaluate phase shift, the spins in the top row, experiencing no phase shift, will all point upward. The spins in the second row (which is experiencing a 180° phase shift) will all be pointing downward (Fig. 13-21).

Thus, whereas the values in the first row will remain unchanged, the values in the second row will be 180° reversed from what they were with no phase shift.

Row 1

1	0	0	1

Row 2 before 180° phase shift

0	0	0	1

Row 2 after 180° phase shift

0	0	0	−1

ASIDE: If we were to have four rows with four phase-encoding steps, the steps would be: 0, 90°, 180°, and 270° phase difference between rows, experiencing a steeper gradient with every successive TR (Fig. 13-22). In our study, with only two rows, we can only have two phase-encoding steps:

1. Zero phase difference (no gradient) between rows.
2. With 180° phase difference, where one row experiences no phase difference and the second row experiences a 180° phase shift from the first row.

This division of phase-encoding steps into equal divisions of 360° all relates to the cosine wave (Fig. 13-23). Therefore, for a phase difference

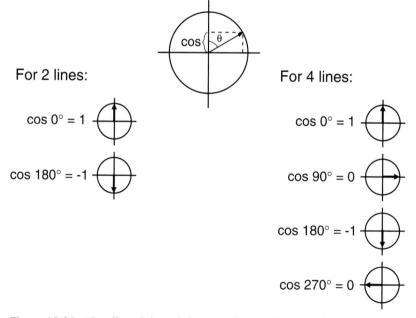

Figure 13-23. The effect of phase shifts on pixel values for two and four rows.

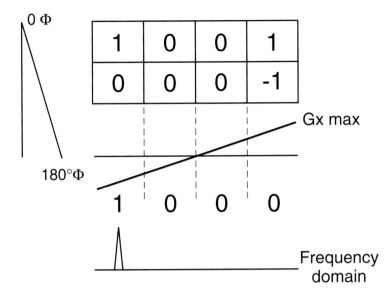

Figure 13-24. The previous 2 × 4 example now exposed to a frequency gradient and a phase gradient (i.e., 180° phase shift).

of 180°, we get the negative value of the original number because cos 180° = −1. For a different phase angle, we would get a fraction of the original value (from 0 to 1, or from 0 to −1, whatever cos θ is).

With this phase-encoding step, let's see what the Fourier transform would be in the frequency-encoding direction (Fig. 13-24). The amplitude in columns 1 to 3 remains unchanged from the 0 phase readings. However, there is a change in the amplitude of column 4:

With zero phase, column 4 adds up to +2 (because 1 + 1 = 2).

With 180° phase, column 4 adds up to 0 (because 1 − 1 = 0).

With the change in phase, the second column is the sum of (+1) and (−1), which is equal to 0. We still don't know what the original value of each pixel was, but we do have a different total value in the Fourier transform of this second line in k-space when we compare it with the first line.

Now, let's do a little mathematics. The following is like solving two equations with two unknowns; solve for a, b, c, and d below:

1	0	0	1
0	0	0	1

0° phase

1	0	0	1
0	0	0	−1

180° phase

a	0	0	c
b	0	0	d

a	0	0	c
−b	0	0	−d

Let's look back at the pixel values in the phase = 0 line and

1. Designate the pixels in the first column (a and b).
2. Designate the pixels in the fourth column (c and d).

Now look at the pixel values in the 180° phase line, and

1. Designate the pixels in the first column (a and −b).
   Note that pixel (a) remains the same as 0 phase line because neither experiences any phase change, but pixel (−b) is negative because it experiences a 180° phase shift compared with pixel (b) in 0 phase line.
2. Designate the pixels in column four as (c and −d).
   Again note that pixel (c) remains the same as 0 phase line because neither experiences any phase change. However, pixel (−d) is negative because it experiences a 180° phase shift compared with pixel (d) in phase = 0 line.

First equations:
$$a + b = 1$$
$$a - b = 1$$

Second equations:
$$c + d = 2$$
$$c - d = 0$$

Add $2a = 2$ Add $2c = 2$

$a = 1$ $c = 1$

$b = 0$ $d = 1$

By using the Fourier transforms of the two lines in k-space, we can determine the amplitude values of each pixel in each column. This is the concept of the **(digital) Fourier Transform (DFT).**

What is k-space in this example? Let's go back to Figure 13-20. The first line in the data space corresponds to the sum of all the signals obtained with 0 phase. With the gradient in the x direction (G_x) causing different phase angles between the columns, the signal will consist of

1. (*cos* of column 1 frequency) with (magnitude = 1), for example, 1 cos t
2. (*cos* of column 4 frequency) with (magnitude = 2), for example, 2 cos $4t$

The sum of these signals will be the signal in the first line of the data space (in this case, cos t + 2 cos $4t$) in time domain. Then the signal is sampled (four times in our example).

The second time around, the second line in the data space corresponding to the 180° phase shift will give us:

1. (*cos* of column 1 frequency) with (magnitude = 1), for example, 1 cos t
2. (*cos* of column 4 frequency) with (magnitude = 0), for example, 0 cos $4t$, which is 0

Thus, we get a different signal in the time domain for the second line in the data space. Then this signal is sampled. Remember that no direct relationship exists between a point in the data space and the same point on the image.

The Fourier transform of the data space contains the four frequencies corresponding to the four samples taken during signal readout using the G_x gradient for frequency encoding. The *magnitude* (amplitude) of the frequencies correlates with the *brightness* on the image. In the x direction, a 1:1 relationship exists between frequency and position on the image. The ampli-

tude at a certain frequency corresponds to the brightness at the corresponding pixel position. In the y direction, a 1:1 relationship exists between the position y and the *phase increment* $\Delta\phi$ (which is related to the gradient strength G_y).

To create the image, we perform a second Fourier transform on the data space. This step is just an additional mathematical step.

Question: How many calculations are necessary to solve the set of equations derived from k-space to create the image (i.e., the number of calculations to solve the DFT)?

Answer: In our example of two rows of k-space with four samples in each row, we had two equations per sample and four samples. So:

$$2 \times 4 = \text{number of calculations}$$

In general, with an N × N matrix, the number of calculations = N × N = N².

Example

In a 256 × 256 matrix:

$256^2 = 2^{16}$ **calculations needed for DFT**

Fast Fourier Transform (FFT)

Fast Fourier transform (FFT) is a signal processing transformation, similar to Fourier transform that solves a DFT in a faster way. The number of calculations for FFT is

$$\text{Number of calculations} = (N)(\log_2 N)$$

Example

For a 256 × 256 matrix:

$$256 \times \log_2 256 = (256)(8)$$

Because 8 is 1/32 of 256, we have cut down the number of calculations by a factor of 32. For $(\log_2 N)$ to be a whole number, the number of frequency-encoding steps has to be a power of 2. This is why frequency-encoding steps are always a power of 2 (i.e., 2^N such as 2, 4, 8, 16, 32, 64, 128, 256, and 512), usually 128, 256, or 512, whenever FFT is used.

Key Points

We have introduced the often intimidating topic of k-space. k-Space can initially be thought of as the "data space" (which can be thought of as an "analog" k-space), with each line in it representing a sampled version of the received signal (the echo). In the data space, the coordinates are in time. (Horizontal scale is on the order of the sampling interval and the vertical scale is on the order of TR.) The Fourier transform of k-space is the desired image.

There is, however, one more step that comes after obtaining the data space and before construction of the true k-space, having to do with the concept of "spatial frequencies," which we shall discuss in Chapter 16.

Questions

13-1 T/F The number of rows in the data space equals the number of phase-encoding steps.

13-2 T/F Each row of data space corresponds to one frequency-encoding gradient strength.

13-3 T/F The center of data space contains maximum signal.

13-4 T/F Each row of data space contains one of the received signals (echoes).

13-5 T/F The axes of the data space are in the time domain.

13-6 T/F There is a direct relationship between the center of the k-space and the center of the image.

13-7 T/F The right half of the data (or k) space is the mirror image of the left half.

13-8 T/F The center of the data space is directly related to the center of the image.

Pulse Sequence Diagram

"A pulse sequence diagram is to an MR scientist as sheet music is to a musician."

Introduction

A **pulse sequence diagram (PSD)** illustrates the sequence of events that occur during magnetic resonance imaging (MRI). It is a timing diagram showing the radio frequency (RF) pulses, gradients, and echoes. Having a good knowledge of the PSD will help the reader follow complicated pulse sequences with more ease and understand the interplay among various scan parameters.

PSD of an SE Sequence

Having been exposed to the concept of gradients, we are now able to illustrate a complete PSD for, say, a spin-echo (SE) sequence (Fig. 14-1).

Everything in the figure looks like what we have discussed before except for a few adjustments in

1. Slice-select gradient (G_z)
2. Frequency-encoding gradient (G_x)
   1a. Once the slice-select gradient (G_z) is applied, then a gradient in the negative direction is introduced in order to *refocus* the spins (Fig. 14-2). Basically, every time we apply a gradient, we dephase the spins. In the case of the G_z gradient, we dephase the spins in order to select a slice. But after the slice is selected, we need to reverse the effect. The purpose of the *refocusing* gradient is to rephase the spins in the slice-select direction. (Alternatively, we can defocus the spins *prior* to slice selection so that

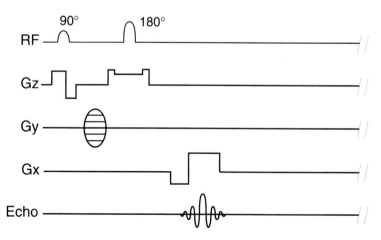

Figure 14-1. A spin-echo PSD.

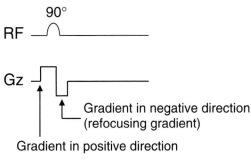

Figure 14-2. The slice-select gradient G_z is followed by a negative lobe to refocus the spins.

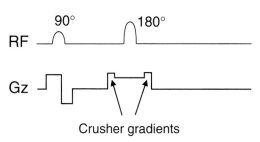

Figure 14-3. Crusher gradients are applied at each side of the slice-selective gradient (applied during the 180° pulse) to achieve more accurate refocusing at time TE.

they come back into phase with the *second* gradient pulse.)

1b. When the 180° pulse is applied, a slice-select gradient may or may not be applied. This is *optional* and depends on whether a single slice or multiple slices are being acquired. But before and after the 180° pulse, we apply a so-called **crusher** gradient so that the 180° pulse has a tri-lobed shape (Fig. 14-3). This is just a triviality. When the 180° pulse is applied, it may have elements that are not exactly 180° leading to unwanted additional transverse magnetization. This may result in the echo not focusing at time TE, as we would expect. So these "crusher" gradients are applied to *offset* that error. (The first lobe is used to balance the third; the second is slice selective; the third destroys the free induction decay [FID] from the unwanted transverse magnetization.)

2. There is an important adjustment in the readout gradient (G_x). If we just apply a gradient while we're reading out the echo, we end up dephasing everything (Fig. 14-4). By the time we get to the middle of the signal, the signal intensity will be decreased because of the dephasing caused by the gradient, and

by the time we get to the end of the signal, there will be maximum dephasing and so much signal loss that there may not be any signal to read!

So we apply a gradient in the negative direction that has an area equal to 1/2 of that of the readout gradient (Fig. 14-5). The length of the readout gradient is the sampling time (T_s). For *stationary spins,* application of a gradient will make the spins go faster and faster and, as they go faster, they'll get out of phase. With the negative gradient, the stationary spins will have a maximum phase difference at the end of the negative gradient. As the gradient is reversed and a gradient in the positive direction is applied, the spins will *rephase* once again. This occurs right at the midpoint of the readout, that is, at time TE. Subsequently, they'll go out of phase again. We can see that at time TE everything is refocused (Fig. 14-5).

If we didn't have the negative gradient lobe, the spins would begin to dephase when the gradient is turned on, and at time TE there would be an undesirable *phase difference*. Phase difference means a smaller signal (Fig. 14-6).

Sometimes, we'll see the notation for the extra G_x gradient illustrated differently (Fig. 14-7). It will be shown as a positive gradient rather than a negative gradient (as we just discussed). You

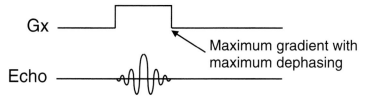

Figure 14-4. If only a constant gradient G_x is applied during readout, we end up dephasing all the spins.

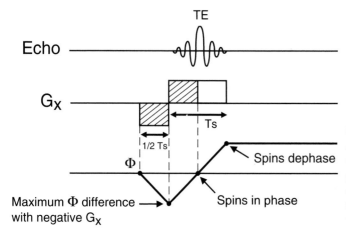

Figure 14-5. Prior to the application of the readout gradient, a negative gradient is applied, resulting in a tri-lobed gradient. The negative lobe causes the spins to get out of phase. Then the spins get back in phase in the center of the echo.

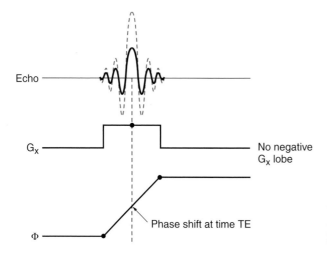

Figure 14-6. In the absence of a tri-lobed G_x, the spins will accumulate a phase in the center of the echo, thus yielding less signal. The dashed line is our desired signal waveform.

might wonder that if the pre-readout G_x gradient is positive, aren't we going to create *more* phase difference with an additional positive lobe?

The answer lies in the fact that in Figure 14-7 the positive pre-readout G_x gradient comes *before* the 180° refocusing pulse. After the G_x pre-readout gradient, we'll have a positive phase difference. This phase difference will stay constant until the 180° pulse is applied (Fig. 14-8).

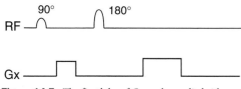

Figure 14-7. The first lobe of G_x can be applied either after the 180° as a negative lobe (as in previous figures) or as a positive lobe prior to the 180° pulse.

After the 180° RF pulse is applied, the phase difference will be reversed. Then it will remain constant until the G_x gradient is applied. Then, the spins will begin going back in phase, reaching a zero phase difference at time TE, and going out of phase afterwards. So, we get the same thing with both the positive and negative pre-readout G_x gradients, depending on where in the pulse sequence the gradient is applied.

Acquisition Time

In previous chapters, we talked about multislice imaging and we said that there was a lot of "dead" time between the end of the echo and the next 90° RF pulse (Fig. 14-9). We can use this "dead" time to our advantage to process other slices.

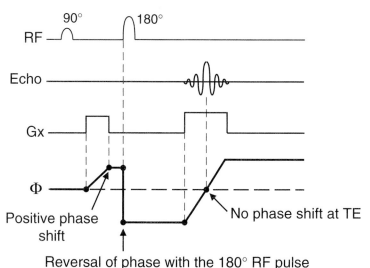

Figure 14-8. This diagram demonstrates how the spins get back in phase at the center of the echo when an additional refocusing positive gradient is applied prior to the 180° pulse.

Question 1: If we manage to fit in all the slices we want within the dead time, what will the acquisition time for the study be?

Answer: It takes TR seconds to fill one line in the data space. Thus, the acquisition time, which is the time it takes to fill the entire data space, is TR times the number of lines in the data space.

Question 2: How many lines (rows) do we have in the data (or k) space?

Answer: The number of lines in k-space equals the number of phase-encoding steps N_p or N_y.

Question 3: Does it help to repeat the sequence all over again?

Answer: We can repeat the whole sequence over again (or repeat each phase-encoding step over again) to average out the noise and increase the signal-to-noise ratio (SNR).

Each cycle is called an **excitation.** The term **NEX** stands for the **N**umber of **EX**citations (also known as **NSA**—**N**umber of **S**ignal **A**verages). So the acquisition time depends on

1. TR (the time to do one line of the data space)
2. N_y (the number of phase-encoding steps)
3. NEX (the number of times we repeat the whole sequence)

$$\text{Acquisition time} = (\text{TR})(N_y)(\text{NEX})$$

This formula is for a conventional SE sequence. Notice that the number of slices doesn't even enter the equation. This is somewhat counterintuitive if one is used to the principles of scan time in CT because, in CT, the more slices we obtain, the longer the sequence will be. This is not necessarily true in MR because of the fact that we can do multiple slices within the time of

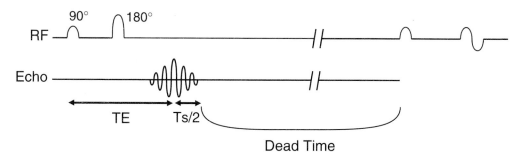

Figure 14-9. There always is a "dead" time between the completion of readout and the next 90° pulse. This dead time can be taken advantage of to acquire other slices.

one TR. Obviously, though, if we decrease the TR, we decrease the number of slices we're able to obtain. So the number of slices is *indirectly* determined by the TR parameter.

Let's say that we want to do a T1-weighted study with a fairly wide coverage. Increasing the TR to allow more slices per TR might be counterproductive because T1 weighting will be reduced. Thus, there is a *trade-off* between increasing coverage and achieving more T1 weighting.

Example 1

$$TR = 1000 \text{ msec}, N_y = 256, NEX = 1$$

$$\text{Acquisition time} = (TR)(N_y)(NEX)$$

$$= (1000 \text{ msec})(256)(1)$$

$$= 256 \text{ sec} \cong 4.27 \text{ min}$$

Let's say that we fit 10 slices in the TR. Then we could obtain the 10 slices in 4.27 min.

Example 2

If, on the other hand, we were only to obtain one slice per TR at a time, we would have to repeat the sequence 10 times to obtain 10 slices, and then the scan time would instead be

$$(10)(1000 \text{ msec})(256)(1 \text{ NEX}) \cong 10 \times 4.27 \text{ min}$$

$$= 42.7 \text{ min}$$

which is, obviously, impractical.

Key Points

We have discussed the topic of pulse sequence diagram (PSD) and illustrated one example for SE imaging. In the chapters to come, we will see examples of more complicated PSDs. Of course, the PSD does not tell us all the parameters used in MR imaging, such as the field of view (discussed in the next chapter), but it offers an algorithm or prescription for performing the study.

Questions

14-1 The acquisition time depends on which of the following? (one or more)

    (a) TR   **(b)** TE   **(c)** N_x

    (d) N_y **(e)** NEX

14-2 **(a)** Calculate the acquisition time for a multiacquisition SE sequence with TR = 2000, NEX = 2, N_y = 128.

    (b) Repeat (a) for single slice acquisition of 10 slices. Is this practical?

14-3 The number of rows in the k-space equals

    (a) N_x **(b)** N_y **(c)** NEX

    (d) N_z **(e)** TR

Introduction

A pulse sequence diagram (PSD) provides a timing algorithm for the sequence of events that is carried out during an MR study. However, the operator must specify the dimensions of the desired part of the body under study. This is the subject of this chapter, namely, the field of view (FOV). As we shall see shortly, there is a limitation as to how small we can make the FOV, depending on the maximum strength of the gradients and the bandwidth of the received signals.

Field of View (FOV)

We're going to discuss the relationship between the following entities:

1. FOV
2. Bandwidth
3. Gradients

Understanding these concepts is important because these features have definite clinical applications.

Let's take an image with its x and y axes (Fig. 15-1). There is an FOV along the x-axis. Normally, we apply a gradient that increases as we move in the x direction (G_x). This means that we create magnetic inhomogeneities along the x-axis in a *linear* fashion. Consequently,

1. At the center point of the FOV, the magnetic field will be $\mathbf{B}_0$.
2. On the right side of the FOV, the magnetic field will be greater than $\mathbf{B}_0$.

3. On the left side of the FOV, the magnetic field will be less than $\mathbf{B}_0$.

The magnetic field along the x-axis is $\mathbf{B}_x$. The value of $\mathbf{B}_x$ is given by the linear equation:

$$\mathbf{B}_x = (G_x)x$$

This equation shows that the value of the magnetic field at any point along the gradient (G_x) is the slope of the gradient (G_x) times the distance x along the x-axis (Fig. 15-2). Let's multiply both sides of the equation by the gyromagnetic ratio γ:

$$\gamma \cdot \mathbf{B}_x = \gamma(G_x)x$$

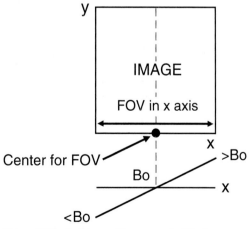

Figure 15-1. An image with axes x and y. The frequency-encode gradient G_x causes the center of the field of view (FOV) to have magnetic field strength $\mathbf{B}_0$ and the right and left ends to have strengths greater and less than $\mathbf{B}_0$, respectively.

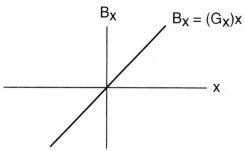

Figure 15-2. The gradient G_x describes a linear equation $\mathbf{B}_x = G_x \cdot x$. Therefore, at $x = 0$, no net magnetic field is added to the system, whereas at a positive value of x, a positive value of magnetic field is added to the main field.

Recall that $(\gamma \mathbf{B}_x)$ is the **Larmor equation,** which relates the magnetic field strength to the frequency:

$$\text{frequency}_x = \gamma \mathbf{B}_x$$

This equation states that the frequency of oscillation at any point along the x-axis is proportional to the magnetic field strength at that point, that is,

$$f_x = \gamma \mathbf{B}_x$$

or

$$f_x = \gamma(G_x)x$$

In other words, the frequency at any point along the x-axis is proportional to the slope of the gradient (G_x) multiplied by the position along the x-axis.

Let's see what happens at each end of the FOV (Fig. 15-3). At the right-side end of the FOV (i.e., at $x = $ FOV/2), the frequency is maximum (call it f_{max}) because the G_x gradient, and therefore the magnetic field strength, is maximum.

The formula for frequency is

$$f_x = \gamma(G_x)x$$

Now, for f_{max}, the distance along the x-axis is ½ FOV. So,

$$f_{max} = \gamma(G_x)\text{FOV}/2$$

Remember this is after we subtract the *center* frequency. Therefore, these measurements are centered around the zero frequency. At the opposite end of the gradient, we have $-f_{max}$:

$$-f_{max} = -\gamma(G_x)\text{FOV}/2$$

What is the **range of frequencies?** The frequency range is from $-f_{max}$ to $+f_{max}$, that is,

$$\text{Frequency range} = -f_{max} \rightarrow +f_{max}$$

$$= \pm f_{max} = 2f_{max}$$

Another term for the range of frequencies is **bandwidth (BW).** Thus,

$$\text{BW} = \pm f_{max} = 2f_{max}$$

If we take the frequency at the right-most side of the image and at the left-most side of the image, we get the range of frequencies, or the bandwidth. We already know that, for maximum frequency,

$$f_{max} = \gamma(G_x)\text{FOV}/2$$

Because

$$\text{BW} = 2f_{max}$$

we can conclude that

$$\text{BW} = \gamma \cdot G_x \cdot \text{FOV}$$

We, therefore, see a dependent relationship among the *field of view, bandwidth,* and *gradient strength.* Let's now solve the equation for the FOV in the x direction:

$$\text{FOV}_x = \frac{\text{bandwidth}}{\gamma(G_x)}$$

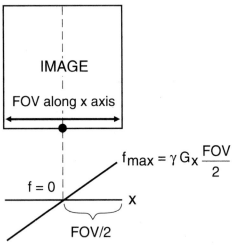

Figure 15-3. At each end of the FOV, the frequency f_x (which is proportional to gradient strength G_x) is maximal. This relationship is given by $f_x = \gamma \cdot G_x \cdot x$, where $x = $ FOV/2 for f_{max}.

This equation shows that the FOV is directly proportional to the bandwidth and that the FOV is inversely proportional to the gradient. Hence, if one wishes to decrease the FOV, one can use either (i) a stronger gradient or (ii) a lower bandwidth.

To ↓ FOV:

1. ↑ Gradient
2. ↓ Bandwidth

There are limits as to how strong you can make the gradient and there are also limits as to how low you can make the bandwidth.

Question: What is the minimum FOV possible?

Answer: It is the minimum bandwidth divided by the maximum gradient:

$$FOV_{min} = \frac{BW_{min}}{\gamma G_{max}}$$

G_{max} and BW_{min} are specific for each machine. For example, for a GE Echospeed Plus 1.5-T scanner,

$$\text{maximum gradient strength} = 23 \text{ mT/m}$$

$$\text{minimum bandwidth} = \pm 4 \text{ kHz} = 8 \text{ kHz}$$

Thus, the minimum FOV is approximately:

$$8 \text{ kHz}/(42.6 \text{ MHz/T} \times 23 \text{ mT/m}) \cong 0.8 \text{ cm}$$

Conversely, to increase the FOV, we can

1. Increase the BW or
2. Decrease the gradient

To ↑ FOV:

1. ↓ Gradient
2. ↑ Bandwidth

(Remember that by increasing bandwidth, we get decreased signal-to-noise ratio.)

Key Points

We have discussed the interesting relationship among the FOV, BW, and gradients:

$$FOV = BW/(\gamma \cdot G)$$

As we saw, there is a limit as to how small one can make the FOV, depending on the minimum allowable BW and the maximum possible gradient strength:

$$FOV_{min} = \frac{BW_{min}}{\gamma \cdot G_{max}}$$

Selecting a smaller FOV may cause an aliasing (or wraparound) artifact, depending on the size of the structure being imaged. More on this is in Chapter 18.

Questions

15-1 If the minimum FOV = 30 cm for a frequency-encoding gradient G_x = 5 mT/m, what would the minimum FOV be for a stronger G_x = 10 mT/m? (i.e., does a stronger G_x reduce or increase the minimum FOV?)

15-2 The min FOV is *inversely* proportional to
   (a) BW
   (b) gradient strength
   (c) TR
   (d) TE

15-3 If the amplitude of a phase-encoding gradient G_y is 0.1 mT/m and its duration is

2 msec, what is the phase shift of the transverse magnetization from a tissue that is 20 mm = 2 cm from the center of the FOV?
   Hint: $\Delta\phi = 360° \times \gamma \times G_y \times$ duration × position, where γ = 42.6 MHz/T.

15-4 The minimum FOV can be reduced by
   (a) increasing the gradient strength
   (b) decreasing the bandwidth
   (c) increasing the sampling interval
   (d) all of the above
   (e) only (a) and (b)

15-5 **T/F** Reducing the FOV minimizes wrap-around artifacts (aliasing).

15-6 What is the minimum FOV for a maximum sampling interval of $\Delta T_s = 10\ \mu\text{sec}$ (i.e., without encountering aliasing) and a maximum frequency gradient of 10 mT/m?
Hint: BW $= 1/\Delta T_s$
   (a) 47 cm
   (b) 23.5 cm
   (c) 47 mm
   (d) 23.5 mm

15-7 The min FOV is *directly* proportional to
   (a) BW
   (b) gradient strength
   (c) TR
   (d) TE

k-Space: The Final Frontier!

Introduction

This chapter will summarize some concepts that we've already discussed and clarify some of the fine points of k-space. Remember that we have, up to this point, referred to the **data space** as an "analog" k-space, and we said that the *Fourier transform* of the data space is the image (Fig. 16-1).

This is, in fact, correct, but there is a problem with this concept: the *matrix* in the data space is very *asymmetric*. In the frequency-encoding direction, the interval between two samples (i.e., the sampling interval ΔT_s) is on the order of microseconds, so that the total time to take all the samples (i.e., the sampling time T_s) is on the order of milliseconds. The time intervals in the phase-encoding direction, however, are each on the order of one TR (i.e., on the order of seconds).

The total time to obtain all the data in the phase-encoding direction is the scan time for one acquisition (on the order of minutes).

Thus, in the data space we have a matrix whose *x-axis* is on the order of *milliseconds* and whose *y-axis* is on the order of *minutes*. This would give us a very asymmetric matrix. The true k-space is the same matrix as the data space, but with a *different* **scale.** Recall that

$$\text{FOV} = \frac{\text{bandwidth}}{\gamma \cdot \text{gradient}} \quad \text{(Eqn. 16-1)}$$

In the last chapter, we talked about the field of view (FOV). We derived Equation 16-1, showing the relationship among the FOV, the bandwidth (BW), and the gradient strength. According to this formula, the FOV is equal to the BW divided by the product of γ and G. We also know from a

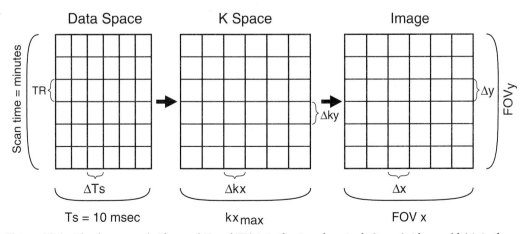

Figure 16-1. The data space (with axes ΔT_s and TR) is in the time domain. k-Space (with axes Δk_y) is in the *spatial* frequency domain and is derived from the data space. The Fourier transform of k-space is the image (with axes x and y), which is in the frequency domain.

previous chapter that the bandwidth is inversely related to the sampling internal (ΔT_s), that is,

$$BW = 1/\Delta T_s$$

From the following two formulas:

$$FOV = \frac{BW}{\gamma G}$$

and

$$BW = \frac{1}{\Delta T_s}$$

we can derive a new formula for the FOV:

$$FOV = \frac{BW}{\gamma G} = \frac{1}{\gamma G \Delta T_s}$$

To calculate this in terms of distance and time, we need to invert both sides of the previous formula to obtain:

$$\frac{1}{FOV} = \gamma \cdot G \cdot \Delta T_s$$

Now consider the FOV in the x and y directions. If we consider the FOV in the x direction, the formula tells us that we need to take the gradient strength and the sampling interval in the x direction.

$$\frac{1}{FOV_x} = \gamma \cdot G_x \cdot \Delta t_x$$

The term ($\gamma \cdot G_x \cdot \Delta t_x$) is denoted Δk_x. If we now look at Figure 16-1, we see that (Δk_x) is the unit interval in k-space in the x direction. Thus,

$$\Delta k_x = \gamma G_x \Delta t_x$$

Let's discuss the units of measurement in the above:

$$\gamma = \text{gyromagnetic ratio} = \text{MHz/T}$$
$$G_x = \text{gradient strength} = \text{mT/m}$$
$$\Delta t_x = \text{sampling interval} = \text{msec}$$

so

$$\Delta k_x = (\text{MHz/T})(\text{mT/m})(\text{msec})$$
$$= (\text{cycles/sec} \cdot \text{T}) \times (\text{T/m}) \times \text{sec}$$
$$= \text{cycles/m}$$

Thus, Δk_x has units of cycles/m or cycles/cm.

The main thing to remember is that Δk_x is 1/FOV in the x direction.

$$\Delta k_x = 1/FOV_x$$

The above formula tells us that the interval in k-space is equal to 1/FOV in the x direction (where the FOV, according to Equation 16-1, depends on the bandwidth and gradient strength in the x direction). This fact is shown diagrammatically in Figure 16-2.

From this, we can see a direct relationship between k-space and the image in that the interval in k-space has an inverse relationship to the FOV of the image. For example, if the FOV of the image is 10 cm, then

$$\Delta k_x = 1/FOV = 1/10 \text{ cm} = 1/0.1 \text{ m}$$
$$= 0.1 \text{ cm}^{-1}(\text{cycles/cm})$$
$$= 10\text{m}^{-1}(\text{cycles/m})$$

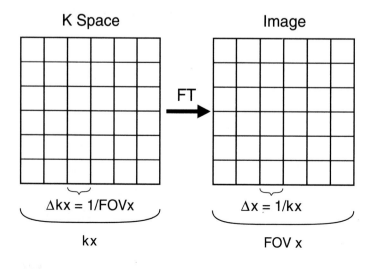

K Space   **Image**

FT

$\Delta kx = 1/FOVx$

kx

$\Delta x = 1/kx$

FOV x

Figure 16-2. The FT of k-space is the image. There is a relationship between the axes in k-space and the image: $\Delta k_x = 1/FOV_x$, $\Delta x = 1/k_x$, where $FOV_x = N_x \cdot \Delta x$ and $k_x = N_x \cdot \Delta k_x$.

Therefore, with an FOV of 10 cm in the image, the pixel size of k-space is 0.1 cm^{-1} or 10 m^{-1}. (Remember that the unit of the axes in k-space is 1/distance or cycles/distance.) The inverse of this is also true:

Δx = pixel size in the image

k_x = sum of the pixels in k-space

In summary:

$$\Delta x = 1/k_x, \Delta k_x = 1/FOV_x$$
$$\Delta k_x = \gamma \cdot G_x \cdot \Delta t_x, k_x = \gamma \cdot G_x \cdot t_x$$

where Δx is the pixel size in the x direction. In essence, this is how we figure out the pixel size in the image.

$$\Delta x = \text{pixel (x direction)} = FOV_x/N_x$$

This formula tells us that the pixel size in the x direction is equal to the FOV divided by the number of pixels in the x direction.

Example

1. Calculate the pixel size for the following situation:

FOV_x = 128 mm

N_x = number of sampling points in the x direction = 128

then the pixel size in the x direction

$$= \Delta x = 128 \text{ mm}/128 = 1.0 \text{ mm}$$

2. Calculate the dimensions in k-space for the above example:

Δk_x = pixel size in k-space = 1/FOV_x

Δk_x = 1/128 mm = 1/12.8 cm

$\cong 0.08$ cm^{-1} = 8 m^{-1}

$k_x = 1/\Delta x = 1/1$ mm = 1 mm^{-1}

$= 10$ cm^{-1} = 1000 m^{-1} = 128Δk_x

The unit in k-space is

Δk_x = cycles/distance

k_x = cycles/distance

Therefore,

k-Space is in the spatial frequency domain.

This is different from the other frequency that we have discussed thus far. Before, we discussed the Fourier transform of a signal that varied with time, with the transform in the frequency domain. Spatial frequency is a different kind of frequency.

The usual frequency = cycles/time
Spatial frequency = cycles/distance

Therefore, when k-space is said to be in the "frequency domain," we are referring to the "*spatial frequency domain*," which, as we just saw, is a mathematical manipulation of the *data space* (which is in the time domain).

Remember that the units of the axes in data space are time: milliseconds and minutes. In k-space, we have converted these axes into "spatial frequencies" that have units of cycles/distance, measured in cm^{-1} (cycles/cm) and m^{-1} (cycles/m). If we Fourier transform k-space, we get the desired image.

Mathematically, we could go straight from the data space, via a Fourier transform, directly to the image. We are simply renaming the variables (i.e., $\gamma G_x \Delta t_x = \Delta k_x$). This renaming is known as an *algebraic manipulation*, but to go through this intermediate mathematical step in k-space allows us to work with a space that is *more symmetric*; now, the distance in the x direction of k-space and the distance in the y direction of k-space are roughly similar (as opposed to the difference between milliseconds and minutes in the x direction and y direction in the data space, respectively).

This same concept in the y direction is somewhat harder to understand, but the same principles hold, namely,

$$\Delta k_y = \frac{1}{FOV_y}$$

The interval k_y in k-space is inversely proportional to the FOV in the y direction.

$$k_y = \frac{1}{\Delta y}$$

The distance in k-space in the y direction is inversely proportional to the pixel size of the image in the y direction.

One more mathematical principle concerns the relationship between phase and frequency:

$$\theta = \int \omega dt$$

In other words, the phase θ is the integral of the frequency with respect to time, where ω (angular frequency) is given by the Larmor equation[1]:

$$\omega = \gamma \mathbf{B} = \gamma \cdot G \cdot x$$

In other words, the frequency ω is proportional to the magnetic field strength which is, in turn, proportional to the gradient strength multiplied by the distance. Thus,

$$\theta_y = \omega_y\, t_y = \gamma \cdot \mathbf{B}_y \cdot t_y = \gamma \cdot G_y \cdot y \cdot t_y$$

or

$$\theta_y = (\gamma\, G_y\, t_y) \cdot y$$

---

[1]You may have wondered why we have been using ω and f somewhat interchangeably in our equations, although these are two separate entities. This practice is all right as long as you keep the right units for the gyromagnetic ratio γ (i.e., MHz/T when dealing with f and 2π MHz/T when dealing with ω).

Remember that:

$$\Delta k_y = \gamma\, G_y\, \Delta t_y$$

and

$$(k_y = \Delta k_y \cdot N_y) \text{ and } (t_y = \Delta t_y \cdot N_y)$$

so

$$k_y = \Delta k_y \cdot N_y = \gamma\, G_y \Delta t_y \cdot N_y$$

Therefore,

$$k_y = \gamma \cdot G_y \cdot t_y$$

so

$$\theta_y = (k_y) \cdot (y)$$

We thus have a very simple relationship between *phase* and *position* along the y direction:

$$\theta_y = (k_y) \cdot (y) = (\gamma\, G_y)\, (t_y)\, (y)$$

In the y direction, the *gradient* at y depends on the position of y. In contrast, we always apply the same gradient in the x direction regardless of what position the x direction is going (i.e., G_x is independent of x). However, in the y direction, we apply different gradients at different points along the y-axis (G_y varies with y: it is 0 at $y = 0$ and gets progressively larger with increasing y).

Key Points

The true k-space is a mathematically manipulated variant of the data space, with axes referred to as "spatial frequencies." Therefore, k-space is in a "spatial" frequency domain. *Spatial frequencies* k_x and k_y are inversely proportional to *distance* (with units of cycles/cm). The Fourier transform of k-space is the desired image.

The spatial frequencies k_x and k_y are expressed as:

$$k_x = \gamma \cdot G_x \cdot t_x$$
$$k_y = \gamma \cdot G_y \cdot t_y$$

with units in cycles/cm.

Questions

16-1 **T/F** Spatial frequencies have units 1/distance (cycles/cm).

16-2 **T/F (a)** The axes in k-space are designated k_x and k_y.

(b) The axes in k-space are in the frequency domain (with units 1/time or cycle/sec).

16-3 **T/F** The Fourier transform of the k-space produces the desired image.

16-4 Δk_x is equal to

(a) $1/FOV_x$ **(b)** $\gamma\, G_x \Delta t_x$

(c) k_x/N_x **(d)** all of the above

(e) only (a) and (b)

16-5 **T/F (a)** The center of k-space contributes to maximum image contrast.

(b) The periphery of k-space contributes to image details.

16-6 **T/F** k-Space can be thought of as a digital (in the spatial frequency domain) version of the data space (which is in the time domain).

17

Scan Parameters and Image Optimization

Introduction

In this chapter, we will discuss all the important parameters in MR imaging that the operator can control and adjust. We will then see how these changes influence the image quality. Every radiologist is comfortable with a particular set of techniques; therefore, "custom-made" techniques can be achieved only if the radiologist is aware of the parameters and trade-offs involved.

Primary and Secondary Parameters

Primary parameters are those that are set directly:

$$\left.\begin{array}{l} \text{TR} \\ \text{TE} \\ \text{TI} \\ \text{FA (flip angle)} \end{array}\right\} \begin{array}{l} \text{contribute to} \\ \textit{image contrast} \end{array}$$

$$\left.\begin{array}{l} \Delta z = \text{slice thickness} \\ \text{Interslice gap} \end{array}\right\} \begin{array}{l} \text{Contribute} \\ \text{to } \textit{coverage} \end{array}$$

$$\left.\begin{array}{l} \left.\begin{array}{l} \text{FOV}_x \\ \text{FOV}_y \end{array}\right\} \begin{array}{l} \text{Contribute to} \\ \textit{resolution:} \end{array} \\ \begin{array}{l} N_x\text{: number} \\ \quad \text{of frequency-} \\ \quad \text{encoding steps} \\ N_y\text{: number} \\ \quad \text{of phase-} \\ \quad \text{encoding steps} \end{array} \left.\begin{array}{l} \Delta x\text{: spacing} \\ \text{in x direction} \\ \Delta y\text{: spacing} \\ \text{in y direction} \end{array}\right\} \begin{array}{l} \text{Contribute} \\ \text{to } S/N \\ \textit{ratio} \end{array} \\ \left.\begin{array}{l} \text{NEX} \\ \text{Bandwidth} \end{array}\right\} \end{array}\right\}$$

From the *primary* parameters above, we can get the *secondary* parameters (which are also used to describe the image):

1. S/N ratio (SNR)
2. Scan time
3. Coverage
4. Resolution
5. Image contrast

Unfortunately, optimization of these parameters may involve some **trade-offs.** To gain some advantage with one parameter, we might have to sacrifice another parameter. Let's start out with the concept of signal-to-noise ratio (SNR).

Signal-to-Noise Ratio. What we want is signal. What we don't want is noise. Although we can't completely eliminate noise, there are ways to maximize the SNR. SNR is given by

$$\text{SNR} \propto \text{(voxel volume)}\ \sqrt{(N_y)\,(\text{NEX})\,T_s} \quad \textbf{(Eqn. 17-1)}$$

which makes sense because $N_y \times \text{NEX} \times T_s$ is the total time the machine is "listening" to the spin echoes.

Since $T_s = N_x \cdot \Delta T_s$ and $\Delta T_s = 1/\text{BW}$, then $T_s = N_x/\text{BW}$.

$$\text{SNR} \propto \text{(voxel volume)}$$
$$\sqrt{(N_y)\,(N_x)\,(\text{NEX})/\text{BW}} \quad \textbf{(Eqn. 17-2)}$$

Therefore, SNR depends on

1. Voxel volume = $\Delta x \cdot \Delta y \cdot \Delta z$
2. Number of excitations (NEX)
3. Number of phase-encoding steps (N_y)
4. Number of frequency-encoding steps (N_x)
5. Full bandwidth (BW)

Let's go through each parameter and see how SNR is affected.

Voxel Volume

If we increase the voxel size, we increase the number of proton spins in the voxel and, therefore, increase the signal coming out of the voxel (Fig. 17-1). The voxel volume is given by

$$\text{Voxel volume} = \Delta x \cdot \Delta y \cdot \Delta z$$

where Δx = pixel size in the x direction, Δy = pixel size in the y direction, and Δz = slice thickness.

NEX (Number of Excitations or Acquisitions). NEX stands for the number of times the scan is repeated. Let's say we have two signals (S_1 and S_2), corresponding to the same slice (with the same G_y). There is constant noise (N) associated with each signal ($N_1 = N_2 = N$). If we add up the signals (assuming $S_1 = S_2 = S$), we get

$$S_1 + S_2 = 2S$$

However, if we add up the noise, we get

$$N_1 + N_2 = (\sqrt{2})N, \text{ where } \sqrt{2} \approx 1.41$$

This formula does not make sense at first glance. Why do we get $\sqrt{2}N$ and not $2N$? The answer has to do with a somewhat complicated statistical concept and the so-called random **Brownian motion** theory, which deals with the *spectral density* of the noise.

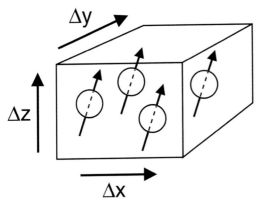

Figure 17-1. A voxel is a three-dimensional volume element with dimensions Δx, Δy, and Δz. The more spins in a voxel, the more signal. Therefore, increasing voxel size increases SNR.

In a simplistic approach, think of the noise as the **variance** (σ^2) of a Gaussian distribution (σ = **standard deviation**). Then, for the sum of the two noise distributions, the variance is additive and given by

$$\sigma_1{}^2 + \sigma_2{}^2 = \sigma^2 + \sigma^2 = 2\sigma^2$$

from which the standard deviation is calculated to be

$$\sqrt{(2\sigma^2)} = (\sqrt{2})\sigma$$

This is where the $\sqrt{2}$ factor comes from. However, you don't need to know the underlying math—you just need to understand the concept. In summary:

$$\frac{S_1 + S_2}{N_1 + N_2} = \frac{2S}{\sqrt{2}N}$$

The resulting signal will be twice the original signal. The resulting noise, however, will be less—it will be the square root of 2 multiplied by the noise $\sqrt{2}N$.

In other words, if we increase the number of acquisitions by a factor of 2, the signal doubles and noise increases by $\sqrt{2}$, for a net $2/\sqrt{2} = \sqrt{2}$; thus, SNR increases by a factor of $\sqrt{2}$.

Therefore, $\uparrow$ NEX by a factor of $2 \rightarrow \uparrow$ SNR by a factor of $\sqrt{2}$.

Think of the NEX as an *averaging* operation that causes "smoothing" and improvement in the image quality by increasing the signal to a greater degree (e.g., factor 2) relative to the increase in the noise (e.g., factor $\sqrt{2}$). As another example, increasing NEX by a factor of 4 results in an increase of signal by 4 and an increase of noise by $\sqrt{4}$ or 2. Thus, SNR increases by 4/2 or twofold.

N_y (Number of Phase-Encoding Steps). The same concept holds for N_y. That is, similar to NEX, there is a 41% ($\sqrt{2}$) increase in SNR when N_y is doubled. As with NEX, when the number of phase-encode steps doubles, signal doubles and noise increases (randomly) by $\sqrt{2}$ (for a net $\sqrt{2}$ increase in SNR).

Bandwidth. An inverse relationship exists between BW and SNR. If we go to a wider bandwidth, we include more noise, and the SNR decreases. If we decrease the bandwidth, we allow less noise to come through, and the SNR increases.

$$\downarrow BW \Rightarrow \uparrow SNR$$

To be exact, decreasing the BW by a factor of 2 causes the SNR to improve by a factor of $\sqrt{2}$.

In general, decreased bandwidth causes the following:

1. Increased SNR
2. Increased chemical shift artifact (more on this later)
3. Longer minimum TE (which means less signal due to more T2 decay). Remember that

$$\text{Bandwidth} = 1/\Delta T_s = N_x/T_s$$

Therefore, a longer sampling time (T_s), which is necessary for a decreased bandwidth, results in a longer minimum TE. With a long TE, increased T2 dephasing results in decreased signal. However, the contribution from reduced noise due to a lower bandwidth outweighs the deleterious effect of reduced signal due to greater T2 decay from increased TE.

4. Decreased number of slices. This decrease is caused by the longer TE. Remember,

$$\text{number of slices} = TR/(TE + T_s/2 + T_o)$$

where T_s is the total sampling (readout) time and T_o is the "overhead" time. A narrower bandwidth is usually used on the second echo of a T2-weighted dual-echo image because, with the second echo, we have a longer TE and we are able to afford the longer sampling time. On the first echo, however, we can't afford to use a narrower bandwidth because we can't afford to lengthen the TE. However, we probably don't need the smaller bandwidth anyway because we already have enough SNR on the proton density-weighted first echo of a long T2, double-echo image. A typical T_s for a 1.5-T scanner is 8 msec, resulting in a BW (for a 256 matrix) of

$$BW = N_x/T_s = 256/8 = 32 \text{ kHz}$$
$$= \pm 16 \text{ kHz} = 125 \text{ Hz/pixel}$$

Note that BW can be described as "full bandwidth" (32 kHz in example above), ± the

Nyquist frequency (which is ± 16 kHz above and defines the FOV) or "bandwidth per pixel" (which is unambiguous if you forget the ±).

A typical "variable bandwidth" option includes

1. A wide bandwidth (±16 kHz) on the first echo, and
2. A narrow bandwidth (±4 kHz) on the second echo, thus increasing SNR and counteracting T2 decay effects.

Question: How does the gradient affect the BW?

Answer: Recall from Chapter 15 that the field of view (FOV) is given by

$$FOV = BW/\gamma G_x \quad \text{or} \quad G_x = BW/\gamma FOV$$

For a given FOV, increasing the gradient G_x causes increased BW and, therefore, decreased SNR.

SNR in 3D Imaging

In 3D imaging, we have the same factors contributing to SNR, plus an additional phase-encoding step in the z direction (N_z):

$$\textbf{3D SNR} \propto \frac{\textbf{(voxel volume)}}{\sqrt{(N_y)(N_x)(N_z)(NEX)/BW}} \quad \text{(Eqn. 17-3)}$$

From this equation, you can see why SNR in 3D imaging is higher than that in 2D imaging. Specifically,

$$SNR(3D) = \sqrt{N_z} \cdot SNR \ (2D)$$

Another way to look at SNR is to say that SNR depends on only two factors:

1. Voxel size
2. Total sampling time

Sampling time (T_s) is the time that we sample the signal. Therefore, it makes sense that the more time we spend sampling the signal, the higher the SNR will be. Let's look again at the formula for SNR (in 2D imaging):

$$SNR \propto \text{(voxel volume)} \sqrt{(N_y)(N_x)(NEX)/BW}$$

Recall that

$$T_s = N_x/BW$$

or

$$1/BW = T_s/N_x$$

so

$$\text{SNR} \propto (\text{voxel volume}) \sqrt{(N_y)(\text{NEX})(T_s)}$$

We know that N_y is the number of phase-encoding steps, which is the number of times we sample the echo corresponding to a particular phase-encoding gradient G_y, and that NEX is the number of times we repeat each phase-encoding step. In essence, the factor

$$T = T_s \cdot N_y \cdot \text{NEX}$$

is the *total sampling time* of all the echoes received for a particular slice. Thus,

$$\text{SNR} \propto \frac{(\text{voxel volume})}{\sqrt{\text{total sampling time of all signals}}}$$

In summary, SNR can be increased by doing the following:

1. Increasing TR
2. Decreasing TE
3. Using a lower BW
4. Using volume (i.e., 3D) imaging
5. Increasing NEX
6. Increasing N_y
7. Increasing N_x
8. Increasing the voxel size

Resolution. Spatial resolution (or pixel size) is the minimum distance that we can distinguish between two points on an image. It is determined by

$$\text{Pixel size} = \text{FOV/number of pixels}$$
$$\uparrow N_y \rightarrow \text{better resolution}$$

If we increase the number of phase-encoding steps, what happens to SNR? Obviously, *better resolution usually means poorer SNR*. However, if we look at Equation 17-2, it appears that by increasing N_y, the SNR should increase! What's the catch? The catch is, we are keeping the FOV constant while increasing N_y. Take, for example,

$$\text{Pixel size along y-axis} = \Delta_y = \text{FOV}_y/N_y$$

By increasing N_y, we are making the pixel size smaller. Now, recall that

$$\begin{aligned} \text{Voxel volume} &= \Delta x \cdot \Delta y \cdot \Delta z \\ &= \text{FOV}_x \cdot \text{FOV}_y \cdot \Delta z/(N_x \cdot N_y) \end{aligned}$$

Incorporating this information into Equation 17-2 gives us another way of expressing SNR:

$$\text{SNR} \propto (\text{FOV}_x)$$

$$(\text{FOV}_y)\Delta z \sqrt{\frac{\text{NEX}}{(N_y)(N_x)(\text{BW})}} \quad \text{(Eqn. 17-4)}$$

This formula allows us to better separate the factors affecting SNR. From this, we can conclude the following:

1. If we keep FOV constant and increase N_y, we will decrease SNR.

$$\uparrow N_y, \text{FOV constant} \rightarrow \downarrow \text{SNR}$$

2. If we increase N_y and increase FOV, thus keeping pixel size constant, then we will increase the SNR. Yet the resolution doesn't change. What is the trade-off here? The answer is the acquisition time, which is proportional to N_y.

$$\uparrow \text{FOV, pixels fixed} \rightarrow \uparrow \text{SNR, } \uparrow \text{time}$$

3. If we increase slice thickness Δz, we get not only more SNR, but also more partial volume artifact.
4. If we increase NEX, we get more SNR at the expense of longer acquisition time. For 3D imaging, Equation 17-4 is modified to

$$\text{SNR (3D)} = (\text{FOV}_x)(\text{FOV}_y)(\text{FOV}_z)$$

$$\sqrt{\frac{\text{NEX}}{(N_x)(N_y)(N_z)(\text{BW})}} \quad \text{(Eqn. 17-5)}$$

Basically, if we want better spatial resolution in a *given* acquisition time, we have to sacrifice SNR. Let's consider a few examples.

1. What happens if we increase the number of pixels with the FOV constant?

   (a) Increase resolution.
   (b) Decrease SNR (refer to Equation 17-4). Therefore, as we decrease the pixel size, we increase the resolution and decrease the SNR.
   (c) Increase scan time (number of pixels increases in phase-encode direction).

2. What happens if we decrease the FOV and keep the number of pixels constant?

   (a) Increase the resolution.
   (b) Decrease SNR.
   (c) Potentially increase aliasing artifact.

3. How do we determine the pixel size (resolution)?

It is determined by dividing the FOV by the number of encoding steps.

Example

For FOV = 250 mm and a 256 × 256 matrix

$$N_x = N_y = 256$$
$$\text{Pixel size } (x) = \text{FOV}_x/N_x = 250/256$$
$$\cong 1 \text{ mm in x direction.}$$
$$\text{Pixel size } (y) = \text{FOV}_y/N_y = 250/256$$
$$\cong 1 \text{ mm in y direction.}$$

In the x direction, there are two ways of increasing resolution (for a given FOV):

1. Increase N_x by reducing the sampling interval ΔT_s (i.e., by increasing the BW) and keeping the sampling time T_s fixed (recall that $T_s = N_x \cdot \Delta T_s$). The advantage here is no increase in TE; the trade-off is a reduction in SNR (due to increased BW).

2. Increase N_x by lengthening T_s and keeping ΔT_s (and thus BW) fixed. Here, the SNR does not change, but the trade-off is an increased TE (due to a longer T_s) and less T1 weighting (this is only a concern in short echo delay time imaging).

Acquisition Time

The acquisition time or scan time, as we have seen previously, is given by

$$\text{Scan time} = \text{TR} \cdot N_y \cdot \text{NEX}$$

where N_y is the number of phase-encoding steps (in the y direction).

For fast spin-echo (FSE) imaging (discussed in detail in Chapter 19), the above is modified to

$$\text{FSE time} = \text{TR} \cdot N_y \cdot \text{NEX/ETL}$$

where ETL = echo train length (4, 8, 16, 32).

For 3D imaging, the scan time is given by

$$\text{Time (3D)} = \text{TR} \cdot N_y \cdot N_z \cdot \text{NEX}$$

where N_z is the number of phase-encoding steps (partitions) in the z direction. In other words,

$$\text{Time (3D)} = N_z \cdot \text{time(2D)}$$

Multiplication by such a large number (e.g., $N_z = 32$ to 64 or 128) might at first seem to result in

an excessively long scan time for 3D imaging, but the TR used in 3D gradient-echo imaging is approximately 100 times smaller (order of 30 msec) compared with the TR used in conventional spin-echo imaging; we can perform a 3D scan in a reasonable time. Recently, 3D FSE imaging (discussed in Chapter 19) has also become feasible.

Example

1. Calculate the acquisition time of an SE sequence with TR = 3000 msec, N_y = 256, and NEX = 1.

   Solution: Scan time = 3000 × 256 msec
   $$= 768 \text{ sec} = 12.8 \text{ min}$$

2. Calculate the acquisition time of an FSE sequence with the above parameters and an ETL of 8.

   Solution: Scan time $= \dfrac{12.8 \text{ min}}{8} = 1.6 \text{ min}$

3. (a) Calculate the acquisition time of a 3D gradient-echo sequence with TR = 30 msec, N_y = 256, NEX = 1, and N_z = 60.

   Solution: Scan time = 30 × 256 × 1 × 60 msec = 460.8 sec = 7.68 min

   (b) If TR = 300 in the previous example, then the scan time = 76.8 min = 1 hr and 16.8 min, which is, obviously, impractical. Hence, 3D techniques use gradient-echo sequences employing a very short TR.

TR. What happens if we increase or decrease TR?

1. Increasing TR:

   (a) increases SNR (according to the T1 recovery curve)
   (b) increases coverage (more slices)
   (c) decreases T1 weighting
   (d) increases proton density and T2 weighting
   (e) increases scan time

2. Decreasing TR:

   (a) decreases SNR
   (b) decreases coverage
   (c) increases T1 weighting

(d) decreases proton density and T2 weighting

(e) decreases scan time

Sometimes an MR technologist will find that, for a certain TR, the required coverage cannot be achieved. Therefore, to increase the coverage, he or she might increase the TR. However, in so doing, T1 weighting is decreased, which may be an undesirable effect.

Coverage

Coverage is the distance covered by a multislice acquisition. It depends on the number of slices and on the slice thickness and the interslice gap (Fig. 17-2). Because

$$\text{number of slices} = TR/(TE + T_s/2 + T_o)$$

then

$$\text{Coverage} = TR/(TE + T_s/2 + T_o) \times (\text{Slice thickness} + \text{gap})$$

where T_s is the sampling time and T_o is the "overhead" time, as we've discussed in previous chapters.

Let's summarize:

1. Coverage is increased if we:

   (a) increase slice thickness

   (b) increase interslice gap

   (c) increase TR or decrease the last TE (i.e., increase TR/TE ratio)

   (d) decrease sampling time T_s (resulting in a lower TE), that is, increase the bandwidth

2. Coverage is decreased if we:

   (a) increase TE

   (b) increase T_s

   (c) increase ETL in FSE imaging (due to longer final TE)

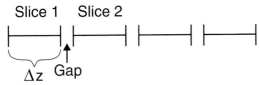

Slice 1   Slice 2

Δz Gap

Figure 17-2. Coverage is determined by slice thickness Δz and by the interslice gap. Coverage = number of slices × (Δz + gap).

3. Increasing interslice gap causes

   (a) increased coverage

   (b) decreased "cross-talk" artifact

   (c) increased SNR (due to increasing effective TR by reducing cross-talk)

   (d) decreased detection of small lesions (which may lie within the gap)

TE (Time to Echo)

Question: What happens if we increase or decrease TE?

Answer:

1. By increasing TE, we:

   (a) increase T2 weighting

   (b) increase dephasing and thus decrease SNR (according to the T2 decay curve)

   (c) decrease number of possible slices (decrease coverage), because number of slices ≈ TR/TE

   (d) no change in scan time (unless, of course, the coverage is not adequate and either longer TR or extra acquisitions are required)

2. The reverse is true for decreasing TE:

   (a) decrease T2 weighting and increase T1 or proton density weighting

   (b) increase SNR (less dephasing). However, if TE is reduced by reducing T_s (i.e., increasing BW), SNR may be reduced!

   (c) increase coverage

   (d) no change in scan time

Question: What causes lengthening of the minimum TE?

Answer:

1. TE should be long enough so that the side lobes of the 180° pulse do not interfere with the side lobes of the FID or the echo (Fig. 17-3). Remember that we need a Fourier transform of the RF pulse with a square shape to be able to get ideal contiguous slices. To do this, the RF must be a sinc wave (sinc t = sin t/t) with as many side lobes as possible. This, in turn, will lengthen the 90° and 180° RF pulse.

2. If TE is so short that it allows interference between the 180° RF pulse and the FID, an

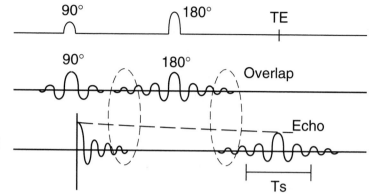

Figure 17-3. To avoid overlapping of the FID and the side lobes of the 180° pulse, you need to increase TE. This increase is one cause of lengthening the minimum TE.

FID artifact (or zipper artifact) will appear along the zero frequency line.

Question: How can TE be shortened?

Answer:

1. One way is to decrease the sampling time T_s. However, this results in a higher BW and therefore a lower SNR (Equation 17-2).
2. There is a limit as to how short TE could be. The factors limiting minimum TE include

   (a) duration of RF pulse (especially the 180° pulse)
   (b) duration of FID
   (c) T_s or BW (which influence the SNR)

3. TE can also be shortened by switching to a gradient-echo sequence because a 180° refocusing pulse is no longer used.

Contrast on a spin-echo technique can be summarized (Table 17-1):

TI (Inversion Time)

As we saw in Chapter 7, inversion recovery sequences employ an additional 180° pulse before the 90° pulse.

Table 17-1		
	TR	**TE**
T1W	Short	Short
PDW	Long	Short
T2W	Long	Long

Advantages

1. Can suppress various tissues by selecting the appropriate TI. More specifically, as we saw in Chapter 7, if

   $$TI = 0.693 \times T1 \text{ (tissue x)}$$

   then tissue x is "nulled" or "suppressed."
2. *STIR* (short TI inversion recovery) sequences suppress fat by selecting

   $$TI = 0.693 \times T1 \text{ (fat)}$$

   Since at 1.5 Tesla, T1 of fat is approximately 200 msec, then to null fat, we must select

   $$TI = 0.693 \times 200 \cong 140 \text{ msec}$$

3. *FLAIR* (fluid-attenuated inversion recovery) sequences suppress fluid by selecting

   $$TI = 0.693 \times T1 \text{ (fluid)}$$

This sequence is used, for example, in the brain to suppress cerebrospinal fluid (CSF) to increase the conspicuity of periventricular hyperintense lesions such as multiple sclerosis plaques. Since at 1.5 T, T1 of CSF is approximately 3600 msec, then to null CSF, we have to select

$$TI = 0.693 \times 3600 \cong 2500 \text{ msec}$$

Disadvantages

1. Decreased SNR
2. Decreased coverage (by a factor of about 2 due to the presence of the extra 180° pulse)

Key Points

In this chapter, we discussed the important and practical factors that influence the quality of MR imaging. To improve the quality of the images, it is crucial to have a firm grasp of the parameters that, directly or indirectly, affect the scan. We introduced the primary and secondary parameters that are used to determine MR images (refer to the *Introduction* in this chapter). In a nutshell, the name of the game is "trade-offs." Often, one cannot gain advantage in one area without sacrificing another.

Questions

17-1 For a TR = 1500 msec, 2 NEX, and a 128 × 128 matrix, calculate the scan time for
(a) a single slice
(b) 10 slices (performed one at a time)
(c) 10 slices performed using a multi-slice (multiplanar) acquisition

17-2 Calculate the maximum number of achievable slices for a TR = 1000 msec, TE = 80 msec, sampling time T_s = 20 msec, and "overhead time" T_o = 10.

17-3 The concept of variable BW: in order to improve SNR, the lowest possible BW is selected. Suppose that the BW is halved:
(a) How is the SNR affected?
(b) What happens to chemical shift artifacts?
(c) How does this affect the maximum number of slices?

17-4 The acquisition time of a single acquisition gradient-echo sequence with TR = 30 msec, TE = 10 msec, NEX = 2, N_y = 256 for acquiring 15 slices is about
(a) 15.36 sec   (b) 153.6 sec
(c) 230.4 sec   (d) 15,360 sec
(e) 230,400 sec

17-5 The SNR in 3D imaging is equal to the SNR in 2D imaging times the factor:
(a) N_z (b) $\sqrt{(N_z)}$
(c) N_y (d) $\sqrt{(N_y)}$

17-6 Increasing TE leads to a decrease in all of the following *except*
(a) T2W   (b) signal
(c) coverage   (d) SNR

17-7 SNR can be increased by
(a) increasing NEX
(b) decreasing BW
(c) increasing N_y

(d) increasing N_x
(e) increasing voxel volume
(f) increasing TR
(g) decreasing TE
(h) all of the above
(i) only (a)−(e)

17-8 Increasing N_y leads to
(a) better resolution
(b) increased SNR (fixed FOV)
(c) increased SNR (fixed pixels)
(d) increased scan time
(e) all of the above
(f) only (a), (c), (d)
(g) only (a), (b), (d)

17-9 For a 128 square matrix and an FOV of 25 cm, the pixel size is about
(a) 0.5 mm   (b) 1 mm
(c) 1.5 mm   (d) 2 mm

17-10 The SNR is proportional to the square root of
(a) $BW/N_x \cdot NEX$
(b) $BW/N_y \cdot NEX$
(c) $N_x \cdot N_y \cdot NEX/BW$
(d) $N_y \cdot BW/NEX$

17-11 Increasing TR leads to an increase in all the following *except*
(a) scan time   (b) SNR
(c) T1W   (d) T2W
(e) coverage

17-12 Minimum TE can be reduced by
(a) reducing the duration of the RF pulses
(b) reducing the sampling time T_s
(c) increasing the bandwidth
(d) using a sequence that doesn't use 180° pulses (as in gradient echo)
(e) all of the above

17-13 The acquisition time in 3D imaging is equal to that in 2D imaging times the factor:

(a) N_z (b) $\sqrt{(N_z)}$

(c) N_y (d) $\sqrt{(N_y)}$

17-14 Coverage is increased by increasing all of the following *except*

(a) slice thickness (b) interslice gap

(c) TR (d) BW

(e) TE

17-15 In STIR, T1 should be set to

(a) 1.44 T1 (fat)

(b) $(1/\sqrt{2})$ T1 (fat)

(c) 2 T1 (fat)

(d) 0.693 T1 (fat)

(e) (1/0.693) T1 (fat)

(f) choices (b) or (d)

17-16 In FLAIR, T1 should be set to

(a) 0.693 T1 (fluid)

(b) (ln 2) T1 (fluid)

(c) (−1ln 0.5) T1 (fluid)

(d) all of the above

17-17 Match (i) STIR; (ii) FLAIR with

(a) dark fluid

(b) dark fat

Introduction

MRI, as with any other imaging modality, has its share of artifacts.

It is important to recognize these artifacts and to have the tools to eliminate or at least minimize them. There are many sources of artifacts in MRI. These are summarized as follows:

1. Image processing artifact

    (a) Aliasing
    (b) Chemical shift
    (c) Truncation
    (d) Partial volume

2. Patient-related artifacts

    (a) Motion artifacts
    (b) Magic angle

3. Radio frequency (RF) related artifacts

    (a) Cross-talk
    (b) Zipper artifacts
    (c) RF feedthrough
    (d) RF noise

4. External magnetic field artifacts

    (a) Magnetic inhomogeneity

5. Magnetic susceptibility artifacts

    (a) Diamagnetic, paramagnetic, and ferromagnetic
    (b) Metal

6. Gradient-related artifacts:

    (a) Eddy currents
    (b) Nonlinearity

    (c) Geometric distortion

7. Errors in the data
8. Flow-related artifacts
9. Dielectric effects

Let's discuss this list in more detail.

Image Processing Artifact

Aliasing (Wraparound). Refer to the discussion on *undersampling* in Chapter 12.

Spin-Echo Imaging. Let's say we're studying the abdomen (Fig. 18-1). If the field of view (FOV) only covers part of the body, we know that we may get **aliasing** (wraparound), but what causes the aliasing?

We have a gradient in the x direction (G_x), with a maximum frequency (f_{max}) at one end of the FOV, and a minimum frequency ($-f_{max}$) at the other end of the FOV. These are the **Nyquist** frequencies (discussed in Chapter 12). Any frequency higher than the maximum frequency allowed by the gradient cannot be detected correctly.

The gradient doesn't stop at the end of the FOV. The gradient is going to keep going because we still have magnetic fields outside the space designated by the FOV. The parts of the body outside the FOV (in this case, the arms) will be exposed to certain magnetic field gradients. One arm will receive a magnetic field that will generate a frequency higher than f_{max} for the FOV. It may be twice the frequency of f_{max}— twice the intended Nyquist frequency. The computer cannot recognize these frequencies above (f_{max}) or below ($-f_{max}$). They will be recognized

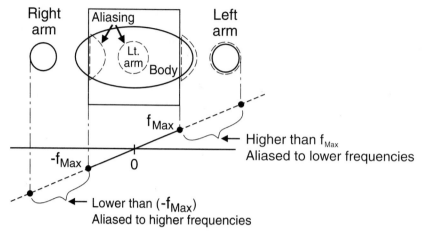

Figure 18-1. For a given FOV and gradient strength, the maximum frequency f_{max} corresponds to the edges of the FOV. Any part outside the FOV will experience a higher frequency. The higher frequencies outside the FOV may be aliased to a lower frequency inside the FOV. This will cause a wraparound artifact.

as a frequency within the bandwidth. The higher frequency will be recognized as a lower frequency within the accepted bandwidth.

For example, if the higher frequency were 2 kHz higher than (f_{max}), it would be recognized as 2 kHz higher than ($-f_{max}$), and therefore its information would be "aliased" to the opposite side of the image—the side of the FOV that corresponds to the lowest frequencies (Fig. 18-1).

The part of the body and arm on the left side of the patient that is outside the FOV and is exposed to a higher magnetic field will have spins oscillating at a frequency higher than (f_{max}). Thus, it will be identified as a structure on the right side of the patient—that side of the image associated with lower frequencies.

Likewise, the arm and body outside the FOV on the right side of the patient will experience spins oscillating at frequencies lower than ($-f_{max}$) and will also be incorrectly recognized by the computer. For example, if the lower frequency were 2 kHz lower than ($-f_{max}$), it would be recognized as 2 kHz lower than (f_{max}), and its information would be "aliased" to the opposite side of the image—the side of the FOV that corresponds to the higher frequencies. This process is also called **wraparound**—the patient's arm gets "wrapped around" to the opposite side.

The computer can't recognize frequencies outside the bandwidth (which determines the FOV). Any frequency outside of this frequency range is going to get "aliased" to a frequency that

exists within the bandwidth. The "perceived" frequency will be the actual frequency minus twice the Nyquist frequency.

$$f(\text{perceived}) = f(\text{true}) - 2f(\text{Nyquist})$$

Why then do we usually see wraparound in the phase-encoding direction? Remember that the number of phase-encoding steps is directly related to the length of the scan time. The phase-encoding steps can be lowered by shortening the FOV in the phase-encoding direction versus the frequency-encoding direction also known as rectangular FOV (see Chapter 23). If the FOV is shortened too much in this direction versus the actual extent of the body then wraparound will occur. Figure 18-2 contains an example of wraparound.

3D Imaging. Wraparound artifact can also be seen in 3D imaging in all three directions.

1. It can be seen along the x and y directions, as with spin-echo imaging.
2. It can also be seen along the slice-select (phase-encoded) direction at each end of the slab (e.g., the last slice is overlapped on the first slice, as in Figs. 18-3 and 18-4).

Example

Suppose the frequency bandwidth is 32 kHz (±16 kHz). This means that if we're centered at zero frequency, the maximum frequency $f_{max} = +16$ kHz and minimum frequency ($-f_{max}$) = −16 kHz (Fig. 18-1). If we have a frequency in the arm (out-

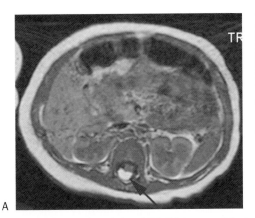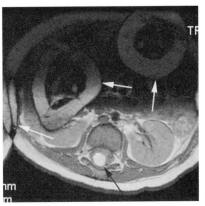

A   B

Figure 18-2. Axial T1 (**A**) and PD (**B**) images of the lumbar spine demonstrate aliasing of the arms in Figure B (*arrows*). Figure B was obtained with a smaller FOV resulting in aliasing artifact. Also note that the patient has a filum terminale lipoma (*black arrows* in **A** and **B**).

side the FOV) of +17 kHz, the perceived frequency will be

$$f(\text{perceived}) = +17\,\text{kHz} - 2(16\,\text{kHz})$$
$$= -15\,\text{kHz}$$

Now, the arm, which is perceived as having a frequency of −15 kHz (rather than +17 kHz), will be recognized as a structure with a very low frequency—only 1 kHz faster than the negative end frequency of the bandwidth—and

will be identified on the opposite side of the image, the low-frequency side.

Remedy. How do we solve this problem?

1. *Surface coil*: The simplest way is to devise a method by which we don't get any signal from outside the FOV. With the patient in a large transmit/receive coil that covers the whole body, we will receive signal from all the body parts in that coil, and those parts outside the FOV will result in aliasing. But

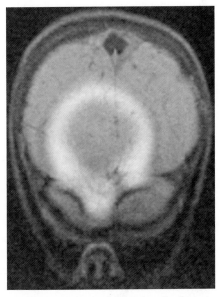

Figure 18-3. 3D gradient-echo T1 image without gadolinium of the abdomen shows slice direction aliasing with the kidneys appearing to be in the lungs (*arrows*). Also note that there is aliasing in the phase-encoding direction (anteroposterior) from the inferior abdominal image's anterior subcutaneous tissue "wrapping around" posteriorly (*arrowheads*).

Figure 18-4. 3D coronal gradient-echo T1 image of the brain shows slice direction aliasing of the anterior skull on to the brain.

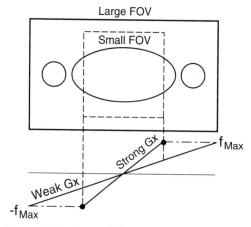

Figure 18-5. To avoid aliasing, increase the FOV.

if we use a **coil** that only covers the area within the FOV, we will only get signal from those body parts within the maximum frequency range, and no aliasing will result. This type of coil is called a **surface coil.** We also use a surface coil to increase the signal-to-noise ratio (SNR).

2. *Increase FOV:* If we double the FOV to include the entire area of study, we can eliminate aliasing. To do so, we have to use a weaker gradient. The maximum and minimum frequency range will cover a larger area, and all the body parts in the FOV will be included within the frequency bandwidth; therefore, no aliasing will result (Fig. 18-5). To maintain the resolution, double the matrix with a weaker gradient (G_x). The maximum and minimum frequency range will still be the same as the stronger gradient. They will just be spread out over a wider distance. Remember, to increase the FOV, we have to use a weaker gradient.

3. *Oversampling:* Two types are discussed:

   (a) Frequency oversampling (no frequency wrap [NFW])
   (b) Phase oversampling (no phase wrap [NPW])
      (a) *Frequency oversampling (NFW):* Frequency oversampling eliminates aliasing caused by **undersampling** in the frequency-encoding direction (refer to the sampling theorem in Chapter 12). **Oversampling** can also be performed in the phase-encoding direction by increasing

the number of phase-encoding gradients.

   (b) *Phase oversampling (NPW):* We can double the FOV to avoid aliasing and, at the end, discard the unwanted parts when the image is displayed (Fig. 18-6). This is called **no phase wrap** (NPW) by some manufacturers. It is also called **phase oversampling** by other manufacturers. Because N_y is doubled, NEX is halved to maintain the same scan time. Thus, the SNR is unchanged. (The scan time might be increased slightly because **overscanning** performs with slightly more than ½NEX.) An example of this is seen in Figure 18-7.

4. *Saturation pulses:* If we saturate the signals coming from outside the FOV, we can reduce aliasing.
5. *3D imaging:* In 3D imaging, if we see this artifact along the slice-select axis, we can simply discard the first and last few slices.

Chemical Shift Artifact. The principle behind the chemical shift artifact is that the protons from different molecules precess at slightly different frequencies. For example, look at fat and H_2O. A slight difference exists between the precessional frequencies of the hydrogen protons in fat and

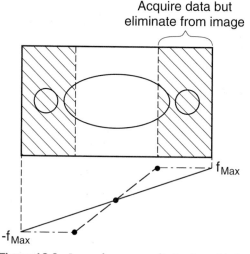

Figure 18-6. In no phase wrap, aliasing is avoided by doubling the FOV in the y direction and, at the end, discarding the unwanted part of the image.

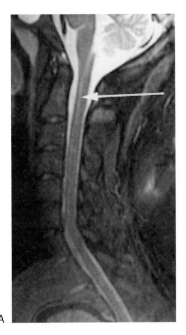
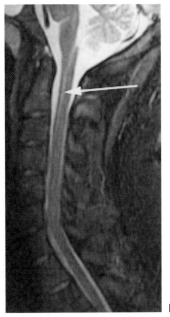

A   B

Figure 18-7. Sagittal STIR image (**A**) of the cervical spine with craniocaudal phase-encoding direction demonstrates aliasing of the brain onto the upper thoracic spine. (**B**) The same image after no phase wrap was applied. Truncation artifact is also seen (*arrows*).

H_2O. Actually, the protons in H_2O precess slightly faster than those in fat. This difference is only 3.5 ppm. Let's see what this means by an example.

Example

Consider a 1.5-T magnet. The precessional frequency is as follows:

1. Frequency $= \omega_0 = \gamma B_0$
   $= (42.6 \text{ MHz/T}) (1.5 \text{ T})$
   $\approx 64 \text{ MHz} = 64 \times 10^6 \text{ Hz}$
2. 3.5 ppm $= 3.5 \times 10^{-6}$
3. $(3.5 \times 10^{-6})(64 \times 10^6 \text{ Hz}) \cong 220 \text{ Hz}$

In other words, at 1.5 T, the difference in precessional frequency of the hydrogen protons in fat and in H_2O is 220 Hz.

Example

We now have a 0.5-T magnet. The precessional frequency of protons in a 0.5-T magnet is 1/3 of a 1.5-T magnet. The frequency difference is then

$$1/3(220 \text{ Hz}) = 73 \text{ Hz}$$

Therefore, at 0.5 T, the difference in precessional frequency of the hydrogen protons in fat and in H_2O is only 73 Hz. In other words, if we use a weaker magnet, we will get less chemical shift.

How does this affect the image? Chemical shift artifacts are seen in the orbits, along vertebral endplates, in the abdomen (at organ/fat interfaces), and anywhere else fatty structures

abut watery structures. In a 1.5-T magnet, the sampling time (T_s) is usually about 8 msec. Let's take 256 frequency points in the frequency-encoding direction.

$$\text{BW} = N/T_S$$
$$= 256/8 \text{ msec}$$
$$\text{BW} = 32 \text{ kHz}$$

These formulas show that the entire frequency range (i.e., bandwidth) of 32 kHz covers the whole length of the image in the x direction. Because we have the FOV of the image in the x direction divided into 256 pixels, each pixel is going to have a frequency range of its own, that is, each pixel has its own BW:

$$\text{BW/pixel} = 32 \text{ kHz}/256$$
$$\therefore \text{BW/pixel} = 125 \text{ Hz}$$

(This representation of BW on a "per pixel" basis is used by Siemens and Philips. It has the advantage of less ambiguity than the ± 16 kHz designation, should the "$\pm$" be deleted.) Thus, each pixel contains 125 Hz of information (Fig. 18-8). Stated differently, the pixel **bin** contains 125 Hz of frequencies. Now, because fat and H_2O differ in the precessional frequency of hydrogen by 220 Hz at 1.5 T, how many pixels does this difference correspond to?

$$\text{Pixel difference} = 220 \text{ Hz}/125 \text{ Hz/pixel}$$
$$\approx 2 \text{ pixels}$$

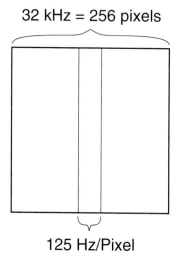

32 kHz = 256 pixels

125 Hz/Pixel

Figure 18-8. At 1.5 T with a BW of 32 kHz and 256 pixels, there will be about 125 Hz/pixel (32 kHz/256 = 125 Hz), that is, there is 125 Hz of information in each pixel. This may be a better way of describing the BW of a scanner because there is no ± confusion.

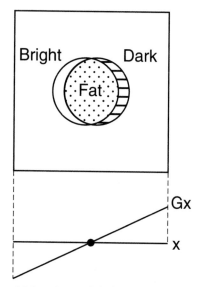

Figure 18-9. Chemical shift effect between fat and water causes a bright band toward the lower frequencies (due to overlap of fat and water at lower frequencies) and a dark band toward the higher frequencies (due to lack of fat and water signals).

This means that fat and H_2O protons are going to be **misregistered** from one another by about 2 pixels (in a 1.5-T magnet using a standard ±16 kHz bandwidth). (Actually, it is *fat* that is misregistered because position is determined by assuming the resonance property of water.) If pixel size $\Delta x = 1$ mm, this then translates into 2 mm misregistration of fat.

MATH: For the mathematically interested reader, it can be shown that

Chemical shift

$$= \frac{3.5 \times 10^{-6} \gamma \mathbf{B}}{BW/N_x} \text{(in pixels)}$$

$$= \frac{3.5 \times 10^{-6} \gamma \mathbf{B}}{BW/N_x} \times \frac{FOV}{N_x}$$

$$= \frac{3.5 \times 10^{-6} \gamma \mathbf{B} \times FOV}{BW/N_x} \text{(in mm)}$$

where $\gamma = 42.6$ MHz/T, $\mathbf{B}$ is the field strength (in T), BW is the bandwidth (in Hz), and FOV is the field of view (in cm).

Let's now consider chemical shift artifact visually (Fig. 18-9). Remember that H_2O protons resonate at a higher frequency compared with the hydrogen protons in fat. With the polarity of the frequency-encoding gradient in the x direction set such that higher frequencies

are toward the right, H_2O protons are relatively shifted to the right (toward the higher frequencies), and fat protons are relatively shifted to the left (toward the lower frequencies). This shifting will result in overlap at lower frequency and signal void at higher frequency. This in turn leads to a *bright band* toward the lower frequencies and a *dark band* toward the higher frequencies on a T1-weighted (T1W) or proton density (PD)-weighted conventional spin-echo (CSE) image. (On a T2W CSE, fat is dark, so the chemical shift artifact is reduced. Unfortunately, on a T2W FSE [fast spin echo—see Chapter 19], fat is bright, and the chemical shift artifact *is* seen.) We will see this misregistration artifact anywhere that we have a fat/H_2O interface. Also remember that this fat/H_2O chemical shift artifact only occurs in the frequency-encoding direction (in a conventional spin-echo image or in gradient-echo [GRE] imaging).

Example—Vertebral Bodies

With frequency-encoding direction—in this case, going up and down (and "up" having higher frequency)—the fat in the vertebral body would be misregistered down, making the lower endplate

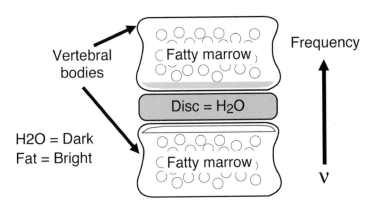

Figure 18-10. Chemical shift artifact in the vertebral endplates produces a dark band in the inferior endplates and a bright band in the superior endplates (assuming the frequency-encoding direction to be upward).

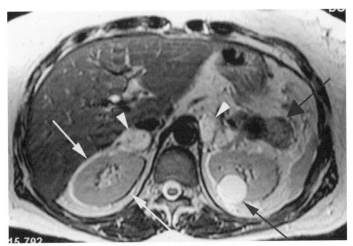

Figure 18-11. Axial T2 FSE image shows alternating bright and dark signal around the kidneys along the frequency-encoding (transverse) direction (*white arrows*). Patient also has bilateral pheochromocytomas (*white arrowheads*), a nonfunctioning islet cell tumor in the tail of pancreas (*wide black arrow*) and a simple cyst in the left kidney (*black arrow*). Patient had von Hippel–Lindau syndrome.

bright due to overlap of water and fat and the top endplate dark due to water alone (Fig. 18-10). If we increase the pixel size, the misregistration artifact will increase.

Figures 18-11 through 18-15 are examples of chemical shift artifact.

Question: What factors increase chemical shift artifact?

Answer:

1. *A stronger magnetic field strength*
2. *A lower BW:*

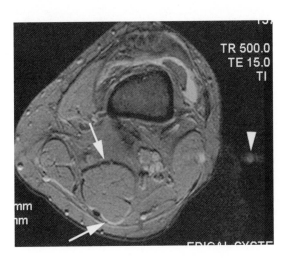

Figure 18-12. Axial T2* gradient-echo image of the knee shows first-order chemical shift (*arrows*) along the frequency direction (anteroposterior). Note that phase-encoding (transverse) direction "ghosting" artifact is also seen (*arrowhead*). A knee effusion is also demonstrated.

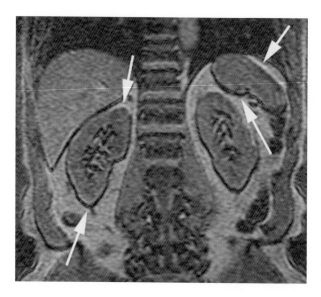

Figure 18-13. Coronal spoiled gradient-echo T1 (TR 93/TE 1.8 msec) image of the abdomen shows the typical alternating bands of dark and bright signal at the fat/water interfaces from chemical shift artifact along the frequency-encoding direction (cranio-caudal).

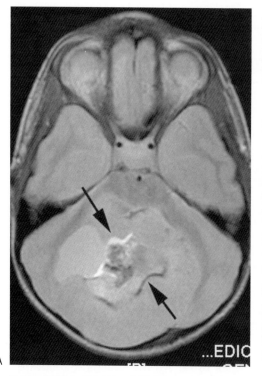

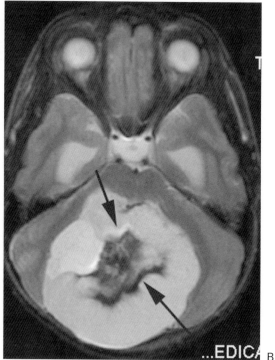

A

B

Figure 18-14. PD (**A**) and T2 (**B**) images of the posterior fossa show alternating bright and dark bands along the frequency-encoding direction (anteroposterior; *arrows*). Notice that the thickness of the artifact is wider in the T2 image secondary to a bandwidth (BW) of ± 4 kHz versus the PD image's BW of ± 16 kHz. Also note that the T2 image shows only the dark band well since the fat has low signal in this CSE T2 sequence, which minimizes the amount of bright signal. Patient had mature teratoma.

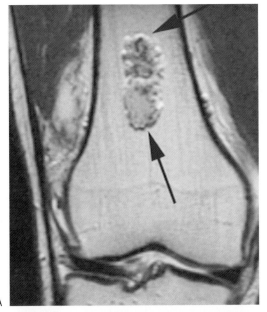

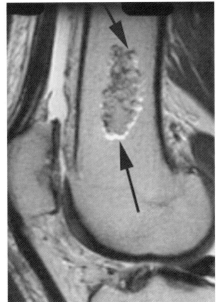

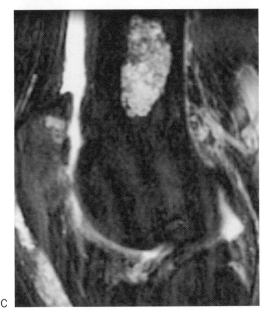

Figure 18-15. Coronal T2 (**A**) of the knee demonstrates chemical shift artifact in the frequency-encoding direction (craniocaudal) secondary to the fatty marrow juxtaposed to an enchondroma. Additional sagittal T2 (**B**) image again shows the artifact; however, now the bright and dark bands have swapped directions due to the frequency-encoding direction swapping (e.g., lower frequencies are superior in the coronal and inferior in the sagittal image). Finally, sagittal T2 image with chemical (spectral) fat saturation (**C**) shows no chemical shift effect.

If we decrease the BW, we have a lower BW per pixel and fewer frequencies/pixel. As an example, if instead of 32 kHz, we have a 16 kHz BW, then

$$BW/pixel = 160 \text{ kHz}/256$$
$$= 62.5 \text{ Hz/pixel}$$

Now, each pixel covers 62.5 Hz, but the chemical shift is still 220 Hz. Consequently,

220 Hz/62.5 Hz/pixel ≅ 4 pixel misregistration

Decreasing bandwidth results in increased chemical shift artifact.

This is one of the side effects of selecting a lower BW on your scanner. Unfortunately, the chemical shift due to field strength and that due to BW are independent and additive; thus, higher field/low BW techniques have the worst chemical shift artifact (Fig. 18-14).

3. Smaller pixels:

If we keep the BW of 32 kHz and the FOV the same but increase the number of frequency-encoding steps to 512 (instead of 256), the pixel bin will have half as many frequencies:

$$\text{Pixel bin} = 32 \text{ kHz}/512$$
$$= 62.5 \text{ Hz/pixel}$$

again leading to a greater chemical shift, as above (i.e., 4 pixels instead of 2).

Solution. How can you fix chemical shift artifacts?

1. Get rid of fat using fat suppression. If there is no signal from fat, there can be no chemical shift. This can be done with a spectroscopic "fat sat" pulse or a STIR sequence (Fig. 18-15).
2. Increase pixel size by keeping FOV the same and decreasing N_x (trade-off: deteriorates resolution).
3. Lower the magnet's field strength (not practical!).

4. Increase bandwidth (trade-off: lowers SNR).
5. Switch phase and frequency directions. This will just change the direction of the chemical shift.
6. Use a long TE (causes more dephasing and less signal from fat).

Chemical Shift of the "Second Kind." This phenomenon applies to GRE techniques (see Chapters 20 and 21). As discussed previously, fat and water protons precess at slightly different frequencies in the transverse plane (220 Hz at 1.5 T). Because water precesses faster, it gets $360°$ *ahead* of fat after a short period of time. Thus, there will be times (TE) when fat and water spins will be totally in phase and times when they will be $180°$ out of phase. At 1.5 T, fat and water are in phase every 4.5 msec. This number is derived by the following:

Frequency difference between fat and water
$= 220$ Hz
Period $= 1$ frequency $= 1/(220 \text{ Hz})$
$= 0.0045$ sec $= 4.5$ msec

In Figure 18-16, fat and water are in phase initially at TE $= 0$ msec, go out of phase at TE $= 2.25$ msec, and are back in phase at TE $= 4.5$ msec. In general, at 1.5 T, fat and H_2O go in and

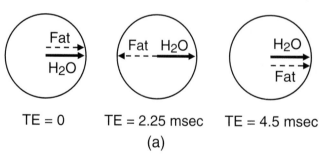

(a)

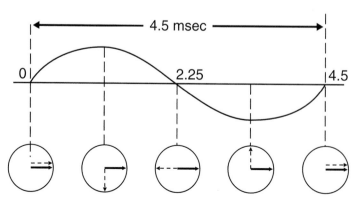

Figure 18-16. Chemical shift effect of the second kind. Fat and water protons get in and out of phase at various values of TE. Specifically, they are in phase at TE of 0, 4.5, and 9 msec and out of phase at TE of 2.25, 6.75 msec, and so on. This effect can be represented graphically by a sine function.

out of phase every 2.25 msec. This is called a **chemical shift effect of the second kind**.

Boundary Effect. If the selected TE is 2.25, 6.75, 11.25, 15.75 msec, and so on, fat and water protons will be out of phase and a dark boundary will be seen around organs that are surrounded by fat (such as the kidneys and muscles). This result is called the **boundary effect, bounce point artifact**, or **India Ink Etching**, which is caused by chemical shift of the second kind. This type of imaging is referred to as **out-of-phase** scanning, referring to the fact that at these TEs, fat and water spins will be 180° out of phase. This phenomenon does not just occur along the frequency-encoding axis (as with the chemical shift artifact of the first kind) because it is a result of fat and water protons phase cancellation in all directions (Fig. 18-17). (Boundary effect does not occur in conventional SE techniques because

of the presence of the 180° refocusing pulse, which is absent in GRE techniques.)

Remedy

1. Make fat and H_2O in phase by picking appropriate TE.
2. Increase the BW (trade-off: decreases SNR).
3. Use fat suppression.

Truncation Artifact (Gibbs Phenomenon). This artifact occurs at high contrast interfaces (e.g., skull/brain, cord/cerebrospinal fluid (CSF), meniscus/fluid in the knee) and causes alternating bright and dark bands that may be mistaken for lesions (e.g., pseudo syrinx of the spinal cord or pseudo tear of the knee meniscus).

The cause is inability to approximate exactly a steplike change in the signal intensity due to a limited number of samples or sampling time. The ripples in Figure 18-18 are responsible for

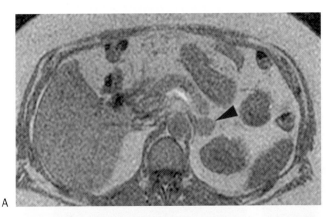

A

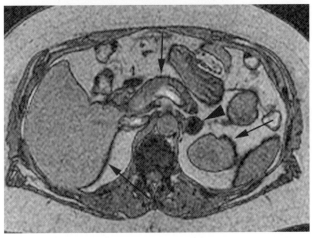

B

Figure 18-17. In-phase (**A**) and out-of-phase (**B**) spoiled gradient T1 images show the "boundary effect" on the out-of-phase images circumferentially at every fat/water interface (*arrows* in **B**). Also note that a left adrenal adenoma loses signal substantially on the out-of-phase image (*arrowhead*).

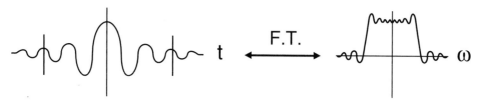

Figure 18-18. Truncation artifact causes a ring-down effect because the FT of a truncated sinc function has ripples at its edges.

the parallel bands seen at such sharp interfaces. This artifact is seen mostly in the phase direction (because we typically have few pixels and lower resolution in phase compared with frequency). Incidentally, the correct term is "truncation artifact." "Gibbs phenomenon" refers to the infinitely thin discontinuity that still persists with an infinite number of pixel elements. Figures 18-7, 18-19, and 18-20 contain examples of truncation artifact.

Remedy

1. Increase sampling time (↓ BW) to reduce the ripples. (Remember, a wider signal in time domain means a narrower one in frequency domain.)

2. Decrease pixel size:
   (a) increasing the number of phase encodes, and
   (b) decreasing the FOV

Partial Volume Artifact. This artifact has the same concept as computerized tomography (CT). To reduce it, decrease the slice thickness (Δz). Figure 18-21 contains an example of partial volume artifact.

Patient-Related Artifact

This artifact is caused by voluntary or involuntary patient motion and by the patient's anatomy. Pulsating motion in vessels is also an

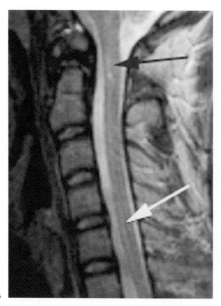

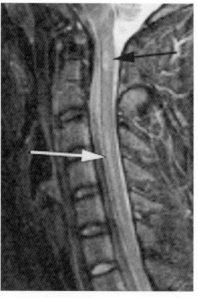

A   B

Figure 18-19. Sagittal fat-saturated T2 image (**A**) shows minimal truncation artifact (*white arrow*); a sagittal STIR image (**B**) shows wider truncation artifact (*white arrow*). The T2 image was obtained with 224 phase-encoding steps, and the STIR used 192 steps. Patient also had a small nonhemorrhagic cord contusion at C1/2 (*black arrows* in **A** and **B**).

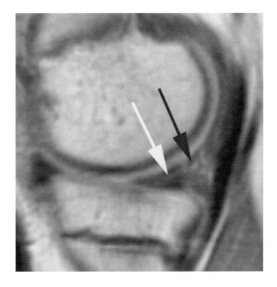

Figure 18-20. Proton density sagittal image of the knee shows truncation artifact mimicking posterior medial meniscus tear (*white arrow*). Note extension of high signal beyond the meniscus (*black arrow*).

interesting source of motion-related artifacts. (More on this in later chapters.)

Motion Artifact. Motion artifact is caused by the patient's (voluntary or involuntary) movements (**random**) or by pulsating flow in vessels (**periodic**). We only get motion artifacts in the *phase-encoding* direction.

Question: Why is motion artifact only seen in the phase-encoding direction?

Answer: The reason is twofold:

1. *First of all, motion along any magnetic field gradient results in abnormal phase accumulation, which mismaps the signal along the phase-encoding gradient.*

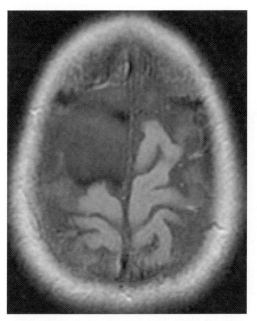

A

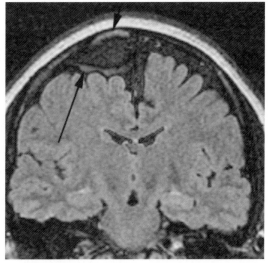

B

Figure 18-21. Axial FLAIR image (**A**) shows some signal within a right convexity lesion that would not be consistent with a simple arachnoid cyst. Additional coronal FLAIR image (**B**) shows the signal to be around, but not in, the lesion (*arrows*). The high signal on the axial image was due to partial volume averaging. The high signal was flow-related enhancement of CSF flowing around the cyst.

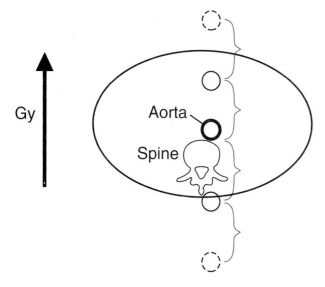

Gy

Aorta

Spine

Figure 18-22. Ghost artifacts are equidistant replica of a pulsating structure, such as the aorta, along the phase direction.

2. *Also, there is a significant asymmetry in the data space (see Chapter 13) so that it takes much less time to sample the signal via frequency encoding (on the order of milliseconds) than to do a single phase-encoding step (on the order of seconds). Thus, most motions experienced during clinical MRI are much slower than the rapid sampling process along the frequency-encoding axis. This disparity between frequency- and phase-encoding periods allows motion artifacts to be propagated mainly along the phase-encoding axis. Motion artifacts along the frequency-encoding axis may occur, but they are insignificant (at best, they may cause minimal blurring).*

Periodic Motion. Periodic motion is caused by pulsating or periodic motion of vessels, heart, or CSF. In the example in Figure 18-22 (also Fig. 18-23), with a cross section of the body through the aorta, and with the phase-encoding in the AP direction, we will get "ghost" artifacts of the aorta equally separated. The artifacts become fainter with increasing distance from the original structure. The separation (SEP) between the "ghosts" is given by

$$SEP = \frac{(TR)(N_y)(NEX)}{T(motion)}$$

Another way of expressing this is

$$SEP = \text{acquisition time}/T(motion)$$

where T(motion) is the period of motion of the object (in this case, the aorta).

Example
The aorta pulsates according to the heart rate. If the heart rate is

$$HR = 60 \text{ beats/min} = 60 \text{ bpm} = 1 \text{ beat/sec}$$

then the period of motion = T(motion) = 1 sec.

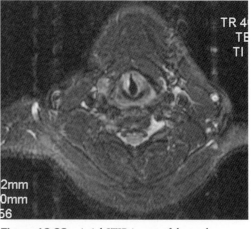

Figure 18-23. Axial STIR image of the neck showed marked ghosting from both arteries and veins in the phase-encoding direction (anteroposterior).

This means that we have a pulsation every 1 sec. For example, if we have a TR = 500 msec = 0.5 sec, NEX = 1, N_x = 256, then

$$SEP = 0.5 \times 256/1 = 128/1 = 128 \text{ pixels}$$

Therefore, we get two ghosts in the image. If the heart rate is 120 bpm, then we get

$$SEP = 128/0.5 = 256 \text{ pixels}$$

and only one ghost.

$$SEP = \frac{(TR)(N_y)(NEX)}{T(\text{motion})}$$
$$= \text{Separation between ghosts (in pixels)}$$

If we multiply this by pixel size, we get the distance between the "ghosts." Therefore, if we increase TR, number of phase-encoding steps, or NEX, we can increase the separation of ghosts so that they won't be so numerous within the body part we're studying. More rapidly pulsating flow (i.e., shorter period) also causes more separation. If the FOV is too small, the "ghost" images outside the FOV might get "aliased" into the FOV. The ghosts may be dark or bright depending on the phase of the pulsating structure with respect to the phase of the background. If they are in phase, they'll be bright, and if they are out of phase, they'll be dark—Figures 18-24 and 18-25.

Remedy

1. Use spatial presaturation pulses to saturate inflowing protons and reduce the artifacts.

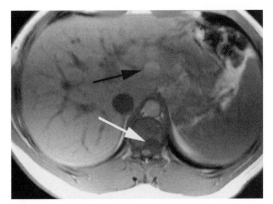

Figure 18-24. Axial spoiled gradient image of the abdomen shows both positive (*black arrow*) and negative (*white arrow*) "ghost" artifacts from the aorta. The negative "ghost" mimics a vertebral body lesion.

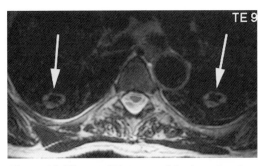

Figure 18-25. Axial T2 image of the thoracic spine shows positive "ghost" artifacts from the CSF that simulate lung nodules.

2. Increase separation between ghosts by increasing TR, N_y, or NEX (which is tantamount to increasing scan time).
3. Swap phase and frequency: although this only changes the direction of the artifacts, it does allow differentiation between a true lesion and an artifact.
4. Use cardiac gating.
5. Use flow compensation.

Random Motion. Random motion is caused by the patient's voluntary or involuntary movements (e.g., breathing, changing position, swallowing, tremors, and coughing). It causes blurring of the image. We may get parallel bands in the phase-encoding direction as well (Fig. 18-26). Although

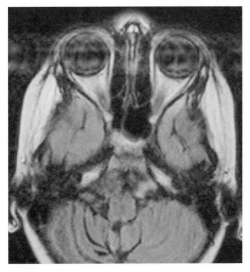

Figure 18-26. Axial FLAIR image shows marked motion artifact in the phase-encoding direction (transverse) from eye movement.

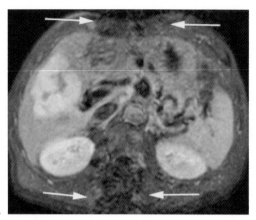 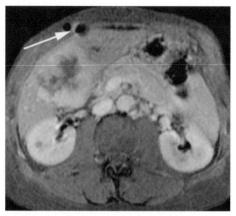

Figure 18-27. Axial CSE T1 image with fat saturation post gadolinium (**A**) shows both periodic and random phase direction (anteroposterior) artifact (*arrows*). A breath-hold spoiled gradient T1 image with fat saturation post gadolinium (**B**) shows near complete resolution of motion artifact. Note that there is increased magnetic susceptibility artifact (*arrow* in **B**) in the gradient-echo image. Patient had a liver hemangioma.

this may simulate truncation artifacts, it is different in that truncation causes *fading* parallel bands.

Remedy

1. Patient instruction: Don't move! (probably the most useful remedy)
2. Respiratory compensation (RC) (uses chest wall motion pattern to reorder scan and minimize motion)
3. Use of glucagon in the abdomen to reduce artifacts due to bowel peristalsis
4. Sedation
5. Pain killers
6. Faster scanning (FSE, GRE, EPI, etc.); sequential 2D rather than 3D scanning (see Fig. 18-27 for an example).

CSF Flow Effects. Dephasing of protons due to CSF motion may sometimes simulate a lesion. Flow compensation techniques can reduce this effect. Examples include the following:

1. Pseudo aneurysm of basilar artery due to pulsatile radial motion of CSF around it (Fig. 18-28).
2. Pseudo MS plaques in the brainstem due to CSF flow in the basal cisterns.
3. Pseudo disc herniation, again secondary to CSF flow.

Remedy

1. Be certain that "lesions" are seen on all pulse sequences (artifacts tend to only be seen on one image).
2. Use cardiac gating.
3. Use flow compensation.

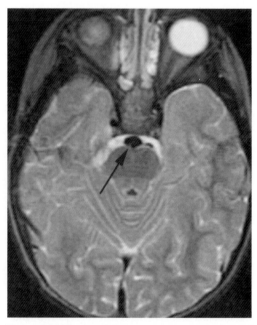

Figure 18-28. Axial T2 image shows marked signal void around the basilar artery mimicking an aneurysm in this 3-year-old patient.

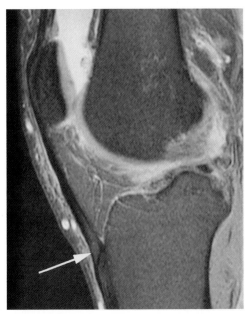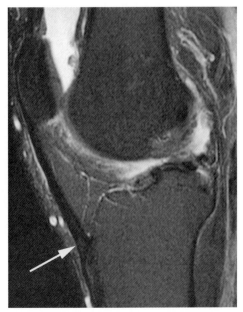

A   B

Figure 18-29. Sagittal PD (**A**) and T2 (**B**) fat-saturated images of the knee show magic angle artifact as seen by increased signal on the short TE PD image (*arrow* in **A**), whereas the tendon itself is not thickened and has dark signal on the T2 image (**B**). Joint effusion is also seen. (Courtesy of D. Beall, MD, San Antonio, Texas.)

Magic Angle Artifacts. In imaging the joints, if a tendon is oriented at a certain angle (55°) relative to the main magnetic field, then the tendon appears brighter on T1- and PD-weighted images, but normal on T2-weighted images. This artifactual increased intensity might potentially be confused with pathology.

Collagen, which is responsible for the majority of tendon composition, has an **anisotropic** structure. This anisotropic structure has properties that vary with the direction of measurement and is responsible for dependence of T2 of tendons on their orientation. (**Isotropic** structures, however, have properties independent of their orientation.)

At the magic angle, the T2 of the tendon is slightly increased. This increase is negligible when TE is long. However, when TE is short (as in T1- or PD-weighted images), the result is increased signal intensity. The mathematics behind this T2 prolongation has to do with some of the mathematical terms in the Hamiltonian going to zero at $\theta = 55°$ (see Figs. 18-29 and 18-30 for examples).

MATH: This **magic angle** effect is the solution to the equation

$$3(\cos \theta)^2 - 1 = 0 \rightarrow (\cos \theta)^2 = 1/3$$

or

$$\cos \theta = \sqrt{1/3}$$

which is calculated to be $\theta \approx 55°$. The above equation comes from a complicated mathematical theory dealing with the so-called **dipolar Hamiltonian.**

RF-Related Artifacts

Cross-talk. We have already discussed this issue in previous chapters. The problem arises from the fact that the Fourier transform (FT) of the RF pulse is not a perfect rectangle but rather has side lobes (Fig. 18-31). We shall use a simpler version of the RF profile, as in Figure 18-32. If we consider two adjacent slices, there will be an overlap in the FT of their RF pulses (Fig. 18-32). Cross-talk causes the effective TR per slice to decrease (due to saturation of protons by the RF signals for adjacent slices). Thus, more

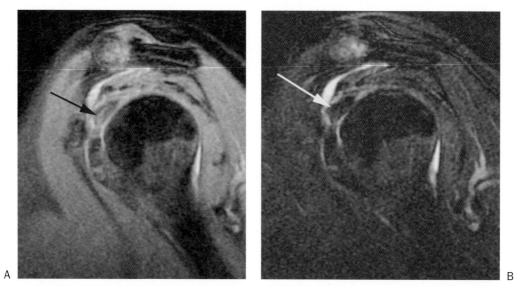

A   B

Figure 18-30. Angled sagittal PD (**A**) and T2 (**B**) fat-saturated images of the shoulder demonstrate magic angle artifact of the intra-articular biceps tendon. There is increased signal on the PD image (**A**), whereas the tendon has dark signal and overall normal appearance on the T2 image. Acromioclavicular joint high signal is from osteoarthritis changes. (Courtesy of D. Beall, MD, San Antonio, Texas.)

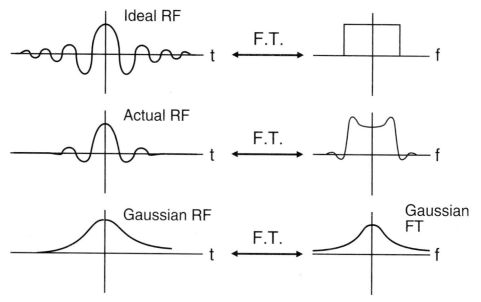

Figure 18-31. The actual RF has a finite time span, yielding side lobes or rings. A Gaussian RF pulse has a Gaussian FT.

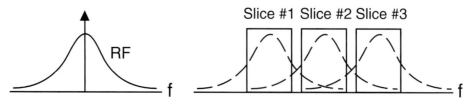

Figure 18-32. Side lobes of the FT of RF pulses (such as in the case of Gaussian curves) may overlap, causing cross-talk.

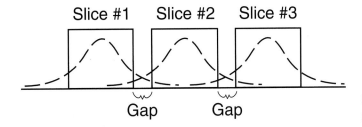

Figure 18-33. To reduce cross-talk, gaps are introduced between slices.

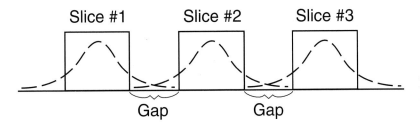

Figure 18-34. The larger the interslice gap is, the less cross-talk is observed.

T1 weighting will result (this is particularly problematic for PD- and T2-weighted images). Also, due to reduced effective TR, the SNR will decrease.

In short, cross-talk causes increased T1 weighting and decreased SNR.

Remedy

1. Gaps can be introduced between adjacent slices (Fig. 18-33).
2. Two acquisitions with 100% gaps can be interleaved.
3. The RF pulse can be lengthened to achieve a more rectangular pulse profile.

Let's discuss these in more detail:

1. If we increase the gap between slices, we reduce cross-talk (Fig. 18-34). The *trade-off* is an increase in the unsampled volume and the increased potential for missing a small lesion located within the gap.
2. It doesn't matter which way we order the slices (we can do slice 1, then slice 3, then slice 2, etc.). Adjacent slices still will be sharing a certain frequency range and cause cross-talk. The only way to eliminate cross-talk is to do two separate sequences each with a 100% gap, such as:

First sequence: odd slices 1, 3, 5, 7, …
Next sequence: even slices 2, 4, 6, 8, …

This is the technique of "true" interleaving. Interleaving within a *single* sequence will not totally eliminate cross-talk, although it might reduce it somewhat. The interslice gap in this case is usually 25% to 50% of the slice thickness and a simple sequence is performed. Interleaving in the true sense, however, will double the scan time because it employs two separate sequences.

Contiguous Slices. The RF pulse on newer scanners more closely approximates a rectangular wave (Fig. 18-35). With this feature, we may have a 10% to 20% interslice gap without significant cross-talk. However, with reduced interslice gap, we reduce coverage and need more slices. Remember, we are talking trade-offs again.

RF Zipper Artifact. This artifact is one form of **central artifacts** (the other form is RF feedthrough,

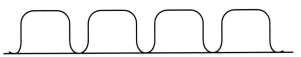

Figure 18-35. The closer the profile of the RF pulse (actually its FT) is to a rectangle, the better we can achieve contiguous slices without encountering cross-talk.

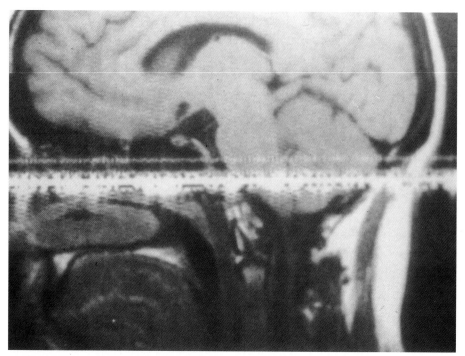

Figure 18-36. Zipper artifact at zero phase.

discussed later). They are referred to as **zippers** due to the formation of a central stripe of alternating bright and dark spots along the *frequency*-encoding axis (at zero phase), as in Figure 18-36. Two sources of zipper artifacts are discussed here.

FID Artifacts. Free induction decay (FID) artifacts occur due to overlapping of side lobes of the 180° pulse with the FID, before it has had a chance to completely decay (Fig. 18-37). This overlapping causes a "zipper" artifact along the *frequency*-encoding direction.

Remedy

1. Increase the TE (increases the separation between the FID and the 180° RF pulse).
2. Increase slice thickness (Δz). This in effect results from selecting a wide RF BW, which narrows the RF signal in the time domain, thus lowering chances for overlap.

Stimulated Echo. This artifact also appears as a narrow- or wide-band noise in the center along the *frequency*-encoding axis. The mechanism is similar to FID artifacts. In this case, imperfect RF

pulses of adjacent slices or imperfect 90° −180° −180° pulses of a dual-echo sequence form a stimulated echo that may not be phase-encoded, thus appearing in the central line along the frequency-encoding axis.

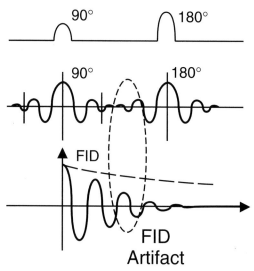

Figure 18-37. FID artifact. The side lobes of the 180° and the FID may overlap, causing a zipper artifact at zero frequency along the phase direction.

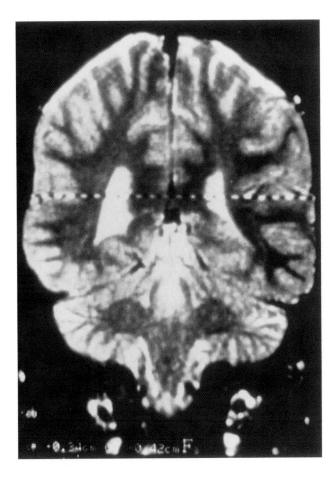

Figure 18-38. RF feedthrough causes a zipper artifact at zero frequency along the phase direction.

Remedy
   1. Use spoiler gradients.
   2. Adjust the transmitter.
   3. Call the service engineer.

RF Feedthrough Zipper Artifact. This artifact occurs when the *excitation* RF pulse is not completely gated off during data acquisition and "feeds" through the receiver coil. It appears as a "zipper" stripe along the *phase*-encoding axis at *zero* frequency (Fig. 18-38).

Remedy. Alternate the phase of the excitation RF pulses by 180° on successive acquisitions; the averaged phase-alternated excitations will essentially eliminate RF feedthrough.

RF Noise. RF noise is caused by unwanted *external* RF noise (e.g., TV channel, a radio station, a flickering fluorescent light, patient electronic monitoring equipment). It is similar to RF feedthrough except that it occurs at the specific frequency (or frequencies) of the unwanted RF pulse(s) rather than at zero frequency (Fig. 18-39).

Remedy

   1. Improve RF shielding.
   2. Remove monitoring devices if possible.
   3. Shut the door of the magnet room!

External Magnetic Field Artifacts

Artifacts related to B_0 are usually caused by magnetic inhomogeneities. These nonuniformities are usually due to improper shimming, environmental factors, or the far extremes of newer short-bore magnets. This can lead to

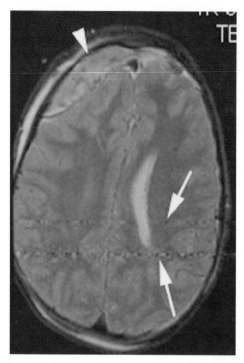

Figure 18-39. Axial T2 image shows RF noise (*arrows*) from monitoring devices in this recent post-operative patient. There is also an epidural hematoma (*arrowhead*).

image distortion (Fig. 18-40). They can be reduced in SE and FSE imaging by using 180° refocusing pulses. They can be a source of image inhomogeneity when a fat suppression technique is used.

In GRE imaging, small spatial nonuniformities cause **moiré fringes** (zebra pattern) due to the overlay of the primary image and aliased overlay (Fig. 18-41).

Remedy. Appropriate **shimming coils (auto shimming)** can minimize the problem.

Magnetic Susceptibility Artifacts

As discussed in Chapter 2, all substances get magnetized to a degree when placed in a magnetic field, and their **magnetic susceptibility** (denoted by the Greek symbol χ) is a measure of how magnetized they get.

There are three types of substances—each with a different magnetic susceptibility—commonly dealt with in MRI: paramagnetic, diamagnetic, and ferromagnetic. These substances were described in Chapter 2 and are briefly reviewed here:

1. **Diamagnetic** substances with no unpaired electrons have negative magnetic susceptibility χ (i.e., $\chi < 0$ and $\mu = 1 + \chi < 1$). They are basically nonmagnetic. The vast majority of tissues in the body have this property.

2. **Paramagnetic** substances contain unpaired electrons, have a small positive χ (i.e., $\chi > 0$ and $\mu > 1$), and are weakly attracted by the external magnetic field. The rare-earth element **gadolinium** (Gd) with seven unpaired electrons is a strong paramagnetic substance. Gd is a member of the **lanthanide** group in the periodic table. The rare-earth element **dysprosium** (Dy) is another strong paramagnetic substance that belongs to this group. Certain breakdown products of hemoglobin are paramagnetic: deoxyhemoglobin has four unpaired electrons and methemoglobin has five. Hemosiderin, the end stage of hemorrhage, contains, in comparison, more than 10,000 unpaired electrons. It is in a group of substances referred to as **superparamagnetic,** with magnetic susceptibilities 100 to 1000 times stronger than paramagnetic substances.

3. **Ferromagnetic** substances are strongly attracted by a magnetic field and have a large positive χ, even larger than that of superparamagnetic substances. Three types of ferromagnets are known: iron (Fe), cobalt (Co), and nickel (Ni). Susceptibility artifacts in MRI occur at interfaces of differing magnetic susceptibilities, such as at tissue–air and tissue–fat interfaces (examples include paranasal sinuses, skull base, and sella). These differences in susceptibilities lead to a distortion in the local magnetic environment, causing dephasing of spins, with signal loss, mismapping (artifacts), and poor chemical fat saturation

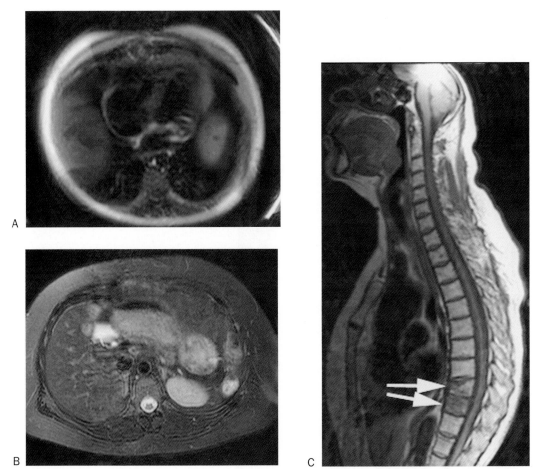

Figure 18-40. Axial T2 fat-suppressed image (**A**) shows distortion of the upper abdomen and lack of effective fat saturation secondary to magnetic field inhomogeneities at the fringe of a short-bore magnet. Comparative slice more inferiorly (**B**) has expected fat saturation and normal appearance without distortion. In another patient (**C**), a sagittal T1 image of the spine shows distortion of the extreme cranial and caudal features in a short-bore magnet. Patient also had two lower thoracic spine compression fractures (*arrows*).

(Figs. 18-42 through 18-44). Ferromagnetic substances (such as metallic clips and foreign bodies), with their large susceptibilities, lead to substantial field distortion and artifacts (Figs. 18-45 through 18-47).

Question: Which MR technique is least sensitive to magnetic susceptibility effects?

Answer: In decreasing order, echo planar imaging (EPI), gradient-echo (GRE) imaging, conventional spin echo (CSE), and fast spin-echo (FSE). FSE is least sensitive to magnetic susceptibility effects due to the presence of multiple refocusing 180° gradients.

Gradient-Related Artifacts

Eddy Currents. Eddy currents are small electric currents that are generated when the gradients are rapidly switched on and off (i.e., the resulting sudden rises and falls in the magnetic field produce electric currents). These currents will result in a distortion in the gradient profile (Fig. 18-48) and in turn cause artifacts in the image.

Nonlinearities. Ideal gradients are linear. However, as in other aspects of life, there is no such thing as an ideal gradient. These nonlinearities cause local magnetic distortions and image

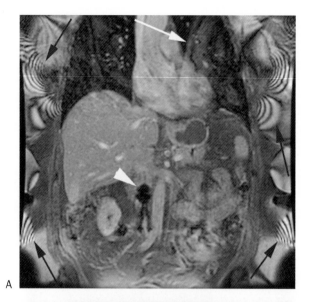

A

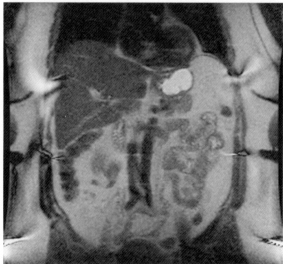

B

Figure 18-41. Coronal postgadolinium spoiled gradient T1 image with chemical (spectral) fat saturation (**A**) shows moiré fringes (*black arrows*). Comparison with single-shot FSE (SSFSE) T2 (**B**) image demonstrates decreased artifact. Also note ghosting on image **A** from the heart and aorta (*white arrow*) and increased magnetic susceptibility from an inferior vena cava (IVC) filter (*white arrowhead*).

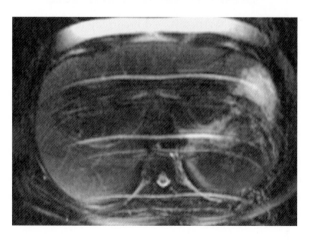

Figure 18-42. Axial T2 FSE with inhomogeneous fat saturation shows "ghosting" artifact from the unsaturated anterior abdominal subcutaneous fat.

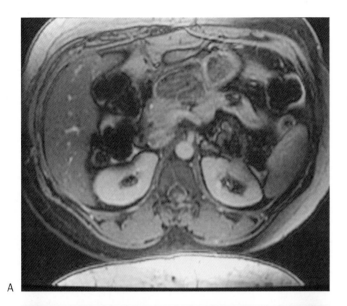

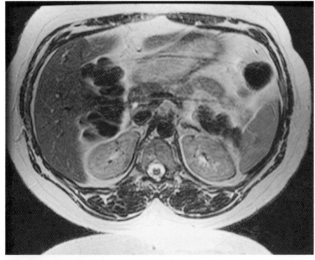

Figure 18-43. Axial postgadolinium fat-saturated gradient-echo T1 image of the abdomen (**A**) shows "blooming" artifact from the interface of the diamagnetic gas and the adjacent soft tissues (best at the splenic flexure). This effect is minimized on the T2 FSE (**B**) image. Note aliasing in the phase-encoding (anteroposterior) direction on both images. Image **A** also has inhomogeneous fat saturation at the diamagnetic interface.

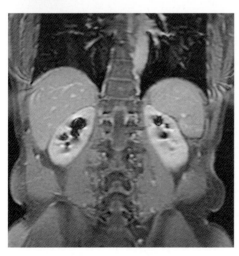

Figure 18-44. Coronal postgadolinium gradient-echo T1 image with fat saturation shows magnetic susceptibility from the densely concentrated paramagnetic substance gadolinium, resulting in dark renal collecting systems with a fringe of bright signal. Also note mild moiré fringes artifact.

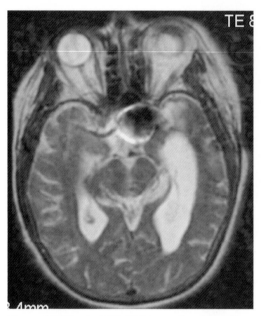

Figure 18-45. Axial T2 FSE image shows metallic susceptibility artifact from an MRI compatible aneurysm clip in the area of the left internal carotid terminus.

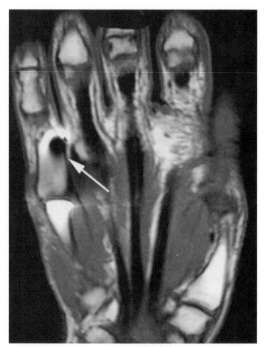

Figure 18-46. Coronal T1 image shows metallic susceptibility from metallic foreign body at the base of the fifth digit.

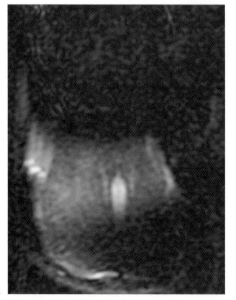

A

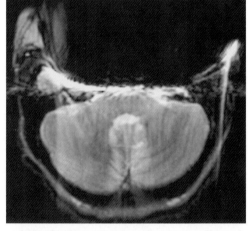

B

Figure 18-47. Axial EPI B_0 (**A**), CSE T2 (**B**), CSE PD (**C**), and FSE T2 (**D**) images show the varying effects of different pulse sequences on metallic susceptibility in a patient with dental braces. The EPI is the worst. The CSE T2 is worse than the PD due to a lower BW (± 4 kHz) for the T2 versus the higher BW (± 16 kHz) for the PD. Finally, the T2 FSE is the best (BW still ± 16 kHz), secondary to multiple 180° refocusing pulses.

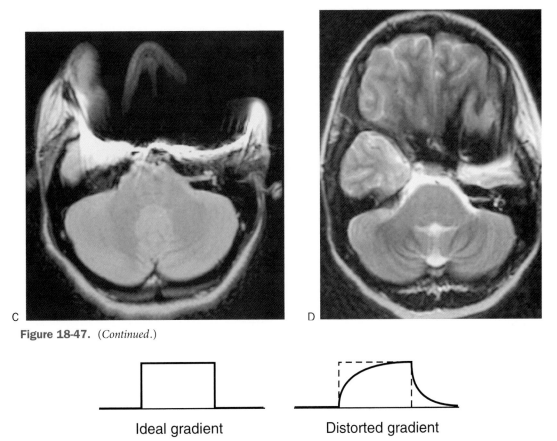

C   D

Figure 18-47. (*Continued.*)

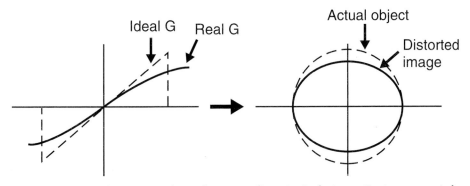

Ideal gradient   Distorted gradient

Figure 18-48. Eddy currents result from rapid on-and-off switching of the gradient and cause distortion in the gradient profile and thus the image.

Figure 18-49. Nonlinearities in the gradient cause distortion in the image. For instance, a circle may appear elliptical.

artifacts. The effect is similar to artifacts related to B_0 inhomogeneities.

Geometric Distortion. Geometric distortion is a consequence of gradient nonlinearities or gradient power drop-off. Figure 18-49 illustrates this concept. The real gradient has dampened peaks, causing image distortion (e.g., a circle may appear elliptical). (Figure 18-50 is an example due to gradient nonlinearities in the more demanding echo planar sequence.) If you find this is a problem, then you need to call your service engineer to fix it.

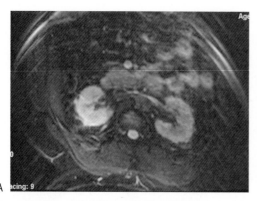
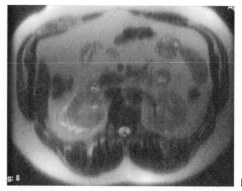

Figure 18-50. Axial T2-weighted EPI image (**A**) of the abdomen shows geometric distortion of the normal ovoid shape of the abdomen. An accompanying SSFSE T2 image (**B**) shows this patient's true shape.

Errors in the Data

Errors in the data are caused by a single calculation error in processing the data related to the k-space of a single slice. The result is a crisscross striation artifact that is present across a single image and not present on any other image. (See Figure 18-51.)

Remedy
1. Delete the discrete error and average out the neighboring data.
2. Simply repeating the sequence solves the problem.

Flow-Related Artifacts

Motion artifacts were discussed previously, including periodic flow artifacts. Other flow-related phenomena are discussed in Chapters 26 and 27.

Dielectric Effects

As the wavelength of the radiowave approaches the dimensions of the body part being imaged, there can be areas of brightening and darkening due to standing waves. This is most pronounced at 3 T and above. Since the body is a conducting medium, the artifact is often called "dielectric effect" (Fig. 18-52). It seems to be worse in large body parts, that is, the abdomen, and seems to be quite common when ascites is present. The solution for dielectric effects is parallel transmission or "transmit SENSE."

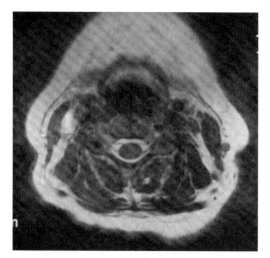

Figure 18-51. Axial T2-weighted image of the cervical spine on a 0.23 T magnet shows diagonal lines coursing throughout the image related to a single data point error in k-space.

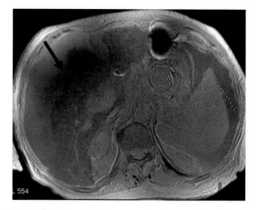

Figure 18-52. 3.0 T proton density–weighted image of the abdomen demonstrates cirrhosis and ascites with regional area of decreased signal intensity due to dielectric effect or "standing waves" (*arrow*).

Key Points

In this chapter, we discussed the most common and important causes of potential artifacts in MR imaging that every MR radiologist should be aware of. For a list of these artifacts, refer to the *Introduction* in this chapter. There are a few other less significant sources of artifacts that were not discussed in this chapter.

Questions

18-1 Regarding chemical shift artifact:
   (a) protons in fat resonate at 3.5 ppm higher than protons in water
   (b) at 1.5 T it is about 220 Hz
   (c) at 1.5 T and for a 32 kHz BW and 256×256 matrix, it is about 2 pixels
   (d) all of the above
   (e) only (b) and (c)

18-2 (a) Determine the chemical shifts (in terms of numbers of pixels) for the following situations (assume 256 frequency-encoding steps):

B_0	0.2 T	0.5 T	1.0 T	1.5 T
BW				
50 kHz				
10 kHz				
4 kHz				

   (b) Repeat this table in terms of millimeters, given an FOV = 24 cm = 240 mm.
   (c) What is your conclusion?

18-3 Periodic motion causes "ghost" artifacts along the phase-encoding direction. The number of *pixels* between two consecutive ghosts is given by (SEP = separation)

$$SEP = TR \cdot NEX \cdot N_y / T$$
$$= \text{acquisition time}/T$$

where T = period of the oscillating motion.
   (a) Calculate SEP for the aortic ghosts (HR = 60 bpm, i.e., T = 1 sec) when TR = 200 msec = 0.2 sec, NEX = 1, N_y = 256.
   (b) What is the maximum number of ghosts you could potentially see along the phase-encoding axis in example (a)?
   (c) What is the effect of increasing NEX?

18-4 Wraparound can be reduced by all of the following *except:*
   (a) using a surface coil
   (b) decreasing the FOV
   (c) using presaturation pulses
   (d) using a no phase wrap option
   (e) using a no frequency wrap option

18-5 Truncation artifacts can be reduced by all of the following *except:*
   (a) decreasing pixel size
   (b) increasing sampling time
   (c) increasing N_y
   (d) increasing FOV

18-6 T/F Chemical shift artifact causes a bright band toward the higher frequency and a dark band toward the lower frequency at a water/fat interface.

18-7 Chemical shift is decreased by all of the following *except:*
   (a) lowering the bandwidth
   (b) using a fat suppression technique
   (c) using a lower field magnet
   (d) using a longer TE

18-8 T/F Fat and water protons get out of phase at TE of odd multiples of 2.25 msec.

18-9 Chemical shift in general can be represented by
   (a) $3.5 \times 10^{-6} \gamma B \cdot N_x / BW$
   (b) $3.5 \times 10^{-6} \gamma B \cdot FOV / BW$
   (c) $3.5 \times 10^{-6} \gamma B / (BW \cdot N_x)$
   (d) both (a) and (b)

18-10 (a) Calculate the separation (in pixels and mm) between aortic ghosts for TR 500 msec, NEX 1, N_y 128, HR 80 bpm, and FOV 20 cm.
   (b) What is the maximum number of ghosts you could potentially see within the FOV?

18-11 Paramagnetic elements include all of the following *except:*
   (a) gadolinium
   (b) dysprosium
   (c) cobalt
   (d) methemoglobin
   (e) both (c) and (d)

18-12 Motion artifacts can be reduced by all of the following *except:*
   (a) fast scanning
   (b) sedation
   (c) 3D imaging
   (d) flow compensation

18-13 CSF flow can lead to all of the following artifacts *except:*
   (a) pseudo MS plaques in the brainstem
   (b) pseudo disc herniation
   (c) pseudo basilar artery aneurysm
   (d) pseudo syrinx

18-14 **T/F** Magic angle artifact demonstrates increased signal on proton density images in a tendon that is positioned perpendicular to the main magnetic field.

18-15 Cross-talk artifact can be reduced by all of the following *except:*
   (a) increasing the gradient strength
   (b) increasing interslice gaps
   (c) double acquisition with 100% gaps interleaved
   (d) improving the RF profile

18-16 The number of ghost artifacts can be reduced by all of the following *except:*
   (a) flow compensation
   (b) presaturation pulses
   (c) decreasing N_y
   (d) increasing TR

18-17 Truncation artifacts include
   (a) pseudo meniscal tear
   (b) pseudo syrinx
   (c) pseudo MS plaques
   (d) all of the above
   (e) only (a) and (b)
   (f) only (a) and (c)

18-18 **T/F** Motion artifacts occur only along the phase-encoding direction.

PART

II

Fast Scanning

Introduction

In this chapter, we will discuss the elegant and cunning technique of fast spin echo. This technique was first proposed by Hennig et al.[1] and was called **RARE** (rapid acquisition with relaxation enhancement). However, it is commonly referred to as **fast spin echo (FSE)** or **turbo spin echo (TSE).** Different manufacturers have different names for it (Table 19-1).

Consider the pulse sequence diagram in Figure 19-1. This pulse sequence can be used for either a CSE or an FSE study.

Conventional Spin Echo

Let's first talk about a conventional spin echo (CSE or SE) study and again see how the lines in k-space are filled in. With a CSE, immediately after the 90° RF pulse, an **FID** (free induction decay) is formed. At a time TE after the first 90° pulse (time TE/2 after the first 180° refocusing pulse—17 msec in our example), we receive the first spin echo. We have a whole train of 180° refocusing pulses, after each of which we get another echo. Each echo is a multiple of 17 msec. Notice that each successive echo has less amplitude as a result of T2 decay.

In a CSE sequence, we can get two echoes, that is, we apply two 180° RF pulses and get back an echo from each pulse, each with a different TE. However, we *could* have as many echoes as

Table 19-1

Manufacturer	Name
GE, Hitachi, Toshiba	Fast spin echo (FSE)
Siemens, Philips	Turbo spin echo (TSE)

we want in a CSE sequence. In our example, we have an eight-echo sequence, all easily occurring within the time of one TR.

With each TR in a CSE, we have a single phase-encoding step. Each of the echoes following each 180° pulse is obtained after a single application of the phase-encoding gradient in CSE. Each echo has its own k-space, and each time we get an echo, we fill in one line of k-space (Fig. 19-1).

In CSE, each k-space will generate a different image, that is, we'll get a first echo image, a second echo image, and so on. With eight 180° pulses generating eight echoes, we'll have eight different k-spaces and eight different images. If we had 256 different phase-encoding steps, we would do this 256 different times. The scan time would be

Scan time = (TR)(number of phase-encoding steps)
(number of excitations [NEX])

Within the scan time, we'll get eight images, one of each TE echo. If we were only interested in the last echo image, we wouldn't have to bother with filling in the k-spaces for the first seven echoes. However, the first seven echoes come "free." We don't save any time by not doing them because we have to wait out the time it takes to

---

[1]Hennig J, Nauerth A, Friedburg H. RARE imaging: a fast imaging method for clinical MR. *Magn Reson Med.* 1986;3:823–833.

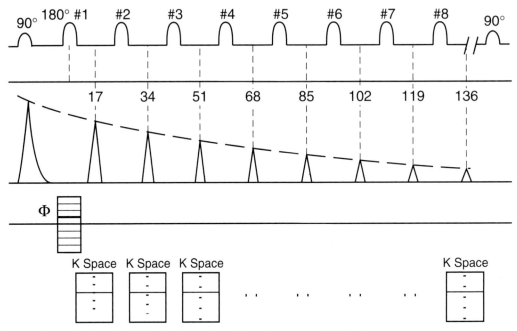

Figure 19-1. A spin-echo PSD with eight echoes. The echo spacing (ESP) is 17 msec.

get to the last echo anyway. In a dual-echo CSE sequence, the first echo is always "free"—it does-n't cost any time. (However, as we shall see later, that isn't true with FSE.)

Thus, for each k-space in CSE, we repeat the TR 256 times (each at a different phase-encoding gradient) and fill in the k-space for each echo with 256 different lines. For an eight-echo train, we get eight different images.

Fast Spin Echo

By using the same example, we can see how FSE works. FSE is a very elegant way of manipulating the CSE technique to save time. Again, we'll start with a train of eight echoes (ETL = 8). However, now we will only have one k-space. We'll fill this k-space eight lines at a time (Fig. 19-2). Instead of having eight separate

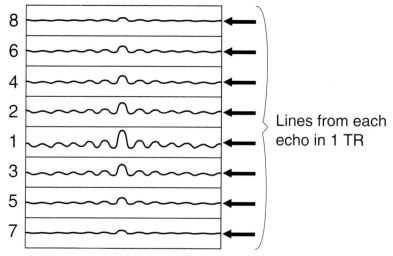

Figure 19-2. In FSE, k-space is filled eight lines at a time in one shot (within one TR).

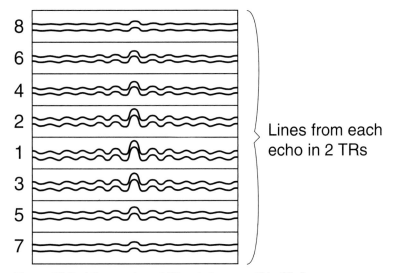

Figure 19-3. After two shots, 16 lines in k-space will be filled.

k-spaces, one for each echo, we will have one k-space using the data from all eight echoes.

Within the time of one TR (one "shot"), we will get eight lines, one from each echo, in the single k-space. With the next TR, we'll accumulate eight more lines, one from each echo, and we'll also put them into the same k-space (Fig. 19-3).

For each shot/TR, we will fill in another eight lines into the single k-space. Because we have a total of 256 lines in k-space, and because during each TR we are filling in eight lines of k-space at a shot, we only have to repeat the process 32 times (i.e., 256/8 = 32) to fill 256 lines of k-space.

In CSE, it took one TR for each line of k-space. Therefore, in a CSE study, we have to repeat the TR 256 times. In this manner, we have cut the time of the study by a factor of eight.

Example
Acquisition time of CSE sequence with TR = 3000 msec, N_y = 256, NEX = 1 is

SE time = (TR)(number of phase-encoding
steps)(NEX)
= (3000)(256)(1)msec
= 12.8 min

This time for the FSE sequence with TR = 3000 msec is

FSE time = (TR)(number of phase-encoding
steps/ETL)(NEX)

= (3000)(256/8)(1)msec
= 1.6 min

In this example, we have shortened the time of the study from 12.8 min to 1.6 min, a factor of eight times faster than the CSE study.

Echo Train Length

Echo train length (ETL) refers to the number of echoes used in FSE. The ETL ranges typically from 3 to 32. The time interval between successive echoes (or between 180° pulses) is called the **echo spacing (ESP)**. A typical ESP is on the order of 16 to 20 msec at a typical high field bandwidth (BW) of 32 kHz (±16 kHz).

Figure 19-4 is an example. Let's say we want an image with contrast reflecting a TE of approximately 100 msec. In FSE, the only TEs we can choose are integral multiples of the ESP (ESP = 17 msec in our example). This is called the **effective TE (TE_{eff}).** We will see shortly that this is *not* a true TE. Therefore, in our example, TE_{eff} = 102 msec (= 6 × 17 msec).

Remember that the center of k-space has maximum signal, and as we go out to the edges of k-space, we get less and less signal. Therefore, if we divide k-space into 8 slabs of 32 lines each (1 slab for each echo), the *center slab* will be assigned to the sixth echo, that is, the echo corresponding to the chosen TE_{eff} = 102 msec (Fig. 19-5).

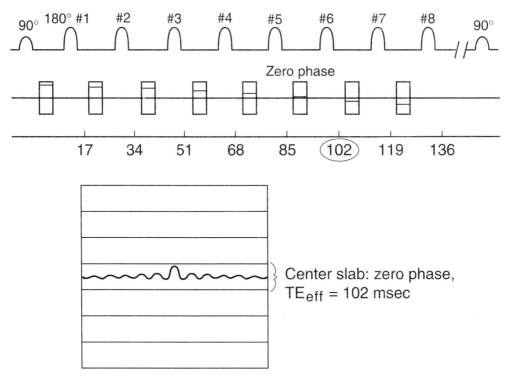

Figure 19-4. An example of FSE with TE$_{eff}$ of 102 msec. The phase gradient corresponding to this echo is minimum. The associated echo is placed in the center row of k-space.

In FSE, before *each* 180° pulse, we place a different value of the phase-encoding gradient. For the 180° pulse before the echo we choose as the TE$_{eff}$ (in this case, 102 msec), we use a phase-encoding gradient with the lowest strength. Each subsequent phase-encoding step will have a gradient with more and more amplitude. This increase will result in the most signal coming from the echo at 102 msec (because this signal is obtained with a minimum phase gradient) and

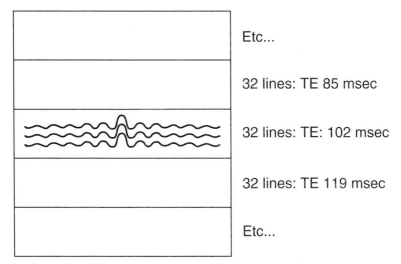

Figure 19-5. The 32 lines in the center of k-space correspond to the echoes associated with the weakest phase gradients.

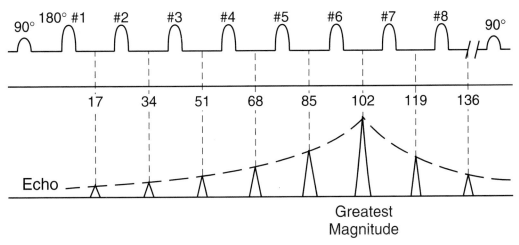

Figure 19-6. The echo corresponding to TE_{eff} of 102 msec has the largest peak.

decreasing signal from all the other echoes because their signals are obtained with increasing phase-encoding gradients (Fig. 19-6).

In the next TR, we again pick a phase-encoding step for the sixth echo that will be close to zero gradient and all the other phase-encoding steps will be close to their previous respective gradient values, so that again the maximum signal during this TR will be obtained from echo 6 (TE = 102 msec) and progressively weaker signals will be obtained from the other echoes.

The signals from the sixth echo (from the 1st to the 32nd TR) will all be placed in the center of k-space (Fig. 19-5). The signals from the other echoes will be placed in the other slabs. The echoes that experience progressively greater phase-encoding gradients (and therefore less signal) fall into slabs further away from the center slab, and those echoes experiencing the weakest phase-encoding gradients (and therefore having more signal) are placed closer to the center slab. k-space is organized so that the greatest amount of signal comes from the center of k-space and the least amount of signal comes from the periphery of k-space.

Therefore, if we choose an ETL of 8 echoes, we will have 8 slabs in k-space, with each slab containing 32 lines from 32 shots. Echo slab corresponds to a different echo. Let's see what the echo looks like (Fig. 19-6).

Because the center slab belongs to the lowest phase-encoding gradient, it will have the least

amount of dephasing. The signal received at TE = 102 msec will have the greatest amplitude. As we go farther away from 102 msec in either direction, the signal amplitude will get progressively smaller because the phase-encoding gradients get progressively larger.

By definition, the maximum signal comes at the TE_{eff} time. But we still get echoes from the other TEs that do not help our contrast. The signals from these other echoes are all in the same k-space. Even though the respective signal amplitudes from the other TEs are progressively smaller, the further away in time they are from the TE_{eff}, they still contribute to the contrast from the TE_{eff}. This is why it is called an **effective TE** and not a true TE.

In a way, what we are doing is *averaging* the echoes, although it is a *weighted average*. By appropriately picking the slabs, we put most of the *weight* on the echo corresponding to 102 msec (the TE_{eff}) and less weight on the other echoes. As we go away from the center slab of k-space, we are reducing the weighting, that is, we are reducing the contribution of the data on that slab to the effective echo.

The previous example gives us a long TR/long TE, which is a T2-weighted image. Now we want to do a proton density–weighted image with a long TR/short TE and a TE_{eff} of approximately 30 msec (Fig. 19-7). In this case, we would assign the center slab of k-space to correspond to the second echo, that is, TE =

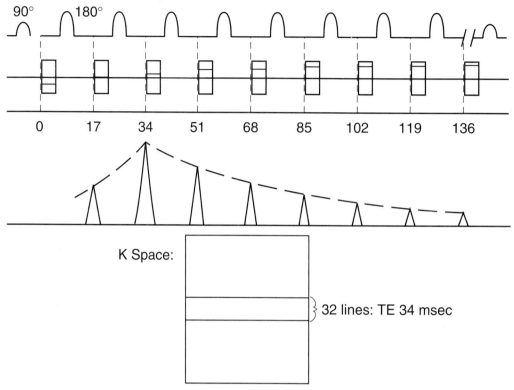

Figure 19-7. Another example with TE_{eff} of 34 msec. Here, the largest echo corresponds to TE of 34 msec.

34 msec. The echo with maximum magnitude will be at a TE of 34 msec, and the magnitude of the signal would fall off progressively with subsequent echoes. This is because, now, the second echo will be assigned the weakest phase-encoding gradients, and the subsequent echoes will have progressively stronger phase-encoding gradients.

Remember that with the TE_{eff} of 34 msec, we are still getting the cumulative signal from the entire echo train of eight echoes. So even information from an echo corresponding to a TE of 136 msec ($8 \times 17 = 136$) is contributing to the signal of the TE_{eff} of 34 msec, which we don't want. Therefore, for a T1-weighted study, we usually pick a smaller ETL such as 4. With an ETL of 4, we would only do four phase-encoding steps. Thus, k-space would only have four slabs, and the longest echo contributing to the contrast of the shortest TE_{eff} (e.g., 17 msec) would be the echo at 68 msec ($4 \times 17 = 68$). This will eliminate the T2 effect on a T1-weighted image caused by the signal contribution of the longer echo times.

Question: What happens to the time it takes to do an FSE study when we decrease the ETL from 8 to 4?

Answer: The time of the study will be increased by a factor of 2.

Question: If we have an ETL of 8, how many lines of k-space do we fill in with each TR?

Answer: We fill in eight lines of k-space with each TR, each line going to a separate slab within k-space.

Question: How many times do we have to repeat the TR to fill up k-space with 256 lines?

Answer: In general, we have to repeat it by the following ratio:

$$\frac{N_y}{ETL} = \frac{number\ of\ phase-encoding\ steps}{echo\ train\ length}$$

Remember that scan time is calculated by the following formula:

$$Scan\ time\ (FSE) = \frac{(TR)(N_y)(NEX)}{ETL}$$

The numerator of the formula is the same as for a CSE study:

$$Scan\ time\ (CSE) = (TR)(N_y)(NEX)$$

The difference in FSE is that the numerator is divided by the ETL. So, in the case of an 8-ETL study, the number of times we would have to repeat the TR (i.e., the number of shots) to complete 256 lines in k-space would be

$$256/8 = 32$$

In the case of a 4-ETL study, we would fill four lines of k-space with each TR. The number of times we would have to repeat the TR to complete 256 lines in k-space is now

$$256/4 = 64\ times$$

Example 1

1. Consider a T2-weighted study with TR = 3000 msec, N_y = 256 and NEX = 1, and let's compare the scan time between CSE and FSE (using a TE_{eff} = 102 msec and ETL = 8).

$$Scan\ time\ (FSE) = \frac{(TR)(N_y)(NEX)}{ETL}$$
$$= (3\ sec)(256)(1)/8$$
$$= 1.6\ min$$

$$Scan\ time\ (CSE) = (TR)(N_y)(NEX)$$
$$= (3\ sec)(256)(1)$$
$$= 12.8\ min$$

2. Repeat the above for a T1-weighted study with TR = 500 msec and FSE using ETL = 4

$$Scan\ time\ (FSE) = \frac{(TR)(N_y)(NEX)}{ETL}$$
$$= (0.5\ sec)(256)(1)/4 = 32\ sec$$

$$Scan\ time\ (CSE) = (TR)(N_y)(NEX)$$
$$= (0.5\ sec)(256)(1) = 128\ sec$$
$$= 2\ min,\ 8\ sec$$

Trade-offs

What are the *trade-offs* of FSE imaging?

Slice Coverage. As we increase the ETL to increase the speed of the exam, we also *decrease* the *number of slices* we can do in a study (Fig. 19-8). In one TR, with eight ETL, we can fit in so many slices. If we use the same TR, but now use an ETL of 16, it will take twice as long to receive the echo (i.e., 16 × 17 msec = 272 msec) because now we have to accumulate data from 16 echoes (each a multiple of 17 msec). Because the time it takes to accumulate 16 lines of k-space is double the time it takes to accumulate eight lines, we can fit in only half the number of slices into one TR.

Therefore, the trade-off is that we decrease the number of slices as we increase the ETL.

$$\uparrow ETL \rightarrow\ \uparrow speed$$
$$\leftrightarrow\ \downarrow coverage(\downarrow number\ of\ slices)$$

One way to get around this is to *increase* TR. Although increasing TR increases scan time, we save so much time by using a long ETL compared with CSE that we can afford a longer TR. We don't need to be limited any more to a TR of 3000 msec. We can go up to 4000 to 6000 msec, get more coverage, and still save time.

Let's say we need a coverage of fifteen 5-mm slices with a 2-mm gap to cover an area of interest (like the brain).

Example 2

Let's choose TR = 3000 msec, ETL = 8, NEX = 1, N_y = 256.

The number of slices we can do in any TR depends on the length of the longest echo (we'll leave out sampling time for now):

$$Number\ of\ slices \leq TR/TE$$

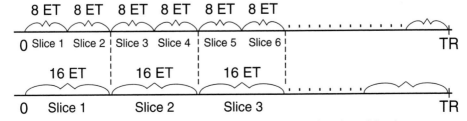

Figure 19-8. Increasing the ETL causes a reduction in coverage (number of slices).

In the case of an ETL of 8, the longest echo is 136 msec (17 × 8 = 136). So,

$$\text{Number of slices} \leq \text{TR/TE}$$
$$= 3000 \text{ msec}/136 \text{ msec}$$
$$\cong 22$$

This formula is regardless of TE_{eff} we pick. The scan time for this example would be

$$\text{Scan time} = \frac{(\text{TR})(N_y)(\text{NEX})}{\text{ETL}}$$

$$= (3000 \text{ msec})(256)(1)/8$$
$$= 1.6 \text{ min}$$

Therefore, we can do 22 slices in 1.6 min with an ETL of 8.

Example 3

Let's now choose a different ETL:
ETL = 16, NEX = 1, N_y = 256, TR = 3000 msec
With an ETL of 16 (since echoes are multiples of 17 msec), the longest echo would be 272 msec (16 × 17 = 272). So,

Number of slices = TR/TE
$$= 3000 \text{ msec}/272 \text{ msec} \cong 11$$

$$\text{Scan time} = \frac{(\text{TR})(N_y)(\text{NEX})}{\text{ETL}}$$
$$= \frac{(3000)(256)(1)}{16} \cong 0.8 \text{ min}$$

With an ETL of 16, we can do only 11 slices, but in 0.8 min. The scan is faster, but we have limited coverage, and we have not accomplished the minimum of 15 slices we needed for the exam.

Example 4

To increase the coverage with an ETL of 16, let's now increase the TR:
TR = 4500 msec, ETL = 16, N_y = 256, NEX = 1
Now,

Number of slices ≤ TR/TE
$$= 4500/272 \text{ msec} \cong 16$$

$$\text{Scan time} = \frac{(\text{TR})(N_y)(\text{NEX})}{\text{ETL}}$$
$$= \frac{(4500)(256)(1)}{16} \cong 1.2 \text{ min}$$

Even though we have limited coverage with an ETL of 16, we resorted to increasing the TR to 4500 msec, which allowed us a coverage of 16 slices (enough to cover the 15 slices we needed for the exam), and we were still able to keep the scan time below the scan time required for an ETL of 8.

Sometimes you'll look at a scan and find that it took twice as long to do the study as you thought it would. What can happen is that the technologist will try to get a coverage that is too wide for the TR chosen. If nothing is corrected, the machine will "default" to performing *two* separate acquisitions to provide the coverage, thus making the exam twice as long. With a simple calculation to allow either increasing the TR slightly or increasing slice thickness slightly, you could rectify the situation more efficiently.

Multi-echo FSE

Consider the case of eight echoes again. With CSE, we would have eight k-spaces, and the first seven echoes would come "free." That's not true for FSE. Every single one of the echoes is used to fill in a line in a k-space. If we want to do double-echo imaging, we have twice as many lines in k-space to fill (in two k-spaces). Thus, we have to either (i) give up half of the echoes per ETL, in which case the scan time is going to be doubled or (ii) repeat the scan twice, and again the scan time is increased. Therefore, regardless of the way we do it, it's going to cost us time.

> **In FSE, the first echo is no longer "free!"**

There are three ways to get a double-echo image with FSE:

1. Full echo train
2. Split echo train
3. Shared echo

Full Echo Train. In a full echo train, all echoes in the train contribute to the image. Thus, the full ETL is completed for effective TE_1 ($\text{TE}_{1\text{eff}}$) before $\text{TE}_{2\text{eff}}$ is performed. In other words, two separate concatenated sequences are acquired. For example, for an

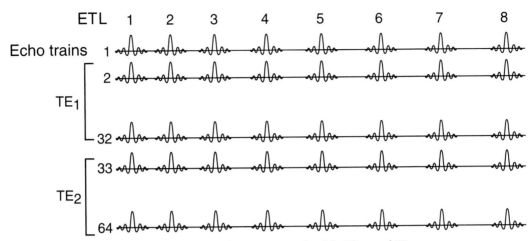

Figure 19-9. In a full echo train, the entire echo train is completed for TE_{1eff} and TE_{2eff}.

ETL of 8 and a 256×256 matrix (Fig. 19-9), 32 echo trains would be required to fill k-space ($8 \times 32 = 256$).

Split Echo Train. In a split echo train, the first half of the echo train contributes to the image with TE_{1eff} and the second half to TE_{2eff} (thus, two k-spaces are created). For example, for an ETL of 8 (Fig. 19-10), only four echoes would be applied to each effective TE. Therefore, 64 trains would be required to fill k-space ($4 \times 64 = 256$).

Shared Echo. In a shared echo approach, the first and last echoes in the train are emphasized for TE_1 and TE_2, respectively, and the echoes in

between are shared for both images. This approach has the advantage of shorter ETL compared with a full or split echo train approach, allowing more slices to be acquired for a given TR (since the number of slices is roughly determined by TR divided by the product of ESP and ETL, i.e., number of slices $\cong$ TR/[ETL $\times$ ESP]).

In Figure 19-11, an ETL of 5 is used and four lines of k-space are filled per TR, three of which are the same for the first and second echo images. (Thus, there is some overlap of the "information" in the two images, compared with the four split echo approach.) Filling four echoes per pass provides the same efficiency as a split echo approach, that is, 64 echo trains will

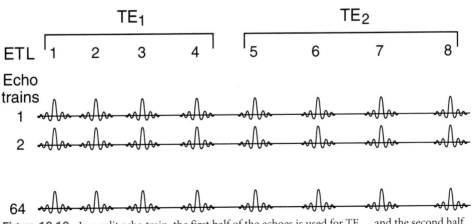

Figure 19-10. In a split echo train, the first half of the echoes is used for TE_{1eff} and the second half for TE_{2eff}.

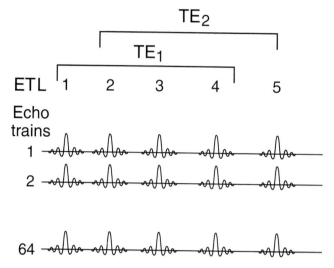

Figure 19-11. In a shared echo approach, the first and last echoes are emphasized for TE_1 and TE_2, respectively, and the rest are shared between the two echoes. In this example, the ETL is 5 and the central three echoes are shared.

be required to fill k-space ($4 \times 64 = 256$). However, the shorter ETL allows 60% more slices to be acquired in the same time. Let's prove this mathematically:

Number of slices (ETL = 5)/
number of slices (ETL = 8)
= [TR/(5 × ESP)]/[TR/(8 × ESP)]
= 8/5 = 1.6 = 100% + 60%

A variant of the shared echo approach is the so-called **keyhole** imaging. In this technique, k-space is covered completely on the first image, but only the central portion (e.g., 20%) of k-space is covered on subsequent images, providing most of the contrast (recall that the center of k-space contains most of the signal). This approach has a disadvantage in that the high spatial frequency outer portion (e.g., 80%) of k-space is shared information; however, it has the advantage of speeding up the subsequent imaging by a factor of 5 (100%/20% = 5). Thus, keyhole imaging is useful when fast repetitive imaging of the same slice is required, for example, for perfusion imaging.

Each of the previous methods has its advantages and disadvantages. The advantages of the **full echo train** approach are full flexibility in selecting the TE_{eff} and the ETL for both the first and the second echoes; the disadvantage is more contrast averaging.

The disadvantage of the **split echo** approach is that the TE_{2eff} is constrained in the second half of the echo train. For example, for an ETL of 16 and an ESP of 17 msec, the minimum TE_{2eff} is

$9 \times 17 = 153$ msec, which might be longer than desired. The advantage is less contrast averaging and crisper images. In general, the split echo train is used for ETLs of 8 or less, whereas the full echo train is used for ETLs greater than 8.

The advantage of the **shared echo** approach is increased coverage (number of slices). The disadvantage is an overlap of information between the two echo images. (Fig. 19-12 gives an example.)

Advantages of FSE

1. The scan time is decreased (which allows faster scanning).
2. The signal-to-noise ratio (SNR) is maintained because we still have 256 phase-encoding steps.
3. The increased speed allows for high-resolution imaging in a reasonable amount of time. An example is 512 × 512 imaging through the internal auditory canals with very long TR.
4. Motion artifacts will be less severe. Because the 180° pulses are evenly spaced, there is a natural **even-echo rephasing** effect. For instance, cerebrospinal fluid (CSF) motion artifacts are much less severe on FSE than on CSE images.
5. The rephasing from the multiple 180° pulses leads to less distortion from metallic objects on FSE images (see Chapter 18; also see the discussion below on magnetic susceptibility).

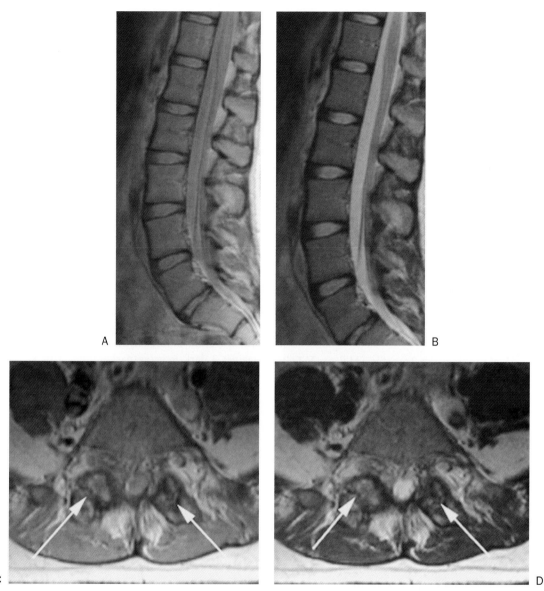

Figure 19-12. Sagittal proton density (**A**) and T2 (**B**), and axial proton density (**C**) and T2 (**D**) images of the lumbosacral spine were acquired using a shared echo approach. Note that the CSF is brighter than would be expected in a CSE proton density acquisition. The fat is bright on the T2 images, which is also typical of the FSE technique. This patient has minimal L5/S1 anterolisthesis that is secondary to bilateral dysplastic facets (*arrows* in **C** and **D**).

6. Similarly, FSE images are much more tolerant of a poorly shimmed magnet than are CSE images.

Disadvantages of FSE

1. Reduced coverage, that is, decreased number of slices.

2. Contrast averaging (k-space averaging) so that

(a) **CSF is brighter on proton density–weighted FSE images.** This is caused by the effect of averaging all the echoes into a single k-space. We are still contributing data from very long TEs into the proton density image, even though the weighting is toward the lower TE. Therefore, we will have some T2 effect (i.e., bright CSF) on a short TE_{eff}. To alleviate this problem, either use a shorter ETL (to exclude longer TEs) or a higher BW (to decrease ESP and the minimum TE_{eff}).

   (b) *Pathology:* **MS plaques and other lesions at the brain/CSF interface may be missed on FSE.** CSF appears brighter on FSE proton density images (as discussed above) and, therefore, the distinction between CSF and periventricular high-intensity plaques is more difficult. As in (a), to alleviate this problem, use a shorter ETL, which helps exclude longer TEs in the echo (fluid-attenuated inversion recovery [FLAIR] has generally solved this problem).

3. **Magnetization transfer (MT or MTC) effect in FSE.** MTC is inadvertently present in FSE. This is caused by the presence of multiple, rapid 180° pulses containing off-resonant frequencies. When MT (discussed in more detail in Chapter 25) is *intentionally* produced, an RF pulse of 500 to 3000 Hz off the bulk water resonance saturates protein-bound water in the broad peaks on either side of the bulk phase water peak. Because the 180° pulses are rapid (in the time domain), they have a broad BW (in the frequency domain), thus containing frequencies off the bulk water resonance frequency. These frequencies suppress protein-bound water like a fat saturation pulse suppresses fat.

4. **Normal intervertebral discs are not as bright on T2-weighted FSE images compared with CSE.** This is caused by the MT effects in FSE previously discussed. They diminish the contrast between desiccated (usually dark) and normal (usually bright) discs.

5. **Magnetic susceptibility effects will be less than with CSE.** This is caused by decreased dephasing from closely spaced (refocusing) 180° pulses that leave little time for spins to dephase as they diffuse through regions of magnetic nonuniformity. In FSE, the signal loss is minimized because of the rephasing effects of multiple 180° pulses. Therefore, T2-weighted FSE images are less sensitive to magnetic susceptibility effects such as metal or hemorrhage (e.g., deoxyhemoglobin and hemosiderin) than are T2-weighted CSE images (Fig. 18-47).

6. **Fat is bright on T2-weighted FSE images.** This is due to suppression of diffusion-mediated susceptibility dephasing caused by the closely spaced 180° pulses[2] (Fig. 19-13). You could do a *fat-saturated* FSE to decrease the intensity of fat.

Example 5

Performing a fat-saturated T2-weighted FSE sequence of the knee to suppress fat in the marrow will allow bone marrow edema to stand out against a dark marrow background. This technique increases the sensitivity of detecting bone bruises (contusions) by about 30%[3] (Fig. 19-14).

Other Features of FSE

More recent versions of FSE with high performance gradients allow other options, such as higher BWs, flow compensation, and three-dimensional (3D) FSE.

   Higher BWs cause a reduction in the sampling time T_s and thus ESP, allowing a lower minimum TE_{eff}. Therefore, the previously hyperintense CSF on supposedly proton density-weighted images can now be made isointense to white matter. Use of a split (versus full) echo train also minimizes unwanted T2 contributions by only averaging the first four echoes of an eight-echo train. (This is the same principle that allows T1-weighted FSEs to be performed, i.e., higher BWs and shorter echo trains.)

---

[2]For more details, refer to Henkelman RM, Hardy PA, Bishop JE, et al. Why fat is bright in RARE and fast spin-echo imaging. *J Magn Reson Imaging.* 1992;2:533–540.
[3]For more details, see Kapelov SR, Teresi LM, Bradley WG, et al. Bone contusions of the knee: increased lesion detection with fast spin-echo MR imaging with spectroscopic fat saturation. *Radiology.* 1993;189:901–904.

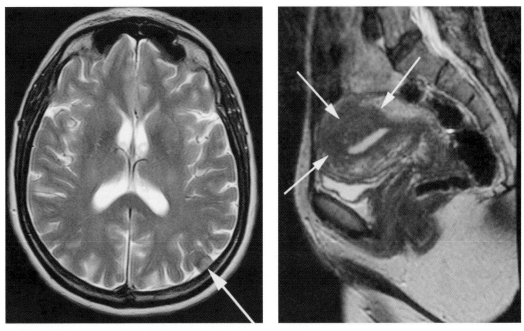

Figure 19-13. Axial FSE T2 image of the brain **(A)** shows an isointense to gray matter meningioma along the left parietal convexity (*arrow*). Sagittal FSE T2 image of the pelvis **(B)** in a different patient demonstrates marked focal thickening of the dark junctional zone (*arrows*) along the fundus and midbody diagnostic of adenomyosis. Note in both examples that the fat is bright.

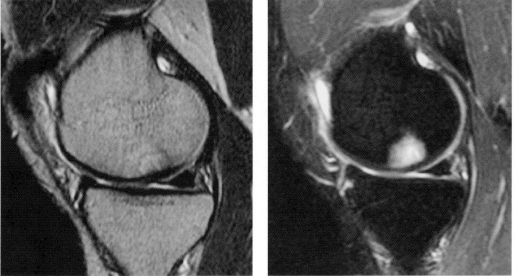

Figure 19-14. Sagittal FSE T2 **(A)** and fat-saturated FSE T2 **(B)** images of the knee demonstrate marked increased conspicuity of focal subchondral bone marrow edema of the distal femur in the fat-saturated image.

Flow compensation is an added feature that is possible with high performance gradients; such gradients allow a higher maximum strength that can be applied over a shorter period. As a result, flow compensation with high performance gradients does not place a large time burden on the cycle.

3D FSE

With the advent of **high performance gradients** (see Chapter 30), 3D FSE imaging in reasonable scan times is available. This imaging is particularly useful for the brain, cervical spine, and lumbar spine where bright CSF (T2-weighted) images are required in more than one plane.

The basic idea in 3D imaging (3D techniques in connection with gradient-echo imaging is discussed in Chapter 20) is to have a phase-encoding gradient not only in the y direction but also in the z direction (Fig. 19-15). Therefore, the multiple slices in 2D FSE are replaced by multiple slabs. **Crusher gradients** (see Chapter 14) are applied before and after every 180° pulse (which is slice selective). Each echo is first phase encoded, then sampled, and finally phase *unwound* (i.e., a **rewinder gradient** is applied—see Chapter 21). Consequently, the scan time will be

$$T(\text{3D FSE}) = (\text{TR} \times \text{NEX} \times N_y \times N_z)/\text{ETL}$$

where N_y and N_z are the number of phase-encoding steps along the y and z axes.

High performance gradients have higher maximum strengths and thus allow a significant reduction in the gradient duration. This, in turn, allows a larger ETL (decreasing scan time) and a reduction in minimum TE (increasing the coverage). Therefore, despite a significant increase in the acquisition time (compared with 2D FSE) caused by the addition of the N_z factor into the previous formula, the scan can still be performed in a reasonable time.

Example 6
What is the scan time for a T2-weighted 3D FSE technique with TR = 3000 msec, ETL = 64, NEX = 1, N_y = 256, and N_z = 32?
Answer:

$$T = 3 \text{ sec} \times 1 \times 256 \times 32/64 = 384 \text{ sec}$$
$$= 6 \text{ min, } 24 \text{ sec}$$

which is very reasonable.

Advantages of 3D FSE

1. Higher SNR (compared with 2D FSE)
2. High (1-mm) isotropic resolution (Fig. 19-16)

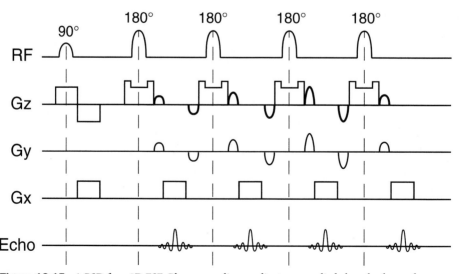

Figure 19-15. A PSD for a 3D FSE. Phase-encoding gradients are applied along both y and z axes.

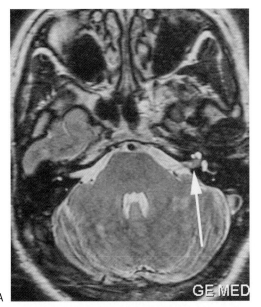 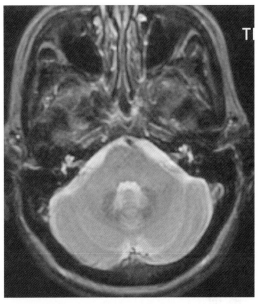

A   B

Figure 19-16. Axial 3D 1.5-mm FSE T2 (**A**) of the internal auditory canals shows a left intracanalicular mass consistent with acoustic schwannoma (*arrow*). **B:** A CSE 5-mm T2 image is shown for comparison. Also note that the subcutaneous fat is bright on the FSE (**A**), whereas it is relatively dark on the CSE T2 (**B**).

3. Less partial volume averaging (due to thinner slices)
4. Capability to perform high-quality reformation in any plane (due to ability to generate *isotropic* voxels)
5. Lower cross-talk (for slab-interleaved approaches)
6. Reduced magnetic susceptibility and field inhomogeneity artifacts (compared with 3D gradient-echo techniques)

Fast IR

By adding a 180° inversion pulse prior to FSE, **fast IR** can be achieved. For more details, refer to the discussion on fast FLAIR in Chapter 25. Fast STIR is similar to fast FLAIR except that the TI is chosen to null fat instead of fluid.

Key Points

FSE imaging provides almost all the advantages of conventional spin-echo imaging at a faster speed. The basic idea behind FSE is utilization of multiple 180° refocusing pulses, which allows filling multiple lines in k-space for a single TR. The ETL is defined as the number of 180° pulses and echoes in the train. As a result, compared with CSE, the acquisition time T in FSE is reduced by a factor of ETL:

$$T(FSE) = T(CSE)/ETL$$

The increased speed also allows for other features not achievable by CSE techniques, such as high-resolution imaging of, for example, the internal auditory canals with very long TRs and, more recently, 3D imaging using FSE.

Questions

19-1 Advantages of FSE include all of the following *except*
  (a) increased speed
  (b) decreased ferromagnetic susceptibility artifacts
  (c) decreased motion artifacts
  (d) increased number of possible slices

19-2 Suppose TR = 4000 msec, TE = 100 msec, NEX = 2, N_y = 256.
  (a) Calculate the scan time for CSE.
  (b) Calculate the scan time for FSE with ETL = 8.

19-3 T/F Increasing ETL leads to increased speed and coverage.

19-4 The scan time for FSE is given by
  (a) $TR \cdot NEX \cdot N_y$
  (b) $TR \cdot N_y \cdot ETL/NEX$
  (c) $ETL/(TR \cdot NEX \cdot N_y)$
  (d) $TR \cdot NEX \cdot N_y/ETL$

19-5 Dual-echo imaging in FSE can be achieved by
  (a) split echo train
  (b) full echo train
  (c) shared echo approach
  (d) all of the above
  (e) only (a) and (b)

19-6 Disadvantages of FSE compared with CSE include all of the following *except*
  (a) brighter CSF on proton density–weighted images
  (b) fat is brighter
  (c) increased magnetic susceptibility effects
  (d) normal intervertebral discs are not as bright

19-7 Calculate the scan time for a 3D FSE technique with TR = 4000 msec, TE = 100 msec, N_x = 128, N_y = 128, N_z = 32, NEX = 1, ETL = 64.

19-8 T/F Given comparable parameters, the scan time of an FSE sequence is equal to that of a CSE divided by the ETL.

Gradient Echo: Part I (Basic Principles)

Introduction

In this chapter, we introduce the **gradient-echo (GRE)** pulse sequence. It is also called **gradient-recalled echo (GRE)**, the reason for which will become clear later in the chapter. The major purpose behind the GRE technique is a significant reduction in the scan time. Toward this end, small flip angles are employed, which, in turn, allow very short repetition time (TR) values, thus decreasing the scan time. Consequently, such techniques are also referred to as **partial flip angle** techniques. One of the most important applications of GRE is the ability to employ three-dimensional (3D) imaging, thanks to the higher speed of GRE due to very short TRs. The major differences between GRE and spin-echo (SE) sequences are explained in this chapter.

Gradient-Recalled Echo

As mentioned in the introduction, the purpose of the GRE technique is to increase the speed of the scan. Recall that the scan time for "conventional" techniques is given by

$$\text{Scan time} = \text{TR} \times N_y \times \text{NEX} \qquad \text{(Eqn. 20-1)}$$

where TR is the repetition time, N_y the number of phase-encoding steps, and NEX the number of excitations. Now, N_y is generally selected to yield a certain resolution (too small an N_y degrades the resolution), and NEX is chosen to yield a certain signal-to-noise ratio (SNR). Consequently, the only parameter in Equation 20-1 that can be controlled to reduce the scan time is TR.

In other words, we wish to select a TR that is as small as possible and still be able to receive a reasonable echo to create an image. If we use 90° radio frequency (RF) pulses, then with very small TRs, the longitudinal magnetization is not given sufficient time to recover to a reasonable value, as depicted in Figure 20-1. This causes a significant reduction in the longitudinal magnetization and the subsequent transverse magnetization (Fig. 20-2). That is, the amplitude of the received signal will be diminished significantly (and, thus, SNR is deteriorated).

To rectify this problem, an RF pulse yielding a smaller flip angle α is used instead of the usual 90° RF pulse. This change causes incomplete flipping of the longitudinal magnetization into the x–y plane, producing transverse magnetization, called, $\mathbf{M}_{xy}$ (Fig. 20-3). In addition, the major component of magnetization remains along the z-axis after the RF pulse (called $\mathbf{M}_z$). Consequently, even with small TRs, there will be sufficient longitudinal magnetization at the time of the next cycle.

MATH: For the mathematically oriented reader, the magnitude of the transverse and longitudinal magnetizations are given by

$$M_{xy} = M_0 \sin \alpha, \, M_z = M_0 \cos \alpha \qquad \text{(Eqn. 20-2)}$$

right after the α RF pulse, where $\mathbf{M}_0$ is the initial magnetization.

After this point, the process of recovery along the z-axis and the process of dephasing in the x–y plane are exactly the same as in its SE counterpart. There is, however, one major difference between GRE and SE sequences. In SE, a 180° refocusing pulse is used to eliminate dephasing

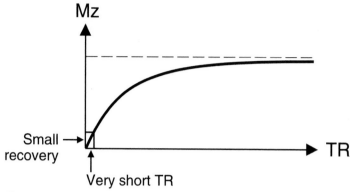

Figure 20-1. After a 90° pulse, longitudinal recovery after a short TR will be very small.

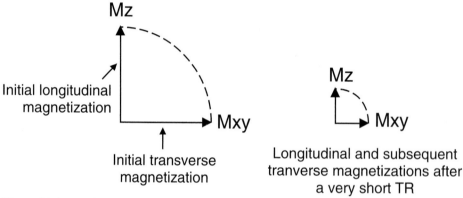

Figure 20-2. **A:** The initial longitudinal and transverse magnetizations. **B:** After a short TR, the subsequent longitudinal and transverse magnetizations will be smaller for a 90° RF pulse.

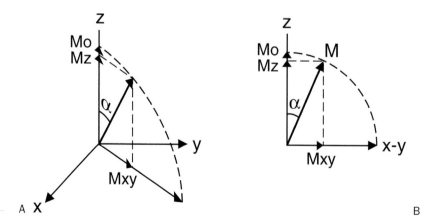

Figure 20-3. **A–B:** If a small flip angle α is used, only a portion of longitudinal magnetization is flipped into the x–y plane, and thus a portion of longitudinal magnetization will remain.

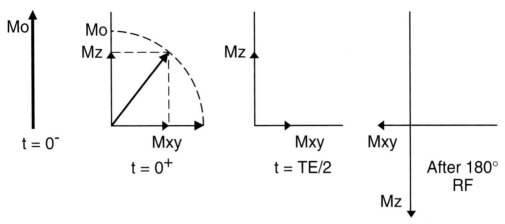

Figure 20-4. After a partial flip angle, longitudinal recovery will no longer be small after a short TR (because partial flip retains a portion of initial longitudinal magnetization). However, a 180° RF refocusing pulse would be counterproductive.

caused by external magnetic field inhomogeneities. This pulse is not used in GRE imaging.

Question: What is the reason for not using a 180° refocusing pulse in GRE?

Answer: Because we use a small flip angle in GRE, there would be a large component in the longitudinal axis at half the echo time (TE/2). (In SE imaging, however, this longitudinal component is insignificant at TE/2 because TE/2 is much smaller than T1 of the tissue.) Let's see what would happen to this longitudinal magnetization if we were to apply a 180° pulse. Although the application of a 180° pulse does yield rephasing in the x–y plane, it also causes M_z to invert and point south (Fig. 20-4). To recover this inverted vector back in the north direction requires a long TR, which is clearly not the desired case in GRE. (The above is not a problem in conventional SE imaging because the longitudinal magnetization at TE/2 is very small and inverting it does not pose any significant loss of signal.)

Question: In the absence of a 180° pulse, how does one form an echo?

Answer: One way is to measure the free induction decay (FID) instead. However, it's impractical to do so because the FID comes on too early and decays more rapidly than we can spatially encode the signal. We need time to apply a phase-encoding gradient and prepare the signal for frequency encoding. We also need time to let the RF pulses and gradients die down before doing anything else. To this end, we will intentionally dephase the FID and rephase (or recall) it at a more convenient time, namely, at TE. This is accomplished via a refocusing gradient in the x direction and is illustrated in Figure 20-5. This gradient has an initial negative lobe that intentionally dephases the spins in the transverse plane and thus eliminates the FID. It is then followed by a positive lobe that rephases the spins, thus restoring the FID in the form of a readable echo. The area under the negative lobe is equal

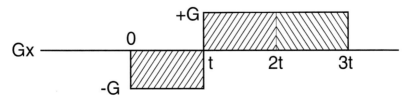

Figure 20-5. Instead of using a 180° pulse, a bilobed gradient is used that has a negative lobe as well as a positive lobe of twice the duration.

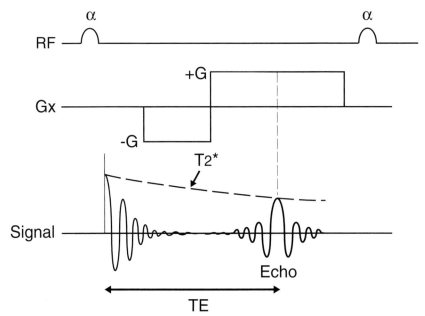

Figure 20-6. The bilobed gradient causes dephasing of the FID and its recalling at time TE (at the center of the positive lobe). Because there is no 180° rephasing pulse, the rate of decay is given by T2* (instead of T2).

to half the area under the positive lobe. The refocusing occurs at the midpoint of the positive lobe. Figure 20-6 illustrates how the FID is refocused at TE. In other words, the FID is first eliminated and then recalled at time TE; hence the name gradient-recalled echo.

Slice Excitation

The other difference between GRE and SE is that in GRE imaging, TR may be too short to allow for processing of other slices. For this reason, short TR GRE techniques may acquire only one slice at a time. This is referred to as *sequential scanning*. (In the next chapter, we will introduce variations of GRE that allow multiplanar imaging by lengthening the TR.) In other words, in a sequential mode (single-slice) GRE, the total scan time is given by

$$\text{Scan time (GRE)} = TR \times N_y \times NEX \times \text{(number of slices)} \quad \textbf{(Eqn. 20-3a)}$$

That is to say, acquisition of additional slices increases the scan time in a sequential mode in GRE imaging.

In the 3D GRE technique (see below), the scan time is given by

$$\text{Scan time (3D GRE)} = TR \times NEX \\ \times N_y \times N_z \quad \textbf{(Eqn. 20-3b)}$$

where N_y and N_z refer to the number of phase-encoding steps in the y and z directions, respectively.

Example

Suppose TR = 50 msec, TE = 15 msec, α = 15°, NEX = 1, and N_y = 128. Then

$$TR \times NEX \times N_y = 50 \times 128 \times 1 \\ = 6400 \text{ msec} = 6.4 \text{ sec}$$

Thus, it takes only 6.4 sec to obtain a single slice. If we were to obtain 10 slices, the scan time would be

$$\text{Scan time (10 slices)} = 6.4 \times 10 = 64 \text{ sec} \\ = 1 \text{ min, } 4 \text{ sec}$$

whereas acquisition of 20 slices would take

$$\text{Scan time (20 slices)} = 6.4 \times 20 = 128 \text{ sec} \\ = 2 \text{ min, } 8 \text{ sec}$$

which is twice as long.

Magnetic Susceptibility

The lack of a 180° refocusing pulse results in greater dephasing of spins compared with conventional SE. This in turn results in greater sensitivity to **magnetic susceptibility** effects. This increased sensitivity can be both problematic (e.g., increased artifact at the air/tissue interfaces) and advantageous (e.g., when searching for subtle hemorrhage), depending on the application (Figs. 20-7 and 20-8).

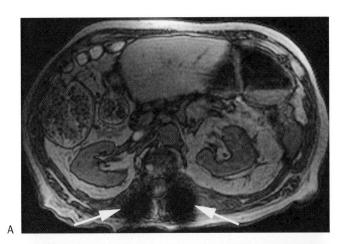

A

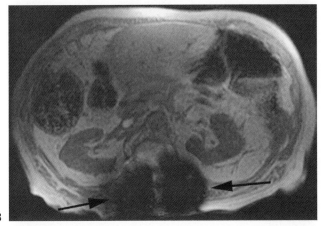

B

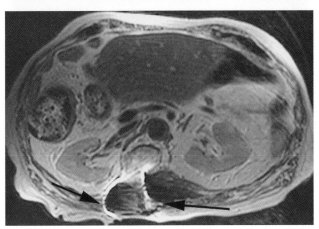

C

Figure 20-7. Axial T1 gradient echo out of phase (TR 110/TE 2) (**A**), and T1 gradient echo in phase (TR 110/TE 4) (**B**) images show marked "blooming" artifact (*arrows*) from the patient's known spinal fixation hardware. The out-of-phase image (**A**) has less artifact than the in phase image (**B**) due to the shorter TE. Axial T2 FSE (**C**) and ½ NEX SSFSE T2

(*continued on next page.*)

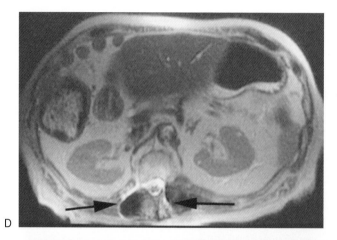

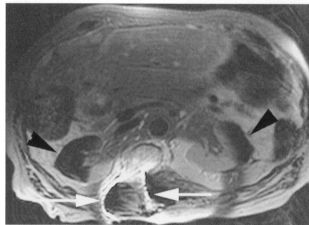

Figure 20-7. *(continued)* **(D)** images have less artifact due to multiple 180° refocusing RF pulses with the SSFSE having the least due to the longest echo train length. Finally, an axial T2 FSE image with fat saturation **(E)** shows ferromagnetic artifact *(arrows)* and magnetic field changes resulting in paradoxical water saturation *(arrowheads)* and very poor fat saturation.

Steady-State Transverse Magnetization

There is one more major difference between GRE and SE pulse sequences. Whereas at the start of each cycle in SE imaging in which there is negligible component of magnetization M_{xy} in the x–y plane, this may not be the case in GRE imaging. In other words, GRE may have **residual transverse magnetization** at the end of the cycle, which will be affected by the next RF pulse. This is because in GRE imaging, TR may be too short to allow for complete dephasing (i.e., T2* decay) of the spins in the transverse plane. (In contrast, in SE imaging, TR is long enough to allow complete dephasing of the spins in the x–y plane.) After a few cycles, this residual transverse magnetization reaches a **steady state**, referred to as M_{ss}. This scheme is

illustrated in Figure 20-9 and is elaborated upon further in the next chapter.

Tissue Contrast

Figure 20-10 depicts a generic GRE pulse sequence diagram (PSD). There are three operator-controlled parameters that affect the tissue contrast: α, TR, and TE. Let's discuss how each of these plays a role in this matter.

First, consider a small flip angle α (e.g., 5° to 30°). As can be seen in Figure 20-11, a small flip angle results in a large amount of (persistent) longitudinal magnetization after application of the RF pulse. This result implies that complete recovery of the longitudinal magnetization to its initial value will take much less time than following the 90° RF pulse of an SE sequence. Consequently, given two tissues with different

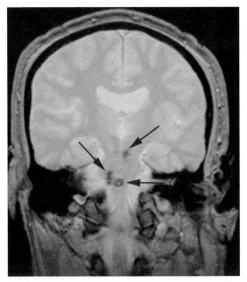

Figure 20-8. Coronal T2* gradient-echo image of the brain shows multiple dark foci in the brainstem from the patient's known multiple cavernous angiomas. This sequence is very sensitive for subtle blood products.

T1 values, a large difference will not exist between their respective T1 curves, and thus T1 recovery plays a minor role. This is better illustrated in Figure 20-12, in which tissue A's and tissue B's T1 curves are drawn for two different flip angles, 10° and 90°. The T1 curves for 10° α start higher on the z-axis owing to the fact that they are only partially flipped into the x–y plane. It can be inferred from this figure that the T1 differences between the two tissues is much less apparent for the smaller flip angle.

> **A small flip angle reduces T1 weighting.**

A small α also implies a small transverse magnetization and thus a small steady-state component, reducing T2* weighting. As shown in Equation 20-2, M_{xy} is directly proportional to M_0; thus, tissue contrast is predominantly affected by proton density. This relationship is

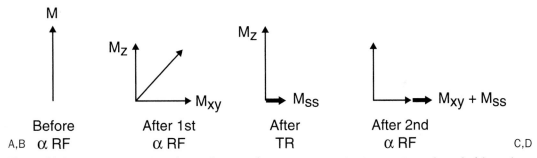

Figure 20-9. A–D: Because TR is short, a fraction of transverse magnetization remains at the end of the cycle, which eventually reaches a steady state, M_{ss}. This steady-state component is affected by the next RF pulse.

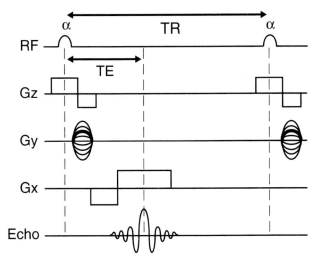

Figure 20-10. A gradient-echo (GRE) PSD.

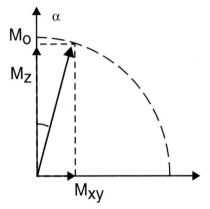

Figure 20-11. A small flip angle results in a large amount of longitudinal magnetization.

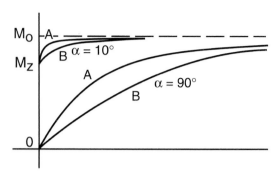

Figure 20-12. When the flip angle is small, it is difficult to discriminate the T1 contrast between two tissues. Thus, small α reduces T1 weighting.

illustrated in Figure 20-13. In this diagram, tissue A (e.g., H_2O) has a higher proton density than tissue B (e.g., fat), that is $N(A) > N(B)$. At time TE, then, the difference between A and B is predominantly explained by their respective proton densities $N(A)$ and $N(B)$.

A small flip angle yields proton density weighting.

Conversely, a large α (e.g., 75° to 90°) allows better differentiation of the T1 characteristics of the two tissues. This should be fairly obvious because in the extreme case when α is 90°, we are in a situation similar to SE, given that TR is not very small. However, if TR is very small, there won't be sufficient time for T1 recovery, thereby reducing T1 weighting (in this case, the large steady-state component that accumulates due to the large α increases T2* weighting—see later text).

A large flip angle (with a large TR) yields more T1 weighting.

For an intermediate α (e.g., 30° to 60°), the result is mixed contrast, although the gain in T1 weighting caused by larger flip angles tends to outweigh the gain in T2* weighting from increased steady state.

Next, consider the TR factor. If TR is very short (say a few milliseconds), then there won't be enough time for complete decay of transverse magnetization before the next α pulse. The residual transverse magnetization ($e^{-TR/T2^*}$) will essentially contribute to the next signal (at low flip angle). Thus, a short TR enhances T2* weighting. More simplistically, for TR < 3T2* (say about 100 msec), contrast depends on T2*.

A short TR (with a small flip angle) increases T2* weighting.

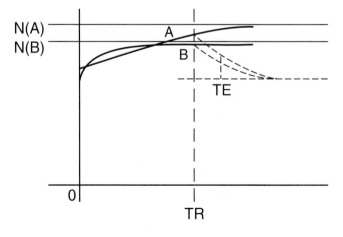

Figure 20-13. Small flip angles also result in small transverse magnetization, and thus poor T2* weighting and enhanced proton density weighting.

Now, consider a long TR. Remember that "long" is a relative term; in GRE, a "long" TR is approximately several hundred milliseconds, which is commensurate with a "short" TR in SE! A long TR allows more recovery of the T1 curves and thus better differentiation of different T1 values. It also causes more T2* decay, reducing the steady-state component and thus reducing T2* weighting.

> **A longer TR enhances T1 weighting.**

Finally, let's discuss the TE factor. This parameter's role in GRE is similar to the SE technique. That is, a short TE reduces T2* weighting and enhances T1 or proton density weighting.

> **A short TE reduces T2* weighting and increases proton density (PD) or T1 weighting. A long TE enhances T2* weighting.**

You might wonder what happens when these parameters are conflicting. For example, what contrast would a large TR and a small flip angle produce? The answer is that ultimately one parameter is going to dominate. In this example, as described previously, a small α predominates and produces a PD–weighted image. How about a short TR and a large α? This combination results in a mixed contrast that is proportional to the T2/T1 ratio of the tissues. (This is the contrast produced by a technique called steady-state free precession (SSFP); see Chapter 21.) Figures 20-14 through 20-16 contain some examples of GRE imaging.

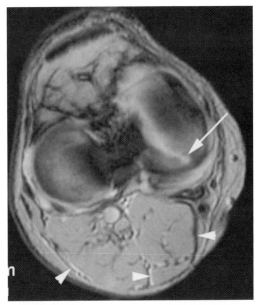

Figure 20-15. Axial T2* gradient-echo (TR 684/TE 20 msec) image of the knee shows high signal in the posterior horn of the medial meniscus diagnostic of meniscal tear (*arrow*). Typical T2 signal is seen. Incidental typical chemical shift artifact is seen in the transverse (frequency-encoding) direction (*arrowheads*).

MATH: Earlier in this book, we introduced a mathematical formula expressing the signal intensity (SI) with respect to TR, TE, T1, T2, and $N(H)$, namely

$$SI = N(H)e^{-TE/T2}(1 - e^{-TR/T1}) \quad \text{(Eqn. 20-4)}$$

Now, with the addition of the flip angle α, this equation is modified as follows:

$$SI = N(H)e^{-TE/T2^*}(1 - e^{-TR/T1})$$
$$[\sin\alpha/(1 - \cos\alpha e^{-TR/T1})] \quad \text{(Eqn. 20-5)}$$

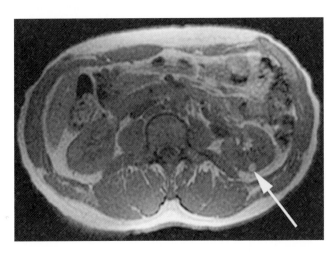

Figure 20-14. Axial T1 gradient-echo image of the abdomen shows typical signal appearance of the abdomen similar to CSE T1 technique. There is a focus of bright T1 signal in the left kidney that represented a hemorrhagic cyst in this patient with von Hippel–Lindau syndrome.

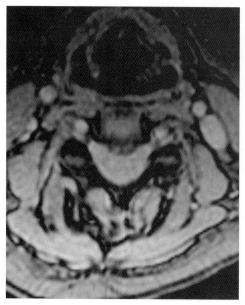
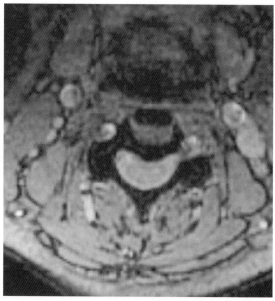

A   B

Figure 20-16. Axial T2* 3D gradient-echo images from the same patient on the same magnet 1 year apart show the second image to have more T2* weighting. The flip angle was constant (5°); however, image **A** had a TR 27/TE 6.9 msec, and image **B** had a TR 35/TE 16 msec. This demonstrates that the longer TE effect predominated versus the effects of a longer TR. Incidental central disc protrusion is seen in both.

Equations 20-4 and 20-5 differ in several ways. The most obvious difference is the term in brackets containing the variable α. Also, note that T2 is replaced by T2*, as is expected in GRE imaging (there is no 180° refocusing pulse).

Equation 20-5 is interesting in the extreme cases, namely, at $\alpha = 0°$ and $\alpha = 90°$. When $\alpha = 90°$ (which is the case in SE), then $\sin \alpha = 1$ and $\cos \alpha = 0$, and the equation becomes

$$SI = N(H)e^{-TE/T2^*}(1 - e^{-TR/T1}) \quad \text{(Eqn. 20-6)}$$

which is the same as Equation 20-4 with T2 replaced by T2*, as expected.

When $\alpha \cong 0$ (i.e., very small) then $\cos \alpha \approx 1$ and $\sin \alpha \cong \alpha$, and Equation 20-5 becomes

$$SI \cong N(H)e^{-TE/T2^*}(1 - e^{-TR/T1})[\alpha/(1 - e^{-TR/T1})]$$
$$= N(H)\alpha e^{-TE/T2^*} \quad \text{(Eqn. 20-7)}$$

which is dependent on the proton density $N(H)$ as well as T2*.

Signal-to-Noise Ratio

The SNR in a GRE technique is decreased per echo (compared with SE) due to shorter TRs in GRE; however, more echoes are obtained in GRE per unit time, somewhat compensating for the former effect.

Chemical Shift Artifact of the Second Kind (Dixon Effect)

This phenomenon was discussed in Chapter 18 (Artifacts in MRI) and applies only to GRE techniques. As discussed there, fat and water protons precess at slightly different frequencies in the transverse plane (220 Hz at 1.5 T). Immediately after the RF pulse, fat and water are both tipped (partially) into the transverse plane and are in phase. At various TEs later, fat and water spins will be in phase or out of phase. At 1.5 T, fat and water get back into phase every 4.5 msec after the RF pulse. This number is derived by the following formula:

Frequency difference
between fat and water = 220 Hz
Period = 1/frequency = 1/(220 Hz)
     = 0.0045 sec = 4.5 msec

Thus, fat and water are in phase initially at TE = 0, go out of phase at TE = 2.25 and back in phase at TE = 4.5, etc. In general, at 1.5 T, fat and H_2O go in and out of phase every 2.25 msec after the RF pulse (refer to Fig. 18-16). This is referred to as **chemical shift of the second kind.**

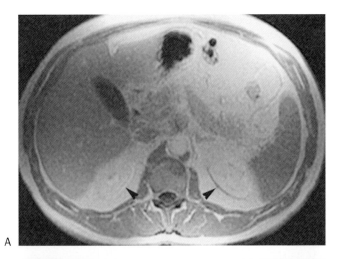

A

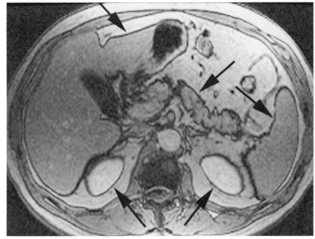

B

Figure 20-17. Axial postgadolinium T1 gradient-echo images obtained in phase (TR 93/TE 4.5 msec) (**A**) and out of phase (TR 93/TE 2.2 msec) (**B**) demonstrate the "boundary effect" at the interface of fat and water protons (*arrows* in **B**). Also note subtle typical chemical shift in the in phase image (*arrowheads*) along the transverse (frequency-encoding) direction.

If the selected TE is 2.25, 6.75, 11.25, 15.75 msec, etc., a dark boundary is seen around organs that are surrounded by fat (such as the kidneys and muscles). This is referred to as a **boundary effect**, which is not observed in SE imaging because of the presence of refocusing 180° pulses. This type of imaging is referred to as **out-of-phase** scanning, referring to the fact that at these TEs, fat and water spins will be 180° out of phase and cancel each other out. It should be remembered that GRE especially at lower bandwidths will also demonstrate standard chemical shift. Figure 20-17 is an example of both types of chemical shift.

To overcome the **boundary effect**, we can do the following:

1. Make fat and H_2O in phase by picking appropriate TE.

2. Suppress fat.
3. Decrease pixel size.

The **Dixon method**[1] takes advantage of this phenomenon to create solely "water excitation" or "fat excitation" images. To understand how this is done, suppose that the signal intensities from fat and water are designated F and W, respectively. Then, the signal intensities of the image with fat and water in phase (I_{ip}) and out of phase (I_{op}) are given by

$$I_{ip} = W + F$$
$$I_{op} = W - F$$

[1]From Dixon WT. Simple proton spectroscopic imaging. *Radiology.* 1984;153:189–194.

Thus,

$$W = (I_{ip} + I_{op})/2$$
$$F = (I_{ip} - I_{op})/2$$

allowing only water (W) or fat (F) imaging. This is the method of Dixon, which is particularly useful for spectroscopic fat saturation at low field strengths.

3D GRE Volume Imaging

3D imaging with contiguous thin slices is feasible by using GRE techniques. This type of imaging is accomplished by an addition of a phase-encoding step (N_z) in the slice-select direction (z-axis). Consequently, the total scan time is now

$$\text{Scan time} = TR \times N_y \times NEX \times N_z \quad \text{(Eqn. 20-8)}$$

where N_z is the number of phase-encoding steps in the z direction. N_z is usually a power of 2 (namely, 32, 64, and 128), but because the addition of a phase-encoding step in the z direction may cause wraparound artifacts in this direction as well, a few of the slices at each end are discarded and the number of slices displayed is slightly less (e.g., 28, 60, and 120). This provides a **slab** of slices.

You may wonder how it is possible to achieve 3D imaging in a reasonable time given the large multiplicative factor N_z. The answer lies in the extremely short TR.

Example
Calculate the scan time for a 3D GRE technique in the C-spine with the following parameters:

$$\text{TR 30/TE 13/}\alpha 5°/\text{NEX 2/256} \times 192/N_z 64$$
$$\begin{aligned}\text{Scan time} &= (TR)(NEX)(N_y)(N_z)\\ &= (30)(2)(192)(64)\\ &= 737280 \text{ msec}\\ &= 737.28 \text{ sec} = 12 \text{ min, 17 sec}\end{aligned}$$

A typical PSD is shown in Figure 20-18. The major difference here is the addition of an RF pulse for selection of a slab (i.e., a **slab-select gradient**), as well as application of phase-encoding steps in the z direction (i.e., **slice encoding**). This is depicted in Figure 20-19.

Volume imaging can be performed using **isotropic** (*cubic*, with $\Delta x = \Delta y = \Delta z$) voxels or **anisotropic** (noncubic) voxels. The advantage of the former is the ability to perform high-quality reformation in any plane of choice. 3D imaging is now also possible using newer FSE techniques that employ high performance gradients. More on this is in a later chapter.

Advantages of 3D GRE

1. Rapid volume imaging of thin contiguous slices without cross-talk (Figs. 20-20 and 20-21)
2. Reformation capabilities (especially if isotropic)

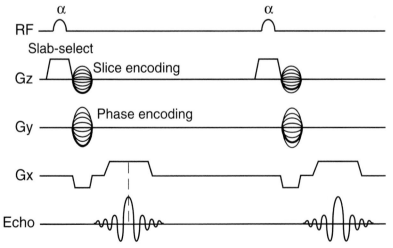

Figure 20-18. A PSD for a 3D GRE. Phase-encoding gradients are applied along both y and z directions. The slice-select gradient is also replaced by a *slab*-select gradient.

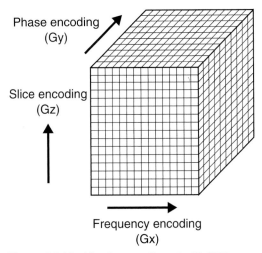

Figure 20-19. The three gradients in 3D GRE are illustrated here.

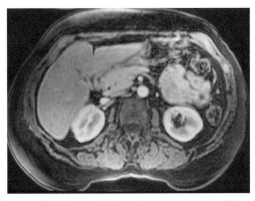

Figure 20-21. Axial T1 gradient-echo image of the abdomen acquired with 3D technique shows normal enhancement of the visualized organs. It was performed with chemical (spectral) fat saturation (see Chapter 23 for details).

3. Increased SNR, because

$$SNR \propto \sqrt{N_z}$$

Advantages of GRE

1. Increased speed
2. Increased sensitivity to magnetic suscepti- bility effects of hemorrhage (allowing bet- ter detection compared with SE)

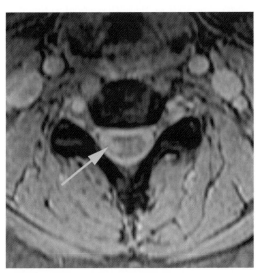

Figure 20-20. Axial T2* gradient-echo image of the cervical spine acquired with 3D technique shows abnormal bright signal in the right lateral aspect of the cord from multiple sclerosis (*arrow*).

3. 3D imaging (e.g., in the cervical spine) in a reasonable time
4. Imaging of flowing blood (i.e., MR angiog- raphy)

Disadvantages of GRE

1. Decreased SNR caused by (a) small α, reducing the transverse magnetization, and (b) very short TR, not allowing suffi- cient recovery of the longitudinal magneti- zation.
2. Increased magnetic susceptibility artifacts (caused by lack of a 180° refocusing pulse), most noticeable at air–tissue interfaces such as in the region of the paranasal sinuses or the abdomen (Fig. 18-43).
3. T2* decay because there are no 180° rephasing pulses. This results in increased sensitivity to magnetic field inhomo- geneities, intravoxel dephasing, and mag- netic susceptibility artifacts (Fig. 18-41).
4. Compared with FID imaging, the GRE technique (which is really an FID-recalled technique) uses a longer TE, thus reduc- ing the SNR caused by increased T2* decay.
5. Introduction of chemical shift effects of the second kind, resulting in a dark band around organs with water–fat interfaces, such as the kidneys, liver, spleen, etc.

Key Points

1 The objective of GRE techniques is to reduce the scan time.

2 Scan time is proportional to TR; a very small TR is possible in GRE imaging.

3 Because a small TR does not allow reasonable recovery of the longitudinal magnetization (thus significantly diminishing SNR), a partial flip angle α (<90°) should be used.

4 Because TR may be too short to allow complete dephasing of the spins in the transverse plane, a residual transverse magnetization may remain before the next cycle.

5 A refocusing gradient (readout direction) is employed that eliminates the original FID and later *recalls* it at the echo time TE (hence the name gradient-*recalled* echo, or GRE).

6 Because TR may be too short to acquire other slices within one TR period, GRE techniques often perform one slice at a time. (In the next chapter, we will discuss multiplanar GRE techniques.)

7 As a result, the scan time is also proportional to the number of slices obtained, that is, scan time = TR $\times$ N_y $\times$ NEX $\times$ (number of slices)

8 The tissue contrast is a function of the flip angle α, the repetition time TR, and the echo time TE. A simplified way of presenting the results is summarized in Table 20-1.

Table 20-1

	Small	Large
α	↑ PDW	↑ T1W
TR	↑ T2*W	↑ T1W
TE	↑ PDW	↑ T2*W

Questions

20-1 **T/F** Regarding chemical shift of the second kind, at 1.5 T, fat and water protons get out of phase at TE = 2.2, 6.7 msec, etc.

20-2 **T/F** A smaller flip angle increases PD weighting and reduces T1 weighting.

20-3 **T/F** GRE techniques often acquire one slice at a time.

20-4 **T/F** In general, GRE techniques use a partial flip angle because very short TRs are used to reduce the scan time.

20-5 **T/F** In the absence of a 180° pulse, a bilobed refocusing gradient is used in GRE.

20-6 **T/F** The longer the TR, the more T2* weighting will be achieved.

20-7 Calculate the scan time for a GRE with TR = 30 msec, NEX = 2, N_y = 256, for (a) a single slice and (b) 15 slices.

20-8 **T/F** Magnetic susceptibility is less with GRE than with CSE.

20-9 **T/F** The reason a 180° pulse is not used in GRE is to reduce the scan time.

20-10 The SNR in 3D GRE is equal to the SNR in 2D GRE times the factor:
(a) N_z
(b) $\sqrt{N_z}$
(c) N_y
(d) $\sqrt{N_y}$

20-11 **T/F** GRE sequences use a partial flip angle because the TR is too small to allow adequate recovery of the longitudinal magnetization to allow sufficient SNR.

Gradient Echo: Part II (Fast Scanning Techniques)

Introduction

In the last chapter, the technique of gradient-echo imaging was introduced. In this chapter, several gradient-echo techniques will be discussed, including **GRASS** (gradient-recalled acquisition in the steady state)/**FISP** (fast imaging with steady-state precession), **SPGR** (spoiled GRASS)/**FLASH** (fast low-angle shot), and **SSFP** (steady-state free precession)/**PSIF** (opposite of FISP). Although every manufacturer uses a different acronym, the underlying concepts are the same. We will also discuss a multiplanar (MP) variant of these GRE techniques (e.g., MPGR-MP FISP, MPSPGR/MP FLASH). Finally, faster versions of these techniques are introduced (e.g., Fast GRASS [FGR]/Turbo FISP, Fast SPGR [FSPGR]/Turbo FLASH) as well as their MP versions (e.g., FMPGR/Fast MP FISP and FMPSPGR/Turbo MP FLASH).

Nomenclature

Table 21-1 contains a summary of the important acronyms used by three major manufacturers: General Electric (GE), Siemens, and Philips. Also refer to the list of abbreviations in the Glossary. As an example, GE uses the prefix "*Fast*" and Siemens uses "*Turbo*" to denote similar fast scanning techniques, be it gradient-recalled echo or spin echo. (The acronyms are spelled out in the Glossary.)

GRASS/FISP

It was mentioned in the last chapter that, in contrast to SE, in GRE there may be **residual transverse magnetization** at the end of each cycle remaining for the next cycle. This residual magnetization reaches a steady-state value after a few cycles and is denoted $\mathbf{M}_{ss}$.

This residual, steady-state magnetization is added to the transverse magnetization created by the next α radio frequency (RF) pulse and thus increases the length of the vector in the x–y plane (Fig. 21-1). This then yields more T2* weighting. In other words, tissues with a longer T2 have a longer $\mathbf{M}_{ss}$ than do tissues with shorter T2.

Actually, to preserve this steady-state component, an additional step needs to be taken in the pulse sequence. A so-called **rewinder gradient** is applied in the phase-encoding direction at the end of the cycle to reverse the effects of the phase-encoding gradient applied at the beginning of the cycle (i.e., it "*unwinds*" the former effect). In other words, the rewinder gradient is nothing but the opposite of the phase-encoding gradient (Fig. 21-2). For instance, if gradient +3 is applied for phase encoding, the rewinding gradient would be −3.

SPGR/FLASH

The word "**spoiling**" refers to the elimination or "spoiling" of the steady-state transverse

Table 21-1

GE	Siemens	Philips
GRASS	FISP	TFE
SPGR	FLASH	T1 FFE
SSFP	PSIF	T2 FFE
FSPGR	Turbo FLASH	T1 TFE

Abbreviations: TFE, turbo field echo; FFE, fast field gradient echo.

magnetization. There are various ways of accomplishing this task:

1. By applying RF spoiling
2. By applying variable gradient spoilers
3. By lengthening TR

RF Spoiling. RF spoiling is the method used in SPGR and is illustrated in Figure 21-3. In this scheme, a phase offset is added to each successive RF pulse. This causes a corresponding phase shift in successive M_{ss} vectors. By maintaining a constant phase relationship between the transmitter and the receiver (achieved via a **phase-locked circuit**), successive M_{ss} vectors cancel each other out. A pulse sequence diagram (PSD) for SPGR is shown in Figure 21-4. In this scheme, rewinder gradients are naturally not used because their purpose is to preserve the steady-state magnetization, thus defeating the purpose of spoiling. An example is seen in Figure 21-5.

Variable Gradient Spoilers. Spoiling can also be achieved by using gradient spoilers. This is accomplished by introducing an additional

gradient with variable strengths from cycle to cycle (Fig. 21-6).

Lengthening TR. The last method to achieve spoiling of M_{ss} is by lengthening TR. When TR is sufficiently large (generally over 200 msec), there is enough time to allow complete dephasing of the spins in the transverse plane (because $TR \gg T2^*$). This is similar to the SE pulse sequence.

> *Question:* For a long TR (e.g., 500 msec), what is the difference between GRASS (or FISP) and SPGR (or FLASH)?
>
> *Answer:* There isn't any! A TR of 500 msec in GRASS effectively allows transverse magnetization to decay away over each cycle, that is, it eliminates the steady-state component (M_{ss}). Consequently, GRASS/FISP and SPGR/FLASH would have similar properties for any given TE and α when TR is long.

SPGR/FLASH Tissue Contrast. By eliminating the steady-state component, only the longitudinal component affects the signal in the SPGR/FLASH technique. Thus, this technique lends itself to reduced T2* weighting and increased T1 weighting. This is true provided α is also relatively large. When α is small, however, the T1 recovery curves play a minor role, and proton density (PD) weighting is increased.

> In SPGR, a long TR and a large α yield T1 weighting. A large TR and a small α yield PD- or T2*-weighted images depending on TE.

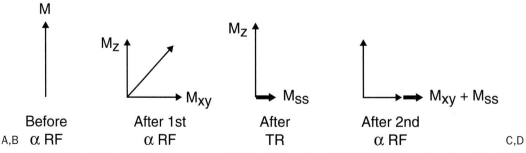

Figure 21-1. **A–D** A residual transverse magnetization that reaches a steady state M_{ss} remains after a short TR.

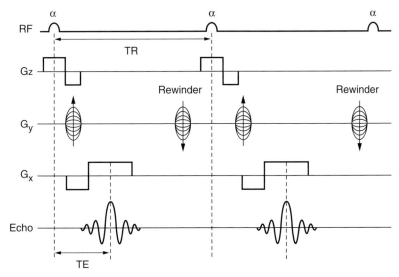

Figure 21-2. A PSD for GRASS/FISP. A "rewinder" gradient is applied along the y-axis at the end of the cycle to reverse the effect of phase-encoding gradient.

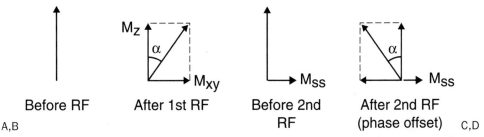

Figure 21-3. **A–D** Spoiling of the steady-state transverse magnetization can be done via RF spoilers (as in SPGR), in which a phase offset is added to each successive RF pulse.

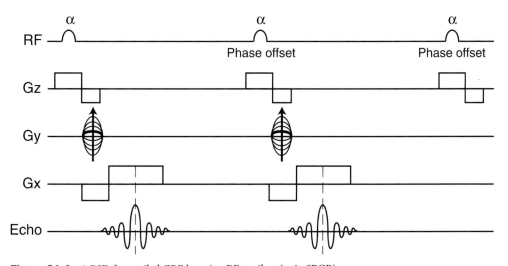

Figure 21-4. A PSD for spoiled GRE by using RF spoilers (as in SPGR).

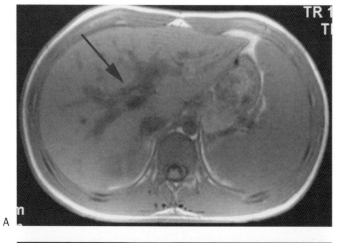

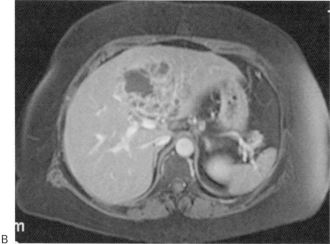

Figure 21-5. Axial spoiled gradient-echo T1 images of the abdomen. **A:** Without contrast-showing periportal edema (*arrow*) secondary to patient's hepatitis. **B:** Postgadolinium with chemical (spectral) fat saturation in a different patient that shows a multiloculated lesion in the medial segment of the left lobe consistent with pyogenic abscess.

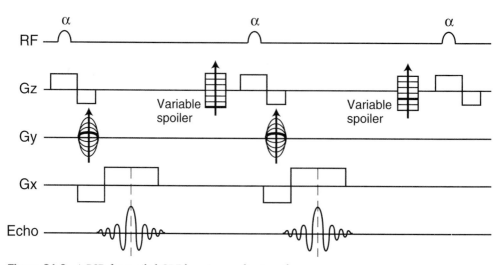

Figure 21-6. A PSD for spoiled GRE by using gradient spoilers.

Disadvantages of SPGR (FLASH)
1. Increased dephasing caused by inhomogeneities in $\mathbf{B}_0$
2. Increased magnetic susceptibility artifacts
3. Increased chemical shift artifacts (dark bands)

SSFP/PSIF

This technique is harder to comprehend. It yields heavily T2 (not T2*)-weighted images. The PSD is shown in Figure 21-7. The idea here is that each α RF pulse contains some 90° and some 180° pulses embedded in it. Therefore, in Figure 21-7, α_1 acts like a 90° excitation pulse and α_2 like a 180° rephasing pulse. This yields a pulse sequence similar to spin echo (SE) whereby an echo is formed at α_3. Because it is difficult to read a signal and transmit α_3 at the same time, the echo is actually recalled 9 msec prior to α_3 by using an appropriate gradient. Note that the echo corresponding to α_1 is formed between α_2 and α_3.

Interestingly, in this scheme, TE is larger than TR (and smaller than 2TR by 9 msec), which is somewhat counterintuitive. The rewinder gradients are also shown in the diagram. The rewinder gradient is one cycle ahead of the phase-encoding gradient due to the mechanism described in the foregoing discussion. (In this technique, any two successive RF pulses can be employed to create an SE.)

SSFP/PSIF Tissue Contrast. The SSFP sequence provides heavily T2 (not T2*)-weighted images with increased scan speed without the use of dedicated excitation and rephasing pulses.

Advantages of SSFP/PSIF
1. Decreased dephasing due to inhomogeneities in $\mathbf{B}_0$ compared with GRASS and SPGR
2. Decreased magnetic susceptibility artifacts compared with GRASS and SPGR
3. Decreased chemical shift artifacts (dark bands) compared with GRASS and SPGR

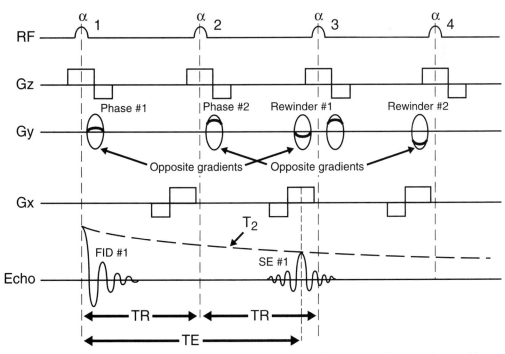

Figure 21-7. A PSD for SSFP/PSIF. Each α pulse contains some 180° pulse embedded in it that acts like a refocusing pulse. This, in turn, will result in a spin echo (SE) at the time of the next α pulse. Hence, contrast is determined by T2 (not T2*).

Disadvantages of SSFP

1. Decreased signal-to-noise ratio (SNR) secondary to the use of longer TEs (TE > TR)
2. Increased sensitivity to nonstationary tissue

Multiplanar Techniques

The GRASS and SPGR sequences can be performed using an MP technique by selecting a long TR (several hundred milliseconds). These are termed MPGR (multiplanar GRASS or multiplanar gradient recalled)/MP FISP and MPSPGR (multiplanar SPGR)/MP FLASH. As mentioned previously, this long TR causes spoiling of the steady-state component in the transverse plane, thus making GRASS and SPGR possess similar features.

We can still achieve both T1 and PD/T2* weighting depending on the flip angle α, as discussed previously. To reiterate, a small α yields PD weighting, whereas a large α yields T1 weighting. More specifically, at small flip angles, MPGR and GRASS behave fairly similarly, whereas at larger angles, MPGR tends to be more T1 weighted than GRASS because MPGR uses a long TR.

Advantages of Long TR

1. SNR is increased, because the longitudinal magnetization has more time to recover completely.
2. MP scanning is feasible because a long TR allows acquisition of other slices during the dead time within one TR period (similar to SE).
3. It is also possible to perform multiecho imaging (e.g., a short TE and a long TE) similar to the multiecho, MP technique in SE. However, the second echo tends to get degraded in GRE secondary to rapid T2* decay.
4. A long TR, as discussed in Chapter 27, reduces **saturation effects** (seen with very short TRs caused by incomplete recovery of the longitudinal magnetization). Consequently, larger flip angles can be used. Although larger flip angles cause more saturation effects, the presence of a longer TR counterbalances it. Larger flip angles obviously increase the length of the transverse magnetization and thus the SNR.

Fast Gradient-Echo Techniques

This topic might at first appear puzzling. Perhaps you are saying that you thought all GRE techniques were "fast." It is true that GRE techniques are generally faster than SE techniques, although the FSE (fast spin echo)/TSE (turbo spin echo) technique may be equally fast. However, there are additional methods that can further increase the speed of scanning. These methods are called Fast GRASS/Turbo FISP, Fast SPGR/Turbo FLASH, and so on.

The MP variants of these methods are also available and are referred to as Fast MP GRASS/Turbo MP FISP, Fast MP spoiled GRASS/Turbo MP FLASH, and so on. These render multiple slices with increased SNR in a rapid time period.

How can you make an already fast GRE technique faster? The answer lies in employing ultrashort TRs and TEs to reduce the **sequence time**, that is, the time it takes to excite, phase encode, and frequency encode. This is achieved by the use of the following:

1. Fractional echo
2. Fractional RF
3. Fractional number of excitations (NEX)
4. Reduction in the sampling time T_s (vis-à-vis by increasing the bandwidth [BW])

The first three items are discussed in Chapter 23 (Figs. 21-8, 21-9, and 21-10). Basically, by using a fraction of the echo and a fraction of the RF pulse, we can in effect decrease the echo time TE. Increasing the BW from ± 16 kHz (i.e., BW = 32 kHz) to ± 32 kHz (i.e., BW = 64 kHz) results in a reduction of the sampling time T_s from 8 to 4 msec for 256 fre-

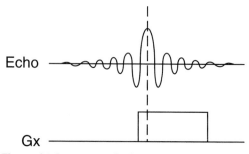

Figure 21-8. Fractional echo.

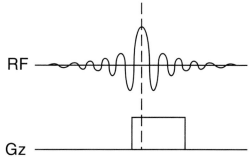

Figure 21-9. Fractional RF.

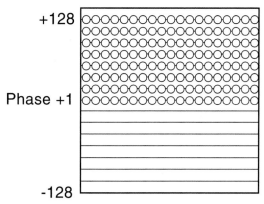

Figure 21-10. Fractional NEX.

quency-encoding steps N_x (Fig. 21-11). The trade-off here is a reduction in SNR because SNR is proportional to $1/\sqrt{BW}$. A wider BW allows more noise through, as shown in Figure 21-11. The active time is now given by

$$\text{Active time} = \text{TE} + T_s/2 + T_o$$

where T_o is the "overhead" time and T_s is the total sampling (readout) time. By minimizing TE and T_s, we can minimize the active time and thus reduce the minimum TR. Employing a fractional NEX decreases the overall scan time because the scan time is proportional to NEX.

In fast MP techniques, a longer TR is used, but multiple slices are acquired within that TR period.

Example

1. Determine the scan time for obtaining 15 slices using Fast SPGR/Turbo FLASH (one slice at a time) when TR = 10 msec, TE = min, N_y = 256, NEX = 1:

   Time = (10)(256)(1)(15)
   = 38,400 msec = 38.4 sec

2. Determine the scan time for obtaining 15 slices using MP Fast SPGR/Turbo FLASH (multislice) when TR = 100 msec, TE = min, N_y = 256, NEX = 1:

   Time = (100)(256)(1) = 25,600 msec
   = 25.6 sec

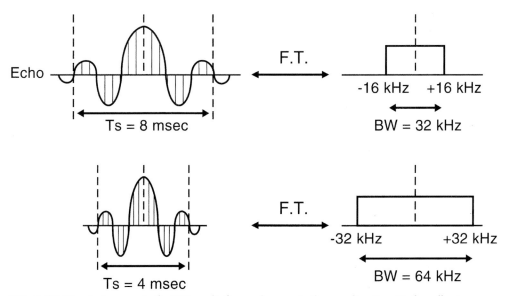

Figure 21-11. An increase in the BW results from a decrease in the sampling time T_s, thus allowing a reduction in TE. The trade-off is a decrease in SNR.

Applications. The technique is useful in applications requiring very fast scanning such as the following:

1. Single breath-hold techniques in the abdomen
2. Imaging of a joint in motion (e.g., temporomandibular joints)
3. Cine imaging of the heart
4. Temporal scanning of the same slice after contrast administration
5. Perfusion images after bolus injection of contrast

Disadvantages

1. Decreased SNR and CNR caused by ultrashort TRs (less so in degree with MP techniques)
2. Increased chemical shift artifacts of the second kind at very low TEs (namely, at TE = 2.2 msec, 6.6 msec, etc.)

Tissue-Prepared Fast GRE Techniques

In fast GRE techniques, ultrashort TRs are employed, so the tissue contrast may be subopti-mal. To help improve the tissue contrast, a technique called magnetization preparation or **tissue preparation** is used (e.g., **MP-RAGE**). Before the α RF pulse (**prep time**), other RF pulses (180° and/or 90°) are applied to the tissue. This prep time allows the tissues to develop a certain contrast (T1 or T2 weighting, depending on the type of application).

Two types of tissue preparation methods are discussed:

1. IR prepared (inversion-recovery prepared)
2. DE prepared (driven-equilibrium prepared)

IR Prepared. First consider the **IR prepared** method. In this scheme (Fig. 21-12), a 180° pulse is applied (prep time) before the α pulse. This method is similar to an inversion-recovery (IR) technique, providing increased T1 weighting and allowing suppression of various tissues depending on the prep time (Table 21-2). Note that the table has prep time values less than we have seen in typical IR sequences; this is because there is less longitudinal magnetization in this partially saturated technique, and hence the inversion time will be less (a similar concept as seen with lower inversion times for lower field strength systems versus longer times for higher

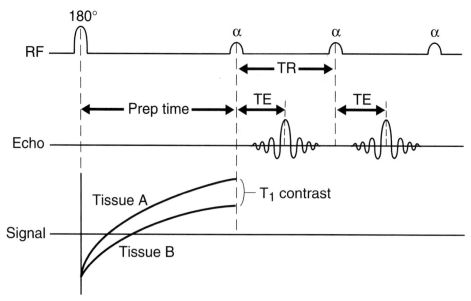

Figure 21-12. In an IR (inversion recovery) preparation Fast GRASS technique, a 180° pulse is applied before the GRE sequence, allowing for better T1 discrimination of two different tissues. This will increase T1 weighting.

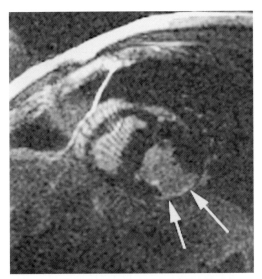

Figure 21-13. Short-axis IR prepared gradient-echo sequence (TR 7/TE 3/TI 150 msec) of the heart 10 min postgadolinium administration (delayed enhancement protocol) shows high signal in the inferolateral wall (*arrows*) diagnostic of myocardial infarction.

field strength). An example can be seen in Figure 21-13.

DE Prepared. The second method is the **DE prepared** technique. It employs a $90° - 180° - 90°$ pulse sequence similar to SE to provide T2-weighted contrast before the α

Table 21-2	
Suppressed Organ	**Prep Time (msec)**
Liver	200–400
Spleen	400–500
CSF	700–800

pulse (Fig. 21-14). The longer the prep time, the more T2 decay occurs and the more T2-weighted the tissue contrast becomes. In other words, tissues with longer T2s are degraded to a lesser degree compared with tissues with shorter T2s, thereby enhancing T2 contrast.

More specifically, referring to Figure 21-14, consider two tissues A and B with different T2 values (tissue A having a longer T2 than tissue B). After the first 90° pulse, both A and B will have similar transverse magnetization vectors. Right before the 180° pulse, tissue B (having a shorter T2) has decayed more than A and thus has a shorter vector in the transverse plane. After the 180° pulses, their direction is reversed by 180° in the transverse plane. The second 90° pulse causes these vectors to be *driven* to the longitudinal axis (hence the name *driven*-equilibrium), but with tissue A (having a longer T2) at a higher value than B. This allows the GRE sequence to start out with a bias toward tissues with longer T2s.

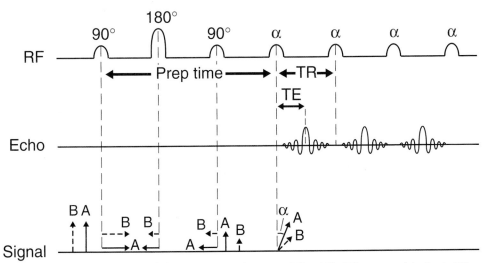

Figure 21-14. In an SE (spin echo) preparation technique, a $90° - 180° - 90°$ sequence (similar to SE) is applied before the GRE sequence, allowing better T2 discrimination. Refer to the text for more details.

Flow Imaging

GRE scanning is generally performed one slice at a time (except in the MP situation); therefore, each slice is an entry slice. Consequently, flow-related enhancement (FRE) applies to every single slice, and vessels appear bright on GRE images.

The basic concept is that no saturated flowing protons enter the slice so that flipping these protons yields maximum signal. This is the basic concept behind 2D or 3D **time of flight (TOF)** MR angiography. This topic is discussed at length in Chapters 26 and 27.

Key Points

1 Several GRE techniques are available: GRASS/FISP, SPGR/FLASH, and SSFP/PSIF (Table 21-1).

2 In GRASS, the residual transverse magnetization is preserved via a rewinder gradient, contributing to increased T2* weighting.

3 In SPGR/FLASH, the residual transverse magnetization is "spoiled" by introducing phase shifts in the successive RF pulses. This causes reduced T2* and increased T1 weighting.

4 Spoiling can also be accomplished via gradient spoilers or by lengthening the TR.

5 In SSFP/PSIF, heavily T2-weighted images are obtained. GRASS/FISP and SPGR/FLASH represent gradient-recalled *FID* sequences, whereas SSFP/PSIF represents a gradient-recalled *SE* (spin-echo) sequence. Interestingly,

in this technique, TE is larger than TR and usually is smaller than 2TR by 9 msec.

6 MP variants of the above are also available (e.g., MPGR/MP FISP and MPSPGR/MP FLASH) by employing a longer TR (over 100 msec).

7 Fast GRE techniques (e.g., FGR/Turbo FISP and FSPGR/Turbo FLASH) provide additional speed. This is accomplished by using a fractional RF, fractional echo, and fractional NEX, as well as a wider BW (shorter sampling time T_s).

8 Combined fast and MP GRE techniques (e.g., FMPGR and FMPSPGR/Turbo MP FLASH) render multiple slices with increased SNR in a fast mode.

9 The characteristics of GRASS/FISP, SPGR/FLASH, and SSFP/PSIF are summarized in Table 21-3.

Table 21-3

GRE Technique	SNR	CNR	Comments
GRASS/FISP	Highest	Best possible T2*	Preserves steady-state component
SPGR/FLASH	Intermediate	Best possible T1W	Spoils steady-state component
SSPF/PSIF	Lower	Provides T2W	Gradient-recalled SE; TR < TE < 2TR

Questions

21-1 Spoiling of the residual transverse magnetization can be accomplished by
  (a) gradient spoilers
  (b) RF spoilers
  (c) long TR
  (d) all of the above
  (e) only (a) and (b)

21-2 Fast GRE techniques may employ
  (a) fractional echo
  (b) fractional RF

  (c) fractional NEX
  (d) narrow BW
  (e) all of the above
  (f) only (a)–(c)

21-3 T/F A rewinder gradient is applied in the phase-encode direction to preserve the residual transverse magnetization M_{ss} (as in GRASS/FISP/TFE).

21-4 T/F Spoiled GRE techniques increase T1 weighting.

22

Echo Planar Imaging

Introduction

In the last three chapters, we discussed some of the fast scanning techniques, namely, the fast spin echo (FSE) and gradient-recalled echo (GRE) techniques along with their "fast" variants. In this chapter, we will discuss the echo planar imaging (EPI) technique, which is the fastest MRI technique available.

Basic Idea in EPI

Unlike other fast scanning techniques that can be achieved via software updates, single-shot EPI requires hardware modifications. More specifically, **high performance gradients** (discussed in Chapter 30) are needed to allow rapid on-and-off switching of the gradients. The basic idea is to fill k-space in one shot (single-shot EPI) with readout gradient during one T2* decay (if longer, T2 blurring will occur) or in multiple shots (multishot EPI) by using multiple excitations. As we shall see shortly, single-shot EPI allows oscillating frequency-encoding gradient pulses and complete k-space filling after a *single* RF pulse. Generally, gradient strengths of over 20 mT/m and gradient rise times of less than 300 µsec are required. Furthermore, extremely fast computers are needed to allow fast digital manipulations and signal processing.

Types of EPI

Two main types exist: **single-shot EPI** and **multishot EPI.** Earlier single-shot EPI techniques used a constant phase-encode gradient. Newer techniques use a "blipped" phase-encode gradient, referred to as "blipped EPI."[1]

Single-Shot EPI. In **single-shot EPI,** all the lines in k-space are filled by multiple gradient reversals, producing multiple gradient echoes in a *single* acquisition after a single radio frequency (RF) pulse, that is, in a single measurement or "**shot.**"

To achieve this, the readout gradient must be reversed rapidly from maximum positive to maximum negative $N_y/2$ times (e.g., 256/2 = 128 times) during a single T2* decay (e.g., 100 msec). Each lobe of the readout gradient above or below the baseline corresponds to a separate k_y line in k-space. Therefore, the number of phase-encode steps N_y is equal to the sum of the positive and negative lobes of the readout gradient. The area under the G_x lobe determines the field of view (FOV)—the larger the area, the smaller the FOV. Apparently, single-shot EPI places tremendous demands on the gradients with respect to maximum strength G_{max} and minimum rise time t_{Rmin} (i.e., the maximum **slew rate** G_{max}/t_R) as well as on the analog-to-digital converter (ADC). In general, ADCs with maximum bandwidths (BWs) on the order of MHz are required rather than the kHz maximum BWs used for conventional spin echo (CSE).

In earlier EPI methods, the phase-encode gradient was kept on continuously (Fig. 22-1)

---

[1]For more details, refer to Edelman RR et al. Echoplanar MR imaging. *Radiology.* 1994;192:600–612.

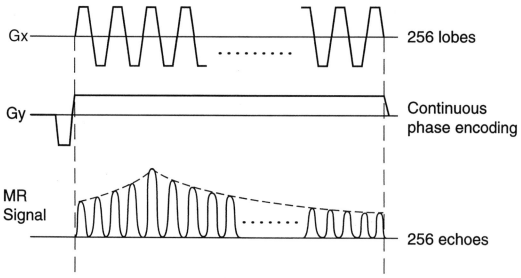

Figure 22-1. A PSD for the original single-shot EPI technique in which a constant phase-encode gradient is applied during readout. The G_x gradient has a sinusoidal shape caused by rapid on-and-off switching of the gradients.

during the acquisition, resulting in the zigzag coverage of k-space (Fig. 22-2). This led to some artifacts during Fourier transformation compared with conventional k-space trajectories. To rectify this problem, the phase-encode gradient was subsequently applied briefly during the time when the readout gradient was zero, that is, when the k-space position was at either end of the k_x axis (Fig. 22-3). This method was referred to as **blipped** phase encoding, as its duration was minimal (200 μsec). Therefore, the same phase-encode gradient is applied briefly N_y number of times (e.g., 256 times). The technique was called **blipped EPI,** and the k-space trajectory (Fig. 22-4) was much easier on the Fourier transformation.

As discussed previously, one of the problems with single-shot EPI is that any phase error tends to propagate through the entire k-space. (This is not a problem in CSE because of the presence of *rewinder gradients*, which reset the phase at the end of each cycle.) The phase errors we are talking about here are not the ones caused by motion (motion artifact is not a problem in the ultrafast EPI) but the errors arising from the variation in the resonating frequencies of protons (e.g., fat and water protons), which lead to mismapping

along the phase-encode axis. Consequently, one of the technical problems of single-shot EPI is magnetic susceptibility artifacts, particularly at air/tissue interfaces around the paranasal sinuses. Also, because of this phase error propagation along the phase-encode axis, chemical shift artifact in EPI is along the phase-encode axis rather than the frequency-encode axis, as in the case of CSE.

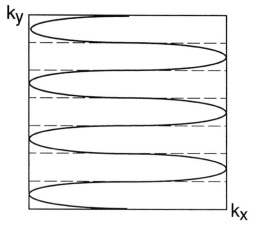

Figure 22-2. Single-shot EPI with constant phase gradient allows traversal of k-space in a zigzag manner after a single RF pulse.

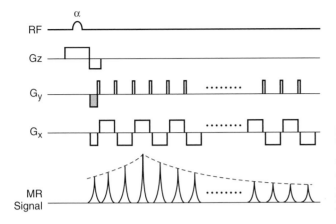

Figure 22-3. A PSD for blipped EPI. The phase-encode gradient is on briefly only while G_x is zero (blipped phase encoding). The signal starts out lower and peaks where it does due to the initial phase offset (G_y) (shaded area).

Multishot EPI. In **multishot EPI,** the readout is divided into multiple "shots" or segments (N_s), so that

$$N_y = N_s \times \text{ETL}$$

where ETL (echo train length) is the number of lines in each segment. Because k-space is segmented into multiple acquisitions, this technique is also called **segmental EPI.**

Advantages of Multishot EPI (Compared with Single-Shot EPI)

1. This technique places less stress on the gradients compared with single-shot EPI.

2. Phase errors have less time to build up compared with single-shot EPI, thus reducing diamagnetic susceptibility artifacts.

Disadvantages of Multishot EPI (Compared with Single-Shot EPI)

1. Multishot EPI takes longer to perform than does single-shot EPI.

2. Because of this fact, multishot EPI is more susceptible to motion artifacts.

Pulse Sequence Diagram in EPI

Figure 22-1 illustrates an example of the original EPI pulse sequence diagram (PSD). The major difference between this sequence and a conventional sequence is the application of a series of sinusoidal-shaped pulse sequences along the readout axis. This series requires rapid on-and-off switching of the gradients to achieve a train of positive and negative gradient pulses. It can be accomplished only with advanced hardware that can support such high performance gradients. The other difference is the application of a constant phase-encoding gradient (remember that k-space is filled in one TR period). (The term TR may not be suitable here because each slice is obtained after a single RF pulse. However, TR could be defined as the time between successive slice-select RF pulses.) The above scheme allows acquisition of raw data for each slice after a *single* RF pulse (unlike routine SE, in which one RF pulse is needed for each phase-encoding step).

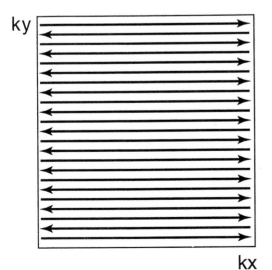

Figure 22-4. The k-space trajectory for blipped EPI in an odd-even manner, which is much easier on the Fourier transformation.

Figure 22-3 provides a PSD for blipped EPI in which the phase-encode gradient is applied briefly N_y number of times when the readout gradient is zero.

k-Space Trajectory in EPI

Unlike CSE, in which data sampling is performed during a constant readout gradient, in earlier single-shot EPI techniques, sampling was carried out during the readout gradient's alternating positive and negative lobes, which caused traversal of k-space in a zigzag or sinusoidal manner (Fig. 22-2). In the case of blipped EPI, k-space trajectory for even echoes is the opposite of that for odd echoes (Fig. 22-4). In multishot (segmental) EPI, data acquisition is carried out in multiple segments in an interleaved manner (Fig. 22-5). Spiral imaging in multishot EPI can also be formed (Fig. 22-6) by using two oscillating gradients.

These trajectories are in contrast to CSE, in which each line of k-space is filled during one TR period (and there are N_y number of such periods).

Scan Time in EPI

Because the entire data acquisition for each slice is accomplished after a single RF pulse,

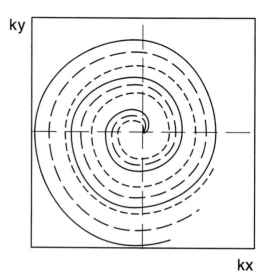

Figure 22-6. A spiral trajectory for multishot EPI using two oscillating gradients.

the scan time for a single slice in single-shot EPI is limited by T2* or T2 decay (on the order of 100 msec).

In general, if **ESP (echo sampling period)** is the time interval between two successive echoes, N_y is the number of lines in k-space, and NEX is the number of excitations (acquisitions), then for single-shot EPI, the scan time is given by

$$T \text{ (single-shot EPI)} = \text{ESP} \times N_y \times \text{NEX}$$

For multishot EPI, the scan time is given by

$$\begin{aligned} T \text{ (multishot EPI)} &= \text{TR} \times N_s \times \text{NEX} \\ &= \text{TR} \times N_y \times \text{NEX/ETL} \end{aligned}$$

which resembles the scan time for FSE (recall that $N_y = N_s \times \text{ETL}$).

Contrast in EPI

Contrast in EPI depends on the **"root" pulsing sequence** (which is similar to preparation prepulses in GRE techniques). For instance, to achieve SE contrast, a 90°–180° SE root sequence is applied before the EPI module. Similarly, a partial flip RF pulse (< 90°) before the EPI module provides gradient-echo contrast. A 180°–90°–180° IR root prior to EPI provides inversion recovery contrast. In addition, diffusion gradients can be added for EPI-diffusion imaging.

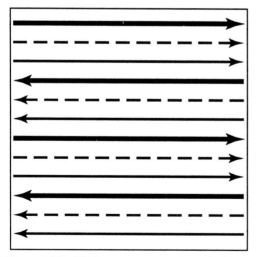

Figure 22-5. The k-space trajectory for multishot EPI. k-Space is divided into multiple segments, which are acquired in an interleaved manner.

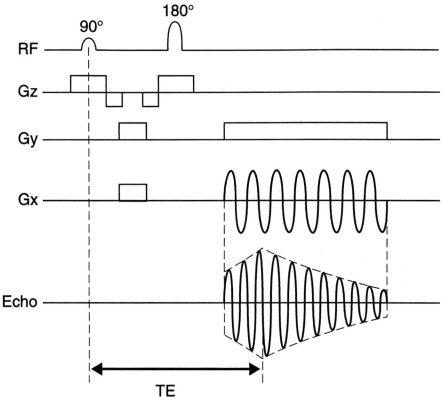

Figure 22-7. An SE-EPI PSD for the original EPI. A 90°–180° root pulsating sequence is applied before the EPI module.

Therefore, we can summarize as follows:

1. SE-EPI (90°–180°-EPI) uses a 180° pulse to overcome external magnetic field inhomogeneities (Fig. 22-7). This technique provides T1 and T2 weighting. Because all the echoes in EPI are acquired with the *same* value of the phase-encode gradient, contrast in SE-EPI is determined from the temporal rephasing of the 180° RF pulse. Contrast in a T2-weighted EPI is very similar to that of CSE, that is, signal is determined by T2 decay and flowing blood is dark.

2. GRE-EPI (α°-EPI) does not employ the 180° pulse, thus providing T2* weighting. This technique is faster and best suited for, say, cardiac cine imaging. Contrast here is determined by the time between the negative phase-encode offset and the EPI readout module.

3. IR-EPI (180°–90°–180°-EPI) allows T1 contrast by applying a 180° inversion prepulse.

Artifacts in EPI

N/2 **Ghost Artifacts.** Even with blipped EPI, phase errors may result from the multiple positive and negative passes through k-space (i.e., alternating polarity of the readout gradient). "Ghost" artifacts of the main image may appear along the phase axis, not caused by motion as in CSE, but by eddy currents, imperfect gradients, field nonuniformities, or a mismatch between the timing of the odd and even echoes. Since the ghosts are derived from half the data (even or odd), they are called *N/2* **ghosts.** See Figure 22-8 for examples.

Remedy. Minimize eddy currents; proper tuning of the gradients.

Susceptibility Artifacts in EPI. Magnetic susceptibility effects in EPI may result in variations in frequencies and phase errors. This effect is reduced for multishot EPI because phase

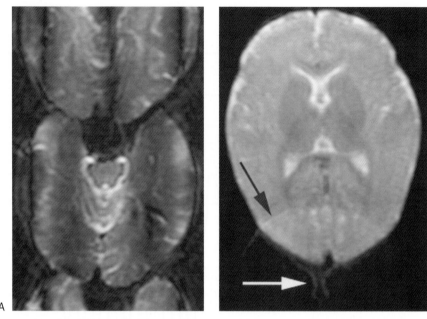

A   B

Figure 22-8. Both **(A)** and **(B)** are b_0 images from an EPI sequence of the brain in different patients. **(A)** has a marked amount of "*N* over 2" artifact, whereas **(B)** has more subtle findings (*arrows*).

errors have less time to build up. Advantages of multishot EPI over FSE is that it has contrast much closer to CSE and it has greater sensitivity to magnetic susceptibility effects such as hemorrhage compared with FSE.

Remedy. Minimized by proper shimming, TE shortening, or use of multishot echo.

Chemical Shift Artifacts in EPI. Because of the presence of phase error propagation along the phase-encode axis, chemical shift artifacts in EPI occur along the phase-encode axis rather than along the frequency-encode axis seen in CSE. These artifacts are much more pronounced than with CSE, so an effective fat suppression technique is necessary.

Remedy. Apply fat suppression.

Functional Echo Planar Imaging

Diffusion Imaging. Diffusion is defined as the process of random molecular thermal motion (also referred to as Brownian motion),

which plays an important role in, for example, cerebrovascular accidents (CVAs). Diffusion-weighted SE-EPI can be accomplished with a pair of diffusion gradients applied before and after the 180° pulse (Fig. 22-9) to dephase and eliminate signals caused by diffusing protons.

Diffusion Tensor Imaging. Diffusion tensor imaging (DTI) is an advanced form of diffusion imaging that quantitates the anisotropy of white matter. (Anisotropy is a property that is different along the three axes in the image, e.g., diffusion.) Instead of a single gradient pulse, a minimum of 6 (and sometimes 55) gradient pulses with a b value of 1000 is applied in addition to the $b = 0$ acquisition, that is, 7 total acquisitions. Three of these acquisitions are the three that are normally performed, that is, Dx, Dy, and Dz. In addition, three combination gradient pulses are performed, corresponding to the off-diagonal elements of the 3×3 tensor matrix (Fig. 22-10).

The theoretical advantage of DTI is that the measured ADC no longer depends on the specific orientation of the x, y, and z gradients of the scanner (true for a point, not a $2 \times 2 \times$ 5-mm voxel). The advantage of DTI is that it

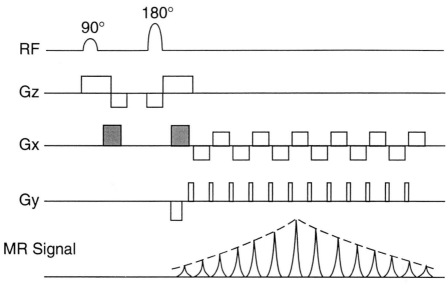

Figure 22-9. Diffusion-weighted SE-EPI. A pair of diffusion gradients (shaded areas) is applied before and after the 180° pulse to dephase and eliminate signals from diffusing protons.

should allow "quantitative diffusion" measurements, which are not dependent on head position in the magnet. In the DTI model, the x, y, and z axes are modified so that the z-axis corresponds to the principal direction of diffusion (typically along the major white matter tract in the voxel). This direction is known as the *principal eigenvector.* The diffusion coefficient in this direction is called the *principal eigenvalue.* In addition to the principal eigenvector and eigenvalues, new eigenvectors (new x and y axes) perpendicular to the new z-axis are

$$D = \begin{pmatrix} D_{XX} & D_{XY} & D_{XZ} \\ D_{YX} & D_{YY} & D_{YZ} \\ D_{ZX} & D_{ZY} & D_{ZZ} \end{pmatrix}$$

Figure 22-10. A diffusion tensor is a 3 × 3 matrix. By performing a mathematical maneuver called a *similarity transform,* the nondiagonal elements in the matrix are eliminated. This amounts to reorienting the z-axis in the voxel so it points along the direction of the principal white matter tract.

described (Fig. 22-11). Diffusion along the three eigenvectors is described by eigenvalues D1, D2, and D3 (Fig. 22-12).

DTI images can be displayed as scalar maps of combinations of D1, D2, and D3 variously called *fractional anisotropy, relative anisotropy,* and *anisotropy index* (Fig. 22-13). Normal white matter has high diffusion anisotropy, that is, diffusion is much greater parallel to than perpendicular to the white matter. Abnormal white matter (due to multiple sclerosis [MS], diffuse axonal injury, or gliosis) has reduced anisotropy. In addition, DTI images can be displayed as principal eigenvector maps, showing the orientation and integrity of white matter in the image (Figs. 22-14 and 22-15).

Perfusion Imaging. Because contrast in GRE-EPI is T2* weighted, it is perfect for performing first-pass **perfusion** sequences with gadolinium. Flowing blood is bright, as with conventional GRE, allowing for EPI magnetic resonance angiography.

Advantages of EPI
1. Scan time is approximately 100 msec or less.
2. Cardiac and respiratory motion won't pose problems any longer.

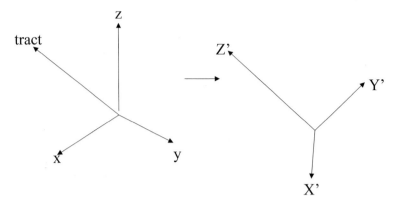

Figure 22-11. Diffusion tensor showing reorientation of coordinate system so new z-axis (z) is parallel to the main white matter tract in the voxel.

3. Proton density-, T1-, and T2-weighted images free of motion artifacts can be achieved.
4. It allows the study of organ function rather than the mere depiction of organ anatomy.
5. Resolution can be improved because time is not a significant factor.

Disadvantages of EPI

1. Because fat-water chemical shift artifacts (of the second kind [Dixon effect]) can be problematic with such short TEs, fat suppression with presaturation techniques is always required for EPI.
2. Because of rapid on-and-off switching of the gradients, there is a potential for generating an electric current or voltage in the patient, thus causing peripheral nerve stimulation where the patient may experience a crawling sensation in the skin

also known as "formication." This shock is caused by the well-known fact in electromagnetic theory that rapid changes in a magnetic field (i.e., $d\mathbf{B}/dt$ for the mathematically oriented reader) induce an electric current (E) in a conductor (in this case the patient).

3. Potential for phase error (caused by slight variations in resonant frequencies) propagation exists. This effect is less for multi-shot EPI as there is less time for phase errors to build up.

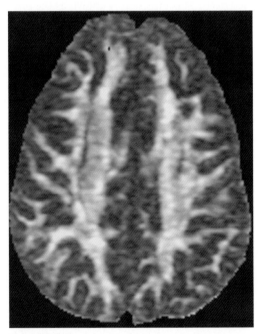

Figure 22-13. Fractional anisotropy map of normal brain. The bright signal in the normal brain indicates the greater anisotropy.

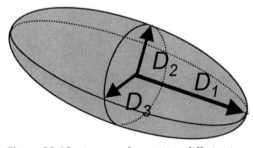

Figure 22-12. A tensor characterizes diffusion in the brain not by a single *apparent diffusion coefficient* but by three diffusion *eigenvalues* (D1, D2, D3) describing diffusion along three *eigenvectors*. The principal eigenvector is parallel to the main white matter tract in the voxel, and diffusion in that direction is characterized by D1.

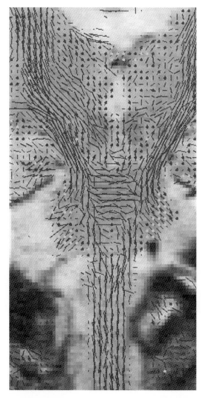

Figure 22-14. Tractography of corticospinal tracts based on plot of diffusion eigenvectors. Lines show projection in plane, and dots show projection perpendicular to plane in image. (Courtesy of Ferenc Jolesz, MD, Boston, MA.)

4. Intrinsic nonuniformities in B_0 and diamagnetic susceptibility effects also result in variable resonance frequencies and increasing phase errors. Again, this effect occurs less in multishot EPI.

Clinical Applications of EPI

1. Diffusion imaging of the brain (by looking at the molecular diffusion of water). This is helpful in early diagnosis of acute CVAs, when routine images are unremarkable, and in distinguishing a CVA from other processes (e.g., neoplasm) (Fig. 22-16).
2. Dynamic perfusion studies of the brain.
3. Cardiac and abdominal imaging free of motion artifacts in an extremely fast mode (Fig. 22-17).
4. Imaging the coronary arteries free of cardiac motion artifacts.
5. Cine cardiac imaging within a single heart beat.
6. Dynamic perfusion study of the myocardium after intravenous administration of gadolinium contrast to assess for ischemic regions (Fig. 22-18).
7. Single breath-hold imaging of the abdomen, providing T1, T2, or PD weighting.

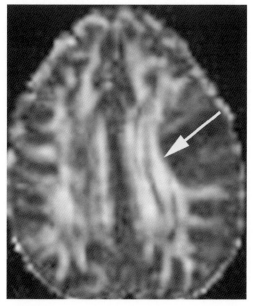

A

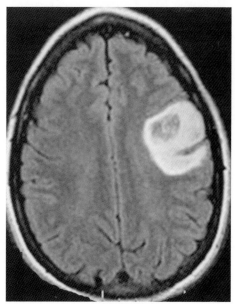

B

Figure 22-15. Anisotropy map **(A)** demonstrates intact white matter tracts subjacent to infiltrating glioma seen in accompanying FLAIR image **(B)**. (Courtesy of Shawn Ma, PhD, Houston, Texas.)

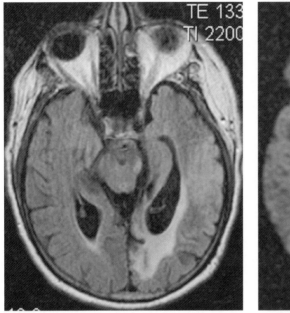 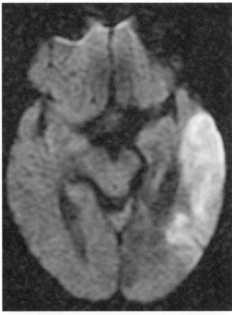

A   B

Figure 22-16. Axial FLAIR (**A**) and DWI (diffusion-weighted image) (**B**) show bright signal on FLAIR in the left occipital lobe with a trace of increased signal in the left temporal lobe. The DWI image confirms that the left occipital lobe signal is due to an old stroke, while showing more clearly the significant new stroke in the temporal lobe.

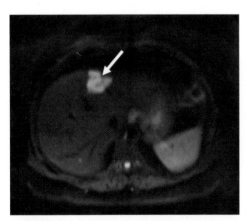

Figure 22-17. Axial EPI DWI image of the liver with a low b value ($b = 50$ sec/mm^2) demonstrates a bright T2 hemangioma (*arrow*). Also note that the low b value provides excellent suppression of signal in the liver vessels. This is a classic example of "T2 shine through."

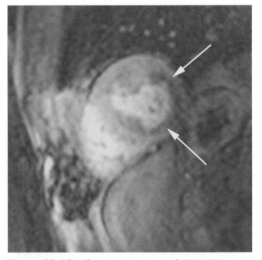

Figure 22-18. Short-axis segmented GRE-EPI dynamic postgadolinium adenosine stress study image shows decreased signal in the inferolateral wall consistent with ischemia (normal signal was seen on the resting study).

Key Points

Echo planar imaging (EPI) is the fastest MR technique that is widely available. It has become particularly important in the imaging of acute CVAs. It employs a train of oscillating frequency-encoding gradients, thus rendering a sinusoidal k-space traversal after a single RF pulse. Consequently, each slice can be imaged in a matter of milliseconds (free of any motion artifact), and the entire study can be accomplished in a matter of seconds.

Questions

22-1 **T/F** Contrast in EPI depends on the root pulsing sequence.

22-2 **T/F** Phase errors are eliminated with blipped EPI.

22-3 Regarding multishot echo, all the following are true *except*

    (a) It places less stress on the gradients compared with single-shot EPI.

    (b) Phase errors have less time to build up compared with single-shot EPI.

    (c) It takes longer to perform than single-shot EPI.

    (d) It is less susceptible to motion artifacts.

22-4 **T/F** In blipped EPI, the phase-encode gradient is constant during the acquisition.

22-5 **T/F** In multishot EPI, k-space is filled after a single excitation pulse.

22-6 **T/F** In single-shot EPI, k-space is traversed in a zigzag fashion.

22-7 *N/2* ghosts are generally seen with

    (a) constant phase EPI

    (b) blipped EPI

    (c) multishot EPI

    (d) none of the above

23

New Scanning Features

Introduction

In this chapter, we discuss some of the more recent techniques used by newer MR scanners with more advanced software. The following is a summary of these features and their functions:

1. To increase speed

   (a) Fractional number of excitations (NEX)
   (b) Fast spin echo (FSE)
   (c) Fast gradient-echo techniques
   (d) Parallel imaging (discussed in the next chapter)

2. To reduce TE

   (a) Fractional echo
   (b) Fractional radio frequency (RF)

3. To increase resolution (without time penalty)

   (a) Asymmetric field of view (FOV)

4. To reduce aliasing

   (a) No phase wrap
   (b) No frequency wrap

5. To increase coverage

   (a) Phase-offset RF pulses

6. To achieve contiguous slices

   (a) Contiguous slices
   (b) 3D acquisition

7. To achieve saturation

   (a) Spatial saturation
   (b) Spectral (chemical) saturation

8. To increase signal-to-noise ratio (SNR)

   (a) Low bandwidth

9. Reduce motion

   (a) Periodically rotated overlapping parallel lines with enhanced reconstruction (PROPELLER)

Remember that FSE and fast gradient-echo techniques are separate pulse sequences, whereas the other features can be added to any pulse sequence.

Fractional NEX

See Figure 23-1, and also refer to Chapter 13.

Mechanism

1. Only a portion of k-space is used (e.g., ½ NEX, ¾ NEX [actually, the number of phase encodes N_y is reduced, not NEX]). Reconstruction is based on inherent symmetry of k-space along the phase axis.
2. Slightly more than half of k-space is used (called **overscan**) for phase correction.
3. The center of k-space is usually included because it contains the strongest signals.

Advantages

1. Increased speed (caused by reduced N_y)

Disadvantages

1. Decreased signal-to-noise ratio (SNR)
2. May increase artifacts

Applications

1. Used for localizer (scout) images

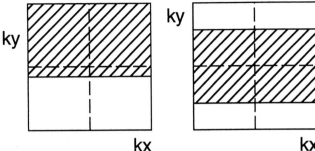

Figure 23-1. Fractional NEX.

2. Used when speed is more important than SNR
3. Body imaging and magnetic resonance cholangiopancreatography (MRCP)

Fast Spin Echo

For more detailed discussion, refer to Chapter 19.

Mechanism

1. Use of multiple 180° refocusing pulses
2. Filling the k-space with multiple lines per TR (per "shot")
3. Echo train length (ETL) denotes the number of 180° pulses (e.g., 2, 4, 8, 16, etc.)

Advantages

1. Reduces scan time by a factor of ETL (2, 4, 8, 16, etc.)
2. Spin-echo contrast without reduction in SNR (SNR can actually be increased by using a very large TR)
3. Decreased magnetic susceptibility—useful in imaging near metal (particularly at higher bandwidth [BW])

Disadvantages

1. Reduced coverage (caused by the presence of long TEs).
2. Cerebrospinal fluid may be bright on proton density images. This is a result of *weighted averaging* effect of later echoes. To reduce this undesirable effect, use a shorter ETL (e.g., ETL = 4), shorter TE (higher BW).
3. Fat is bright on T2-weighted images because of elimination of diffusion-mediated dephasing caused by the closely spaced 180° pulses as spins diffuse through regions of different magnetic field strength (e.g., fat and water).
4. Magnetic susceptibility effects (e.g., hemorrhage) are reduced because of decreased dephasing from closely spaced (refocusing) 180° pulses, which leave little time for spins to dephase as they diffuse through regions of magnetic nonuniformity.
5. May increase heating as a result of rapid train of RF pulses.

Applications

1. Fast scanning
2. High resolution (e.g., internal auditory canals)
3. Increase SNR with reasonable acquisition time
4. Single breath-hold technique
5. Isotropic T2-weighted data set (e.g., 3D FSE)

Fractional Echo

See Figure 23-2.

Mechanism

1. Only a fraction of the received echo is sampled (feasible because of the symmetry of the echo about TE and symmetry of k-space along frequency axis).

Advantages

1. TE can be reduced
2. SNR is improved in early echoes (less T2 decay)
3. Improves T1 weighting (reduces T2 effect)
4. May decrease flow artifacts and susceptibility effects

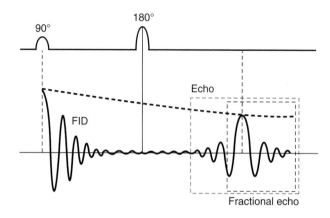

Figure 23-2. Fractional echo. Note outer dashed box is the full echo while the inner dashed box represents the fractional echo.

Applications
1. T1-weighted images
2. To reduce flow artifacts and magnetic susceptibility effects

NOTE: Using a higher bandwidth can also result in a lower minimum TE, however, at a SNR loss.

Fractional RF (90°, 180°, or Partial Flip)

See Figure 23-3.

Mechanism
1. Same principles as in fractional echo (a fraction of the RF pulse is included in the pulse cycle because of the symmetry in the pulse).
2. TE can be reduced accordingly.

Features. The features are similar to those of fractional echo.

Asymmetric FOV

See Figure 23-4.

Mechanism
1. Rectangular FOV is used (FOV is typically reduced in phase direction because N_y is typically less than N_x).
2. May get square or rectangular pixels.

Advantages
1. With rectangular FOV, we can obtain resolution of, say, 512×512 matrix in the time it takes to perform a 512×256 acquisition.
2. Increases speed while maintaining resolution.
3. Useful when the anatomy being imaged is asymmetric (smaller) in phase direction (e.g., the spine).

Disadvantages
1. Reduced SNR compared with full FOV
2. May cause wraparound in phase direction

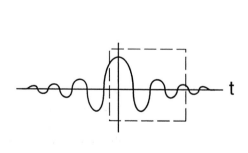

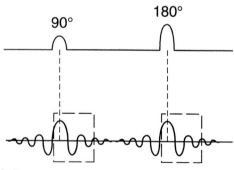

Figure 23-3. Fractional RF (90° or 180° or partial flip).

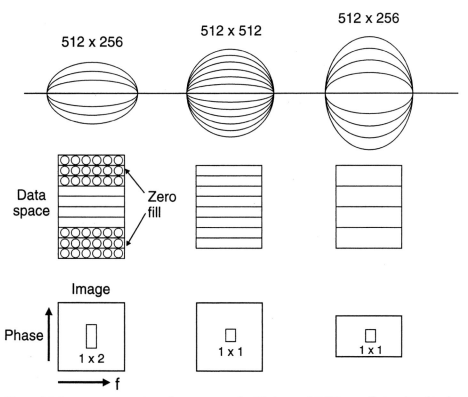

Figure 23-4. Asymmetric FOV. When a rectangular FOV is used, FOV typically is reduced in the phase direction. By acquiring more phase-encoding steps, a higher resolution can be achieved. In this example, you can acquire 256 phase-encoding steps and still get a 512 resolution.

Applications
1. Spine
2. Extremities
3. Abdomen

No Phase Wrap (Phase Oversampling)

See Figures 23-5, 18-7 and 18-8.

Mechanism
1. Doubles the number of phase-encoding steps and the FOV.
2. Discards one half of FOV at each end to maintain the specified FOV.
3. NEX is reduced by one half to keep time constant.

Advantages
1. Reduces or eliminates wraparound (aliasing)
2. No change in SNR or scan time

Disadvantages
1. If 1 NEX is used, scan time is doubled.

Applications
1. Small FOV (may cause wraparound)
2. Extremities

No Frequency Wrap (Frequency Oversampling)

Mechanism
1. The echo is **oversampled,** thus ensuring that the *Nyquist frequency* requirement is satisfied (e.g., 512 samples are obtained by the analog to digital convertor [ADC] even though N_x may read 256). Remember that the Nyquist law requires that the sampling frequency ω_s be at least twice as high as the maximum frequency present in the signal (ω_{max}). Stated differently, at least two samples are needed per

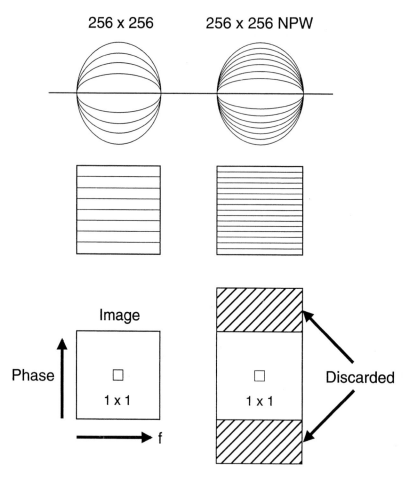

Figure 23-5. No phase wrap. To avoid wraparound in the phase-encoding direction, you can select this feature to double the FOV in that direction and automatically discard the unwanted portions at the end. In this example, you can acquire 512 phase-encoding steps and get a 256-step resolution.

cycle corresponding to the highest frequency waveform.

2. Various low-pass filters (LPFs) and band-pass filters (BPFs) are also used to get rid of unwanted high frequencies in the signal.

Advantages

1. Avoids wraparound in the frequency-encoding direction
2. No increase in the scan time

Disadvantages

1. May decrease SNR because, by increasing the number of samples, the sampling interval is reduced and thus the BW is increased (remember BW $= 1/\Delta T_s$ and SNR $\propto \sqrt{1/\mathrm{BW}}$).
2. This is done internally, that is, the operator has no control over it.

Applications

1. Almost always automatically turned on during routine scanning

Phase-Offset RF Pulses

See Figure 23-6.

Mechanism

1. Simultaneously excites two slices with two RF pulses that have a phase offset

Advantages

1. Doubles the number of slices per TR (without increasing time)
2. Can achieve more T1 weighting by reducing TR

Disadvantages

1. May increase wraparound artifact

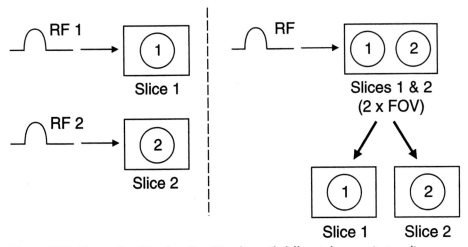

Figure 23-6. Phase-offset RF pulses. Two RF pulses with different phases excite two slices simultaneously.

Applications

1. When a short TR is desired, and a large area is studied.
2. Gadolinium-enhanced studies in which shorter TR enhances paramagnetic effects of contrast.

Contiguous Slice Option

See Figure 23-7.

Mechanism

1. Employs longer RF pulses that have a more rectangle-shaped frequency transform, reducing cross-talk.
2. This eliminates/minimizes the need for interslice gaps.

Advantages

1. Can achieve (almost) contiguous slices

2. Eliminates the need for interleaving (which doubles the scan time when correctly performed with two acquisitions)

Disadvantages

1. Increases TE (longer RF pulses)
2. Fewer slices per TR

Applications

1. When gaps are not desirable

3D Acquisition

Mechanism

1. Gradient-echo (GRE) technique over a 3D volume.
2. 3D FSE T2 is an option.
3. Requires a *phase*-encoding gradient along the slice-select z-axis.
4. Contiguous slices (zero gaps).

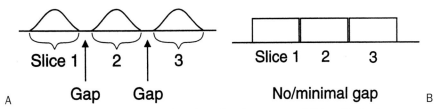

Figure 23-7. Contiguous slices can be achieved with an improved RF profile that better approximates a rectangle.

Advantages

1. Increased SNR (due to acquisition from larger volume)
2. Allows thin, high-resolution contiguous slices and/or overlapping slices
3. Allows for high-quality reformation in any plane

Disadvantages

1. May introduce wraparound artifacts at each end of the volume (end of the slab) caused by the presence of phase encoding in the z direction (Figs. 18-3 and 18-4).
2. Scan time now incorporates the number of phase-encoding steps along the z-axis (e.g., 28, 60) into the formula as well. That is to say,

$$
\begin{aligned}
\text{Acquisition time(3D GRE)} \\
&= T(\text{3D GRE}) \\
&= \text{TR} \cdot \text{NEX} \cdot N_y \cdot N_z \\
&= N_z \cdot T(\text{2D GRE})
\end{aligned}
$$

but because TR is very short, this is acceptable. For 3D FSE, this formula becomes

$$
\begin{aligned}
\text{Acquisition time(3D FSE)} \\
&= T(\text{3D FSE}) \\
&= \text{TR} \cdot \text{NEX} \cdot N_y \cdot N_z/\text{ETL} \\
&= N_z \cdot T(\text{2D FSE})
\end{aligned}
$$

where ETL can be chosen to be very large.

Applications

1. C-spine
2. MR angiography (e.g., circle of Willis)
3. Dynamic gadolinium abdomen

Spatial Saturation Pulses (Sat Pulses)

See Figure 23-8.

Mechanism (also see Chapter 25)

1. Ninety-degree saturation pulses are applied on either side of selected volume (can be applied in any direction: anterior/posterior, superior/inferior, and right/left).
2. Sat bands are usually applied to suppress phase ghosts caused by flow-related phenomena.

Advantages

1. Minimizes phase ghosts
2. Minimizes flow artifacts

Disadvantages

1. May cause signal suppression in the remainder of the FOV
2. May lengthen TR, thus increasing the scan time

Applications

1. Imaging of the spine: Saturation band is placed anterior to the vertebral bodies to suppress artifacts arising from the heart and great vessels.
2. MR angiography: Saturation pulses are placed at one end of a vessel to suppress either venous flow (to obtain MR arteriography) or arterial flow (to obtain MR venography).
3. Abdominal imaging (minimizing artifacts from the aorta or inferior vena cava).
4. Brain (minimizing artifacts from the internal carotid arteries and dural sinuses).

Chemical (Spectral) Presaturation

See Figure 23-9.

Mechanism (also see Chapter 25)

1. A frequency-selective presaturation pulse is applied before the RF excitation pulse, thus eliminating the longitudinal magnetization for a specific tissue.
2. The presaturation pulse is applied immediately before the 90° pulse of the SE. The tissue whose Larmor frequency matches the frequency of the presat pulse first sees a 90° spectral presat pulse that flips it into the x–y plane. A short time later, the longitudinal component $\mathbf{M}_z$ has really not had time to recover. Thus, the subsequent 90° excitation pulse that flips this minimal $\mathbf{M}_z$ into the x–y plane generates a minimal signal.

Applications

1. To suppress fat or water by appropriate selection of the frequency

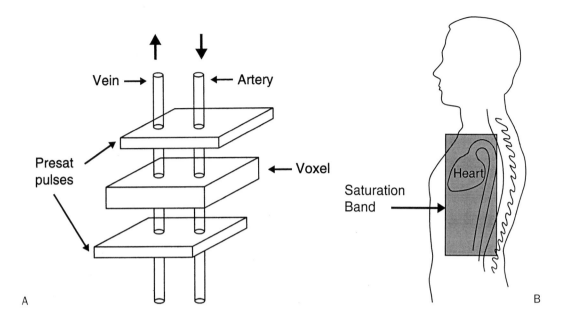

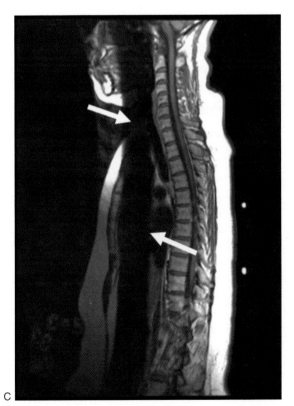

Figure 23-8. **A:** Spatial saturation pulses are placed immediately before or after each slice (outside the FOV) in the case of flow imaging of arteries or veins. **B:** Spatial saturation pulses are placed in front of the spine (within the FOV) to reduce artifacts from perivertebral vessels. **C:** Sagittal T1 image of the spine demonstrates an anterior saturation pulse over the heart resulting in a band of dark signal (*arrows*) and suppression of artifacts from the heart.

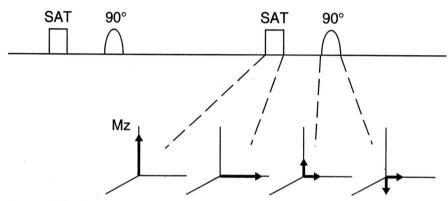

Figure 23-9. Chemical (spectral) presaturation pulses.

Advantages

1. It resolves tissues with similar T1 values (such as fat and gadolinium-enhanced tumors).
2. This technique does not have any influence on the signal from tissues other than the one being suppressed (in contrast, IR affects the contrast of all tissues).

Disadvantages

1. Since this approach employs a frequency-selective technique, it suffers from sensitivity to magnetic field inhomogeneities (see Figs. 18-42, 18-43, and 20-7).
2. Requires extra time (thus lengthening TR and increasing the scan time).
3. Increases the number of RF pulses, causing extra RF heating.

Low Bandwidth (Variable BW)

Mechanism

1. On double-echo SE sequence, the second echo has a lower BW

Advantages

1. Increases SNR (remember that SNR $\propto 1/\sqrt{BW}$) of second echo

Disadvantages

1. Increased chemical shift artifacts (see Fig. 18-14)
2. Decreases allowable number of slices (due to increased TE)

Applications

1. Any study requiring a higher SNR
2. Example: Dual SE of brain—a narrower BW is used on the second echo (to increase SNR, which is decreased because of T2 decay)

Periodically Rotated Overlapping Parallel Lines with Enhanced Reconstruction

Mechanism

1. Periodically rotated overlapping parallel lines with enhanced reconstruction (PROPELLER) (GE) and BLADE (Siemens) cover k-space in a radial (vs. Cartesian) fashion with several lines of k-space included in each fast spin-echo blade. The centers of k-space can be realigned if there is motion between acquisition of the blades.
2. By combining FSE-based PROPELLER with diffusion, the diamagnetic susceptibility artifacts over EPI-based diffusion can also be eliminated.

Advantages

1. Reduces gross motion (Fig. 23-10)
2. Increases SNR

Disadvantages

1. Requires 50% to 60% more time to perform

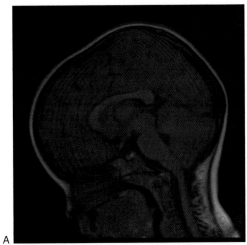 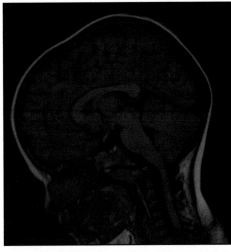

A   B

Figure 23-10. A: Sagittal T1 of the brain in a 3-year-old patient evaluated for seizures demonstrates multiple curvilinear lines from motion artifact. **B:** Sagittal T1 with PROPELLER (BLADE) was then performed to prevent this child from being sedated with resultant elimination of motion artifact and a diagnostic image.

Key Points

Many new MR techniques are reviewed in this chapter. These, along with their major trade-offs, are summarized below.

Advantage	Feature	Disadvantage
Increase speed	Fractional NEX	↓ SNR, ↑ artifacts
	FSE	↓ Coverage, ↑ contrast averaging
	Fast gradient-echo techniques	↓ SNR
	Parallel imaging (discussed further in next chapter)	↓ SNR
Reduce TE	Fractional echo	Both: may ↑ artifacts
	Fractional RF	
Increase resolution (without time penalty)	Asymmetric FOV	↓ SNR and ↑ potential for wraparound
Reduce aliasing	No phase wrap	May slightly ↑ scan time
	No frequency wrap	May ↓ SNR
Increase coverage	Phase-offset RF pulses	May ↑ wraparound
Contiguous slices	Contiguous slices (CS)	May ↑ TE
	3D acquisition	May ↑ scan time
Saturation	Spatial saturation	Both: slightly ↑ scan time
	Spectral (chemical) saturation	Chem Sat: sensitivity to field inhomogeneity
Increase SNR	Low bandwidth (variable BW)	Increased chemical shift artifacts
		Slightly fewer slices
Reduce motion	PROPELLER or BLADE	↑ Scan time by about 50%–60%

Questions

23-1 Speed can be increased by
(a) FSE or GRE techniques
(b) fractional NEX
(c) reducing BW
(d) all of the above
(e) only (a) and (b)

23-2 An asymmetric FOV may result in all of the following *except*
(a) reduced SNR
(b) increased potential wraparound
(c) increased resolution
(d) increased scan time

23-3 A lower BW leads to all of the following *except*
(a) reduces minimum TE
(b) increased chemical shift artifacts
(c) decreases coverage
(d) increased SNR

23-4 T/F Spatial saturation pulses are used to minimize phase ghosts and flow artifacts.

23-5 T/F The SNR is increased in 3D GRE.

23-6 T/F Minimum TE can be reduced by using fractional NEX.

24

Parallel Imaging

Introduction

Parallel imaging is an approach for reducing scan time and includes techniques such as sensitivity encoding (SENSE) and generalized autocalibrating partially parallel acquisition (GRAPPA). Vendor implementations of these techniques are also known as array spatial and sensitivity encoding technique (ASSET), autocalibrating reconstruction for Cartesian sampling (ARC), integrated parallel acquisition technique (iPAT), and rapid acquisition through parallel imaging design (RAPID).

Vendor Name	Technique	Sensitivity Calibration
SENSE (Philips)	SENSE	Prescan
ASSET (GE)	SENSE	Prescan
ARC (GE)	GRAPPA	Auto
GRAPPA (Siemens)	GRAPPA	Auto
mSENSE (Siemens)	SENSE	Auto
RAPID (Hitachi)	SENSE	Auto

Parallel imaging requires the use of phased-array coils. Depending on how many coils are used, time savings (or acceleration factors) of between 2 and 3 are easily achievable, albeit with a similar signal-to-noise ratio (SNR) cost as accompanies other "fast imaging techniques" based on decreasing phase steps or fewer excitations. As a result, parallel imaging is most useful for high SNR situations, for example, CE-MRA and 3T.

Concepts

The "parallel" in parallel imaging refers to the fact that each coil in the phased array receives data at the same time (i.e., in parallel). Recall from Chapter 2 that a phased array is made up of many small coils, with 32 or more available on modern systems.

Parallel imaging works by knowing the local sensitivity of each coil in the phased array. The field of view (FOV) is made intentionally too small in the phase-encoding direction, and the resulting aliasing is unwrapped using this information. The basic concepts were described in the early 1990s, and the first successful clinical implementation was simultaneous acquisition of spatial harmonics (SMASH). SMASH has now been superseded by more sophisticated techniques and the main approaches in clinical use today are SENSE and GRAPPA.

A parallel imaging acquisition with an acceleration factor of 2 acquires data only for every other line of k-space. The corresponding images have a ½ FOV and exhibit aliasing artifact. The SENSE and GRAPPA approaches work either by unwrapping the aliasing in the images or, equivalently, by filling in the missing lines of k-space (Fig. 24-1).

Both approaches make use of the different spatial sensitivities of the coils in the phased array. Due to their distinct spatial locations, each coil has different view of the object (Fig. 24-2). Knowing their spatial locations and sensitivity profiles allows the aliasing to be undone by postprocessing.

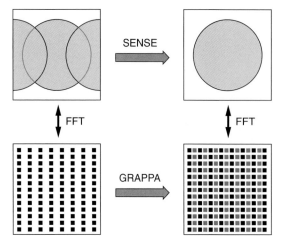

Figure 24-1. Image domain (*top*) and the associated k-space (*bottom*), which indicates how aliasing in the image domain is equivalent to undersampling in k-space. The SENSE method unwraps the aliasing in the image, but the same result can be obtained using GRAPPA to fill in lines of k-space.

Prescan or Autocalibration

There are two common ways to determine the spatial sensitivities of the coils in the phased array. SENSE and GRAPPA differ in the way that spatial sensitivity maps are determined and how the postprocessing is done.

Prescan. A large 3D volume acquisition lasting a few seconds run immediately after the localizers. This gives low-resolution images of the entire region inside the scanner and provides spatial sensitivity maps for all subsequent scans.

Autocalibration. A few extra phase-encoding lines are acquired within each parallel imaging scan. These are used in postprocessing to train the algorithm how to generate missing k-space lines for that specific scan only.

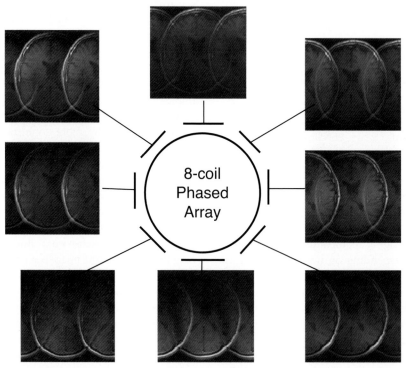

Figure 24-2. Aliased images obtained from an 8-coil phased array. Note each image has the characteristic spatial sensitivity of the coil, such that signals near the coil are strong and those far away are weak. This basic information allows us to work out which signals are in the right location and which signals have been aliased from ½ FOV away.

SENSE Equations

$A_1 = S_{11}O_1 + S_{12}O_2$
$A_2 = S_{21}O_1 + S_{22}O_2$

We have 2 equations and 2 unknowns, which can be solved to give O_1 and O_2.

Key
A_1 = aliased pixels from coil 1
A_2 = aliased pixels from coil 2

S_{11} = sensitivity of coil 1 at location 1
S_{12} = sensitivity of coil 1 at location 2
S_{21} = sensitivity of coil 2 at location 1
S_{22} = sensitivity of coil 2 at location 2

O_1 = object pixel at location 1
O_2 = object pixel at location 2

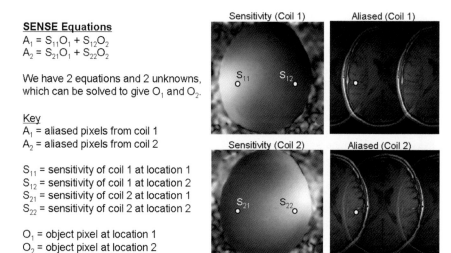

Figure 24-3. Description of the SENSE parallel imaging method. Coil sensitivity maps (*left*) from two coils in the phased array and aliased images (*right*). The equations express the aliased pixels as a sum of two distinct spatial locations weighted by the coil sensitivities.

Advantages/Disadvantages

1. Prescan only needs to run one time so there is little time spent on sensitivity measurements.
2. Autocalibration calibrates on every scan so it can tolerate patient repositioning between scans.
3. Autocalibration costs a few extra phase-encodes so acceleration factors will be slightly lower (e.g., 1.9 rather than 2). Note the SNR decrease is proportionate (e.g., $\sqrt{1.9}$ decrease rather than $\sqrt{2}$).

SENSE. Sensitivity encoding generally uses a prescan to measure sensitivity of the coils. The individual images are divided by a body coil image to remove "contaminating" structure, leaving just the spatial sensitivity of the coils (or sensitivity maps). These are shown in Figure 24-3; for simplicity, only two coils in the phased array are shown.

Since we used an acceleration factor of 2, we know the aliased pixels come from two locations at a distance of exactly ½ an FOV apart. We also know the pixels are weighted by the sensitivity of the coil, for example, pixels close to the coil will have a higher weighting than pixels further away. By knowing the aliasing pattern and the spatial sensitivities, we can write a linear equation and

solve it to obtain the values of the two pixels (Fig. 24-3). The process is repeated for all pixels.

Because the coil sensitivity maps and aliased images are represented in the spatial domain, SENSE is often described as an *image-domain* parallel imaging technique.

GRAPPA. GRAPPA uses autocalibration to provide information about the coil sensitivities. For an acceleration factor of 2, alternate lines of k-space are skipped but a few additional lines are acquired at the center for calibration. The overall acceleration factor is slightly reduced although the calibration data contribute to the SNR so the SNR is proportionate to the overall acceleration factor. A schematic of the k-space data is shown in Figure 24-4.

In GRAPPA, we seek to recreate the missing k-space lines using a combination of its neighbors, often just two neighboring lines. Note the SMASH technique mentioned above uses just one neighboring line.

The key is to work out how to generate missing lines, and this is where the calibration data are needed. If the calibration data consist of (say) line 2, then we need to find what linear combination of lines 1 and 3 can give the closest approximation to line 2. We must also specify a coil, so the full procedure is to determine what

GRAPPA Equations

$$K_{12} = C_{11}K_{11} + C_{13}K_{13} + C_{21}K_{21} + C_{23}K_{23}$$
$$K_{22} = C_{11}K_{11} + C_{13}K_{13} + C_{21}K_{21} + C_{23}K_{23}$$

To calibrate, we have 8 unknowns (C's and D's) and ~256x2 data points (K_{12} and K_{22}).

Key:

K_{11} = coil 1 k-space line 1
K_{12} = coil 1 k-space line 2
K_{13} = coil 1 k-space line 3
K_{21} = coil 1 k-space line 1
K_{22} = coil 1 k-space line 2
K_{23} = coil 1 k-space line 3

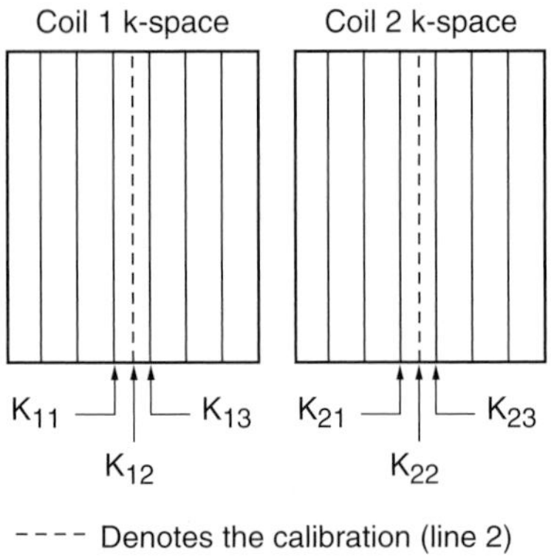

$C_{11}, C_{13}, C_{21}, C_{23}$ = grappa coefficients (coil 1)
$D_{11}, D_{13}, D_{21}, D_{23}$ = grappa coefficients (coil 2)

Figure 24-4. Description of the GRAPPA parallel imaging method. The undersampled k-space from two coils are shown (*solid lines*), along with the calibration data (*dotted lines*). By a computational search, we look for coefficients (*C* and *D*) that minimize the difference between our estimate of the calibration lines, generated by the equations, and the actual acquired calibration line.

combination of lines 1 and 3 *from all coils* gives the best approximation to line 2 *from coil 1*. Similarly, we must determine what combination gives the best approximation to line 2 of coil 2.

Once the coefficients are determined, the missing lines anywhere in k-space can be generated from a combination of the neighboring lines. The final result is a full k-space for each coil, which are then Fourier transformed and combined into a single image using standard methods (e.g., the square root sum of squares).

Because the coil calibration and data are represented in k-space, GRAPPA is often described as a *frequency-domain* parallel imaging technique.

SNR and g-factor. An image produced with half as many phase-encodes has an SNR that is decreased by $\sqrt{2}$; however, the SNR is often significantly worse at higher acceleration factors. This is the result of unfavorable coil geometries, or the "*g*-factor." The overall loss of SNR in a parallel imaging acquisition is the square root of the acceleration factor multiplied by the *g*-factor. So ideally the *g*-factor should be close to 1.

The *g*-factor is a numerical measure of how difficult it is to solve the SENSE (or GRAPPA) equations. Benign *g*-factors (i.e., close to 1) occur when the coils have very different views of the object along the phase-encoding direction. Likewise, poor *g*-factors occur when coils have virtually the

same sensitivity. In terms of the SENSE equation, the latter would occur when $S_{11} = S_{21}$ and $S_{12} = S_{22}$ so there is effectively only one equation. In this case, it is impossible to find a solution and the *g*-factor would be infinite. In practice, coils always have some similarities and some differences. These vary for each pixel in the image and this gives rise to the spatially varying SNR characteristics of parallel imaging.

Figure 24-5 shows images for SENSE and GRAPPA reconstructions. Some points to note are

- The overall SNR is in inverse proportion to the square root of the acceleration factor.
- GRAPPA acceleration factors are slightly lower due to autocalibration.
- Spatially varying SNR is observed, particularly, with higher acceleration factors.
- Generally, little difference is seen between SENSE and GRAPPA images.

There are many ways to alter the SNR in parallel imaging by postprocessing. Mathematically, it is straightforward to constrain the SENSE and GRAPPA images to appear smooth, or to incorporate prior knowledge about how the object should look. Although these may increase the SNR, there is always a trade-off to be made! Often spatial resolution may be compromised or subtle artifacts may be introduced that are hard to understand.

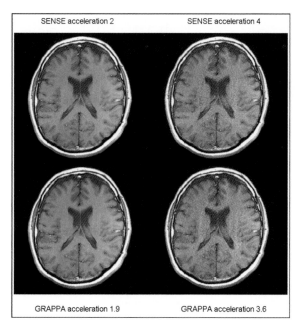

SENSE acceleration 2   SENSE acceleration 4

GRAPPA acceleration 1.9   GRAPPA acceleration 3.6

Figure 24-5. 3T images produced by SENSE and GRAPPA at two comparable acceleration factors, reconstructed from virtually the same data. For most applications, accelerations of 2 perform well, and the SENSE and GRAPPA methods are interchangeable. At higher accelerations, structured noise and artifacts start to become a problem for both.

Key Points

We have looked at the concepts behind parallel imaging, which uses phased-array coils to accelerate scans, and taken a close look at two popular methods, SENSE and GRAPPA. We saw that each coil in a phased array produces an image with a characteristic spatial sensitivity and that postprocessing can undo the aliasing introduced by reducing the FOV in the phase direction, for a corresponding saving in scan time. We noted that acceleration factor of 2 is readily obtainable on current systems; this is likely to increase as special purpose coils for high accelerations are developed.

Questions

24-1 What does the word "parallel" refer to in parallel imaging?
  - **(a)** The need to use fast computers for postprocessing
  - **(b)** The simultaneous data acquisition by the coils
  - **(c)** The blend of phase-encoding and phased-array coils
  - **(d)** The arrangement of the coils needed to make it work

24-2 With 8 coils and an acceleration factor of 2, what will be the SNR change relative to a nonaccelerated scan?
  - **(a)** 1/2
  - **(b)** $\sqrt{1/2}$

  - **(c)** 1/4
  - **(d)** No change

24-3 Which imaging situation is incompatible with parallel imaging
  - **(a)** Diffusion-weighted EPI
  - **(b)** 3T high field
  - **(c)** Large FOV body coil
  - **(d)** 128 channel phased array
  - **(e)** All of the above

24-4 T/F Higher acceleration factors can be obtained by using a more powerful gradient system.

24-5 T/F Parallel imaging is most compatible with applications that have inherently high SNR.

25

Tissue Suppression Techniques

Introduction

One of the beauties of MR, especially with some of the new features, is the ability to image a body part while "suppressing" the signal coming from a certain selected tissue. This suppression allows perturbation of tissue contrast to enhance the signal coming from tissues of greater interest (such as a pathology). Two types of tissues are commonly suppressed in clinical practice: fat and water.

Suppression Techniques

Several suppression techniques are available, some of which are listed below.

1. Inversion recovery techniques
2. Chemical (or spectral) saturation or frequency-selective presaturation
3. Spatial presaturation in the field of view (FOV)

Inversion Recovery (IR) Techniques. This technique was discussed at length in Chapter 7. The IR pulse sequence diagram (PSD) is shown in Figure 25-1. By appropriate selection of TI (time to inversion), we can nullify or suppress a certain tissue. In fact, as we saw in Chapter 7, if

$$TI = (\ln 2) [T1(tissue\ x)] = 0.693\ T1(tissue\ x)$$

then tissue x is nulled. Thus, TI can be chosen to null fat or water or any other desired tissue depending on the application (Fig. 25-2).

STIR (Short TI Inversion Recovery). This is the IR technique that is used to suppress fat.

Example
What is the TI used in STIR? At 1.5 T, T1 of fat is approximately 200 msec. Then

$$TI = 0.693 \times 200 \cong 140\ msec$$

FLAIR (Fluid-Attenuated Inversion Recovery). This is an IR technique that nulls fluid. For example, this sequence is used in the brain to suppress cerebrospinal fluid (CSF) to bring out the periventricular hyperintense lesions, such as multiple sclerosis (MS) plaques (Fig. 25-3).

Example
What is the TI used in FLAIR? At 1.5 T, T1 of CSF is approximately 3600 msec. Then

$$TI = 0.693 \times 3600 \cong 2500\ msec$$

Fast FLAIR. STIR sequences are typically performed with a fast spin-echo (FSE) technique; however, there are some novel changes that must be performed to apply FSE technique to the normally slow FLAIR sequence and achieve CSF suppression in a fast manner.[1] Figure 25-4 depicts a schematic representation for Fast FLAIR. In this scheme, the following parameters are used:

TR = 10,000 msec

TI = 2500 msec

FSE with ETL = 8

TE_{eff} = 112 msec

---

[1] Hashemi RH et al. Suspected multiple sclerosis: MR imaging with a thin-selection fast FLAIR pulse sequence. *Radiology.* 1995;196:505–510.

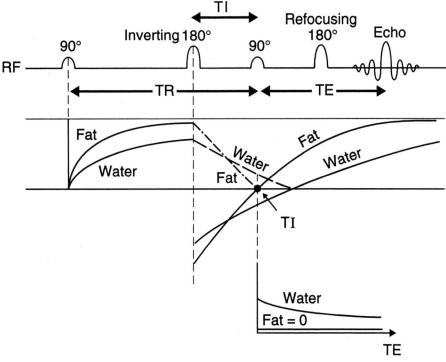

Figure 25-1. Inversion recovery (STIR shown). The recovery curves following the 90° and 180° pulses are illustrated for fat and water.

In Figure 25-4, there are two packets of 15 slices each. During the first 5000 msec, 15 slice-selective 180° inverting pulses are followed 2500 msec (TI) later by 15 slice-selective FSE readout in 2500 msec. During the second 5000 msec, recovery occurs in the first 15 slices (for a total TR of 10,000 msec), and the process is repeated on the second set of 15 interleaved slices. In all, 30 slices are acquired.

A TR of 10,000 msec allows almost complete longitudinal recovery of CSF. This relatively long time period also makes it possible to perform multislice interleaving during inversion and readout. The inversion "period" is the time during which 15 slice-selective 180° pulses are applied. It is the time TI (2500 msec in this case) from the first 180° inverting pulse to the 90° pulse at the beginning of the readout period. FSE readout takes 136 msec (8 × 17 msec) for each slice. The readout "period" is the time (also 2500 msec) during which 15 slice-selective readouts are performed. The recovery period is the time from the slice-selective 90° pulse

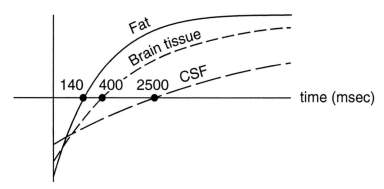

Figure 25-2. TI required to null fat, brain, or CSF.

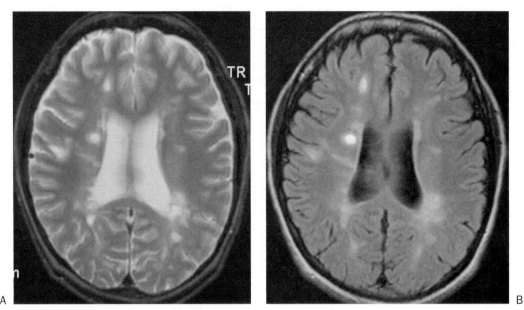

Figure 25-3. Axial T2 (**A**) and FLAIR (**B**) images of the brain demonstrate the different conspicuity between the images of the bright multiple sclerosis lesions.

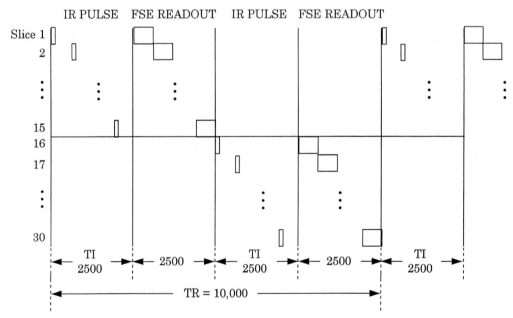

Figure 25-4. A schematic representation for Fast FLAIR. There are two packets of 15 slices each. During the first 5000 msec, 15 slice-selective 180° inverting pulses are followed 2500 msec (TI) later by 15 slice-selective FSE readout, in 2500 msec. During the second 5000 msec, recovery occurs in the first 15 slices (for a total TR of 10,000 msec) and the process is repeated on the second set of 15 interleaved slices. In all, 30 slices are acquired in 8 min.

beginning an FSE readout to the next slice-selective 180° inverting pulse, which is TR–TI (10,000 − 2500 = 7500 msec in this case).

The maximum number of slices that can be acquired in one TR is determined either by the time period TI or by (TR–TI), whichever is shorter. The longer the TR, the more complete recovery of magnetization will be before the next excitation. A long TR will also result in better signal-to-noise ratio (SNR) and increased contrast-to-noise ratio (CNR) between the lesion and gray and white matter.

Unfortunately, when TR is increased, the TI necessary to null CSF does not increase to the same degree. This difference results in inefficient usage of time because (TR–TI) becomes larger and larger, and the number of slices is still limited by TI. Given the TR of 10,000 msec and the TI of 2500 msec used in this study, 5000 msec (i.e., 10,000 − 2 × 2500) would be "wasted" before the next cycle. To increase the efficiency, the sequence takes advantage of this dead time to acquire a second multislice inversion-readout slab.

In this arrangement, the number of slices acquired can be doubled in the same time duration with no dead time when the TR to TI ratio equals 4. As the ratio approaches 6, yet another multislice section can be added, and so on. This approach allows the flexibility to choose TR and TI with little concern for time efficiency.

Advantages of IR

1. No significant extra RF heating (unlike spectral presaturation—see later text—due to the longer TI time vs. the very short time between the spectral presaturation pulse and the root RF pulses)
2. No variability caused by magnetic field inhomogeneities (like spectral presaturation—see below)

Disadvantages of IR

1. Tissues with similar T1 values are all suppressed and thus cannot be differentiated (e.g., fat and blood or gadolinium-enhanced tumors—Figs. 25-5 and 25-6)

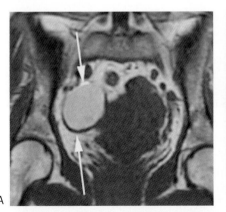

A

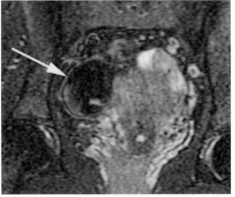

B

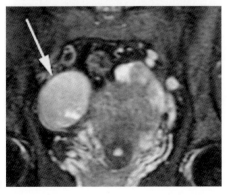

C

Figure 25-5. Coronal T1 (**A**) of pelvis shows bright right adnexal lesion. Coronal STIR (**B**) shows complete loss of signal, which may imply fat, but is nonspecific since the FSE T2 with chemical (spectral) fat saturation (**C**) shows that there is some signal within the lesion, indicating that it is not a fat-containing lesion. Note the chemical shift artifact in the T1 (**A**) lending further evidence that this is not a fat-containing lesion. Diagnosis: endometrioma.

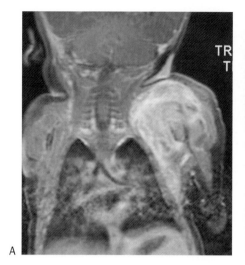

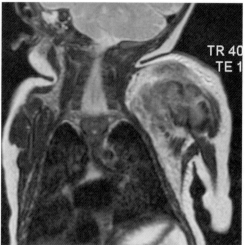

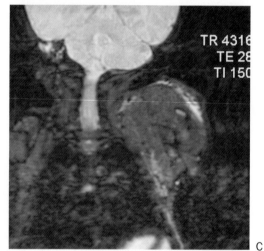

Figure 25-6. Coronal T1 postgadolinium image with fat saturation (**A**) shows a large enhancing hemangioma in the left shoulder of a young patient with Kesselbach–Merritt syndrome. Pregadolinium coronal FSE T2 image (**B**) shows areas of bright signal; however, a postgadolinium STIR image (**C**) shows signal dropout from the T1 shortening effects of gadolinium that make the lesion's T1 equivalent to that of fat.

2. Long acquisition times caused by long TRs
3. Low SNR

Chemical (Spectral) Presaturation. In this technique, a frequency-selective presaturation pulse is applied very shortly before the RF excitation pulse, thus eliminating the longitudinal magnetization for a specific tissue, for example, fat. It can be used to suppress fat or water by appropriate selection of the frequency (based on the Larmor equation, keeping in mind that at 1.5 T, water protons precess 220 Hz faster than fat protons). This scheme is illustrated in Figure 25-7. Here, the presaturation pulse is applied immediately before the 90° pulse of the SE. The tissue whose Larmor frequency matches the frequency of the presat pulse

first sees a 90° spectral presat pulse that flips it into the x–y plane. A short time later, the longitudinal component M_z has really not had time to recover. Thus, the subsequent 90° excitation pulse that flips this minimal M_z into the x–y plane generates a minimal signal (Fig. 25-7). An example is in Figure 25-8.

Advantages
1. Resolves tissues with similar T1 values (such as fat and gadolinium-enhanced tumors, or fat and blood products—Fig. 25-5)
2. No influence on the signal from tissues other than the one being suppressed (in contrast, IR affects the contrast of all tissues)

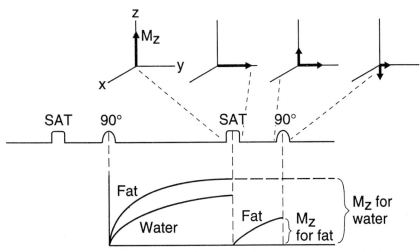

Figure 25-7. Spectral presaturation. A frequency-selective presaturation pulse is applied before the excitation pulse to eliminate longitudinal magnetization for a specific tissue such as fat or water.

Disadvantages

1. Suffers from sensitivity to magnetic field inhomogeneities because it employs a frequency-selective technique (Fig. 25-9)
2. Requires extra time (thus lengthening TR and increasing the scan time)
3. Increases length of RF pulses, causing extra RF heating

Spatial Presaturation. Spatial presaturation is done generally to reduce motion-and-flow-related artifacts of structures adjacent to—or actually within the FOV next to—the region of interest. Examples include

1. Imaging of the spine: a saturation band is placed within the FOV anterior to the vertebral bodies to suppress artifacts arising from the heart and great vessels (Fig. 23-8).
2. MR angiography: saturation pulses are placed outside the FOV at one end of a vessel to suppress either venous flow (for achieving MR arteriography [MRA]) or arterial flow (for achieving MR venography [MRV]).

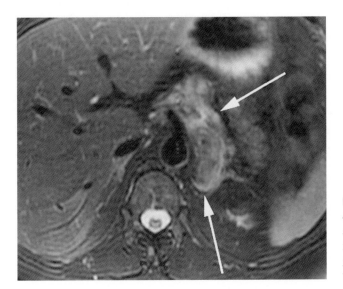

Figure 25-8. Axial T2 FSE image with chemical (spectral) fat saturation shows suppression of fat signal. There is an intermediate brightness left adrenal ganglioneuroma (*arrows*), which extends toward the midline.

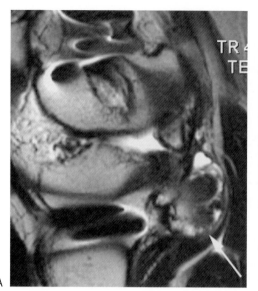
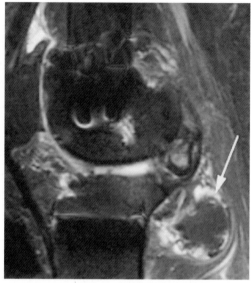

A

B

Figure 25-9. Sagittal T2 FSE image with fat saturation (**A**) of the knee shows marked field distortion and inhomogeneous fat saturation due to metallic susceptibility artifact. Sagittal fast STIR (**B**) shows homogeneous fat saturation and less distortion and reveals a mild amount of bright signal in the distal femur. There are also advanced patellofemoral osteoarthritis changes and a large loose body posterior to the tibia (*arrow*).

Spatial presaturation is accomplished by applying an extra 90° pulse before the 90° pulse of the SE sequence. This additional sat pulse saturates tissues, including moving structures, within the slice, eliminating signal (and thus associated artifacts). For more details, refer to the discussion on saturation in Chapter 23.

Magnetization Transfer (MT). Magnetization transfer (MT) is a technique that suppresses protein-bound water. The idea behind MT is that protons in protein-bound water exhibit a resonant frequency that is approximately 500 to 2500 Hz away from that of bulk water protons (Fig. 25-10). MT saturation pulses are simply off-resonant pulses with their center frequency 1000 to 2000 Hz removed from the Larmor frequency of protons and a bandwidth (BW) of several hundred to several thousand hertz, as shown in Figure 25-10A, thus allowing suppression of these protons. The result is shown in Figure 25-10B. Note that the off-resonant protein-bound water is saturated. Because the protein-bound protons and the bulk water protons

are in rapid exchange, the saturation is transferred to the bulk phase protons. Thus, the peak amplitude of bulk water is reduced. MT is somewhat similar to spectral fat suppression techniques except that here, the off-resonant frequency is up to 2000 Hz (2 kHz) as opposed to 220 Hz in the case of fat suppression.

This technique is used, for example, in time of flight (TOF) MR angiography (see Chapter 27) as a means of suppressing the background brain tissue to enhance visualization of smaller, more peripheral vessels.

Magnetization Transfer Effect in FSE. As discussed in Chapter 19, MT is inadvertently present in FSE because of the presence of multiple, rapid 180° pulses. These rapid 180° pulses have a broad BW that contains frequencies off the bulk water resonance frequency that tend to suppress protein-bound water.

Clinical Applications of Fat Suppression
   1. To differentiate between fat and methemoglobin (chemical saturation).

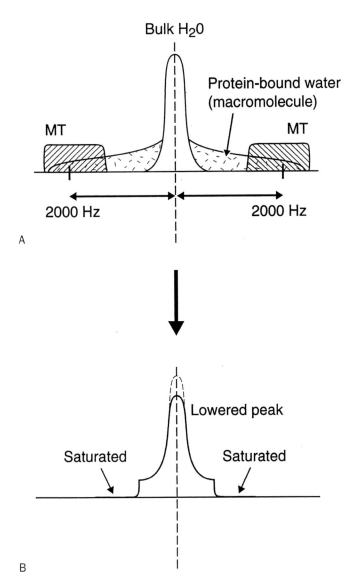

Bulk H$_2$0

Protein-bound water
(macromolecule)

MT   MT

←——— 2000 Hz ———→ ←——— 2000 Hz ———→

A

Lowered peak

Saturated   Saturated

B

Figure 25-10. Magnetization transfer. **A:** Protein-bound water has a resonant frequency of about 500 to 2500 Hz off that of bulk water. **B:** Spectral saturation of these off-resonant frequencies will result in suppression of protein-bound water. This technique is used, for example, in MRA for background suppression.

2. *Musculoskeletal:* to minimize fat signal in the marrow to bring out the signal from marrow edema (e.g., due to bone contusion, tumor, and infection; chemical saturation or inversion recovery—Fig. 25-11).

3. *Orbits:* to suppress the retro-orbital fat to allow detection of enhancing retro-orbital pathology on a contrast-enhanced study (chemical saturation—Fig. 25-12).

4. *Neck:* to suppress fat in order to detect, and better evaluate the extent of, a mass (chemical saturation or inversion recovery).

5. *Body:* to identify macroscopic fat-containing lesions such as angiomyolipomas, mature teratomas, and myelolipomas (chemical saturation).

Clinical Applications of Water Suppression.
Brain: to suppress CSF to bring out periventricular high intensity lesions such as MS plaques, thus increasing their detectability (FLAIR).

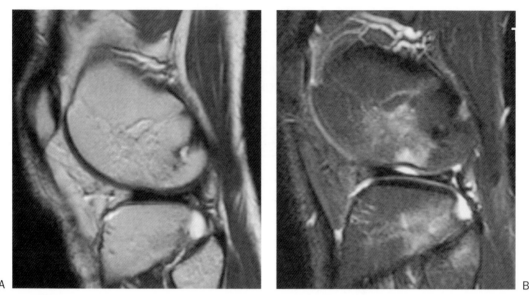

A   B

Figure 25-11. Sagittal T2 FSE (**A**) and sagittal fast STIR (**B**) images demonstrate better conspicuity of the bone marrow edema with the STIR fat suppression technique. (Chemical saturation could be used as well.)

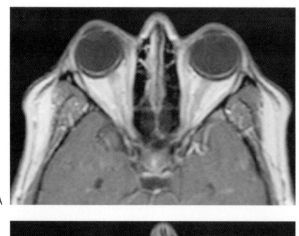

A

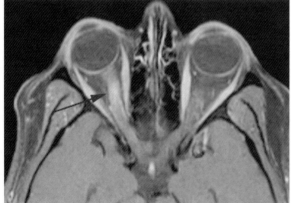

B

Figure 25-12. Axial postgadolinium T1 images without (**A**) and with fat saturation (**B**) show marked increased conspicuity of the enhancing right optic nerve (*arrow* in **B**) in this patient with optic neuritis.

Key Points

Tissue suppression is an important feature of MRI—it allows improved tissue contrast and enhanced lesion detectability. Generally, two tissues are subject to suppression: fat and water. The two major suppression techniques are inversion recovery (IR) and chemical (spectral) saturation. Each technique has its own advantages and disadvantages. The selection of the type of technique depends on the clinical application. Other tissues may be saturated (e.g., protein-bound water and flowing blood).

Major fat suppression techniques include

1 STIR

2 Chemical (spectral) fat sat

Major fluid suppression techniques include

1 FLAIR

2 Chemical (spectral) water suppression

Techniques for suppression of protein-bound water include

1 MT technique for background suppression

2 MT effect in FSE

Effects of presaturation technique in the FOV include

1 Saturation bands reduce flow artifacts (e.g., in spine imaging)

2 Saturation pulses remove venous or arterial flow (e.g., in MRA or MRV)

Questions

25-1 In an IR sequence, the TI to null a tissue is given by
(a) 0.693 T2
(b) 0.693 T1
(c) (1/0.693) T1
(d) (1/0.693) T2

25-2 The T1 of CSF at 1.5 T is about 3600 msec. What is the approximate TI to null CSF?
(a) 2500
(b) 5000
(c) 140
(d) 249.48

25-3 **T/F** Protons in protein-bound macromolecules have a resonant frequency that is about 220 Hz removed from that of bulk water.

25-4 **T/F** Magnetization transfer techniques saturate the off-resonant protein-bound water protons.

25-5 **T/F** Fast or Turbo FLAIR is currently the most sensitive MR sequence for detection of periventricular white matter disease.

25-6 Major water suppression techniques include
(a) STIR
(b) Spectral water suppression
(c) FLAIR
(d) all of the above
(e) only (b) and (c)

25-7 Major fat suppression techniques include
(a) STIR
(b) Spectral fat suppression
(c) FLAIR
(d) all of the above
(e) only (a) and (b)

25-8 **T/F** FSE demonstrates an inherent magnetization transfer property.

26

Introduction

Unlike computerized tomography (CT) (with or without contrast), in which the appearance of flowing blood in a vessel is predictable, the appearance of flowing blood in MRI is much more complicated. Flowing blood or cerebrospinal fluid (CSF) can appear dark or bright depending on numerous factors, including, but not limited to, the following:

1. Velocity
2. Pulse sequence (e.g., spin echo [SE] vs. gradient echo [GRE])
3. Position of the slice containing the vessel relative to the rest of the slices
4. Contrast (TR and TE)
5. Echo number (even or odd)
6. Slice thickness
7. Flip angle
8. Gradient strength and rise time
9. Use of gradient moment nulling techniques
10. Use of spatial presaturation pulse
11. Use of cardiac gating
12. Chance of cardiac gating (pseudogating)

Types of Flow

In Chapter 18, we discussed two types of motion: random and periodic. Blood and CSF flow have a periodic-type motion. Furthermore, flow of blood can be divided into the following:

1. Laminar flow
2. Plug flow
3. Turbulent flow
4. Flow (stream) separation/vortex flow

These types of flow are depicted in Figure 26-1. Let's discuss these separately.

Laminar Flow. This type of flow is seen in most normal vessels and has a parabolic profile. If the lumen radius is R, then the velocity v at position r would be

$$v(r) = V_{max}(1 - r^2/R^2)$$

where V_{max} is the maximum velocity in the center of the lumen. Therefore, the average velocity in the lumen is given by

$$V_{ave} = V_{max}/2$$

Plug Flow. This type of flow is usually seen only in large vessels (aorta) with high velocities. The velocity across the lumen is constant, thus yielding a flat velocity profile:

$$v(r) = V_{max} = V_{ave} = constant$$

Turbulence. This phenomenon is observed in abnormal vessels (e.g., distal to stenosis) or at bifurcations during which a random motion of fluid elements is observed. **Vortex flow** and large-scale recirculation zones (i.e., **eddies**) are other terms that refer to such random motions.

Flow (Stream) Separation. This phenomenon is observed near the wall of a vessel (e.g., in the proximal internal carotid artery) in which some of the flow is separated from the main streamline.

Question: What determines laminar versus turbulent flow?

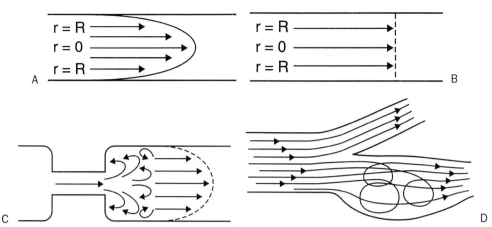

Figure 26-1. Types of flow. **A:** Laminar flow. **B:** Plug flow. **C:** Turbulent flow (distal to stenosis). **D:** Flow (stream) separation.

Answer: A dimensionless number called the Reynolds number (Re) can predict the type of flow. It is given by

$$Re = (density \times velocity \times diameter)/viscosity$$

where density is in g/cm^3, velocity is in cm/sec, diameter is in cm, viscosity is in centipoise or g/cm-sec, and Re has no units. If Re < 2100, then flow is laminar. If Re > 2100, then flow is turbulent.

Question: What is a typical blood flow velocity?

Answer: It depends on the vessel. Table 26-1 gives some examples.

The blood velocity may be much higher in abnormal conditions, such as in an arteriovenous fistula (AVF).

Question: What is the difference between flow and velocity?

Answer: A mathematical relationship exists between bulk or volumetric flow in a vessel lumen and the velocity of flow:

$$v = Q/A$$

where v is the average velocity (in cm/sec), Q is the bulk or volumetric flow (in cm^3/sec), and A is the cross-sectional area of the vessel (in cm^2).

Normal Appearance of Flowing Blood. Most flow effects can be attributed to one of the following:

1. Time-of-flight (TOF) effects
2. Motion-induced phase changes

TOF effects can lead to the following:

1. Signal loss (*high-velocity signal loss* or *TOF loss*)
2. Signal gain (*flow-related enhancement* [FRE])

Flowing blood can appear bright or dark. Three main independent factors result in each case:

1. ↓ SI of flowing blood

   (a) high velocity
   (b) turbulent flow
   (c) dephasing

2. ↑ SI of flowing blood

   (a) even-echo rephasing
   (b) diastolic pseudogating
   (c) FRE

Let's discuss each of these separately.

Table 26-1	
Vessel	**Blood Flow Velocity (cm/sec)**
Aorta	140 ± 40
Superficial femoral artery	90 ± 13
Vertebral artery	36 ± 9
Venous flow	<20

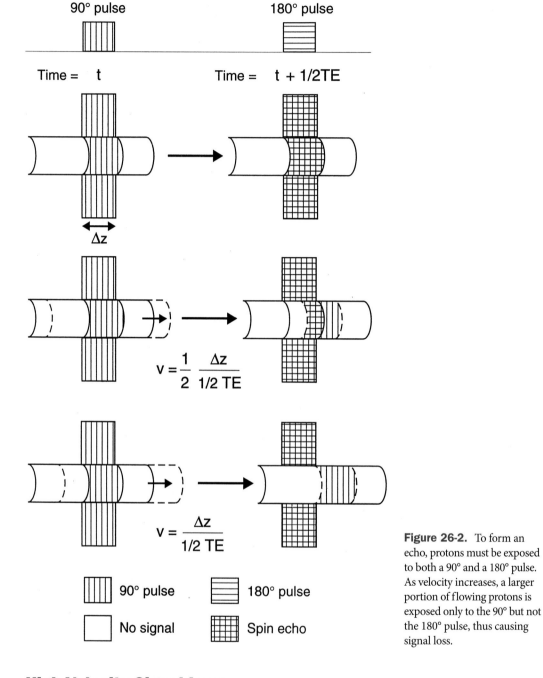

Figure 26-2. To form an echo, protons must be exposed to both a 90° and a 180° pulse. As velocity increases, a larger portion of flowing protons is exposed only to the 90° but not the 180° pulse, thus causing signal loss.

High-Velocity Signal Loss

In SE imaging, the protons must be exposed to both a 90° and a 180° radio frequency (RF) pulse to give off a signal. High-velocity signal loss or **TOF** loss occurs when flowing protons do not remain within the selected slice long enough to be exposed to both RF pulses.

Figure 26-2 illustrates how the magnitude of signal loss is a function of the velocity. To see how this works, first recall the simple relationship among time, distance, and velocity:

$$\text{Velocity} = \text{distance/time}$$

or

$$v = d/t$$

The distance each proton in flowing blood has to travel within a slice is the slice thickness Δz. The time between a 90° pulse and a 180° pulse is one-half TE.

Thus, if the velocity of flowing blood is

$$v = \Delta z/(1/2\ \text{TE})$$

then protons flowing into the slice would be exposed only to the 90° pulse, and not to the 180° pulse, thus forming no signal or SE. Let's give this velocity an arbitrary name v_m, that is,

$$v_m = \Delta z/(1/2\ \text{TE})$$

However, if the velocity were 0 (i.e., for stagnant blood), then an SE would be formed. If the velocity falls in between, only a fraction of the protons would form an SE. The fraction of protons escaping the 180° pulse is given by

$$v/v_m = v(1/2\ \text{TE})/\Delta z$$

Thus, the fraction of protons receiving both RF pulses is

$$1-v/v_m = 1-v(1/2\ \text{TE})/\Delta z$$

The signal intensity is, therefore, proportional to

$$I \propto 1-v(1/2\ \text{TE})/\Delta z$$

Figure 26-3 illustrates the linear relationship between signal intensity (I) and velocity v. It is clear from this graph that if the velocity of flowing blood is at least equal to v_m (i.e., $v \geq v_m$), then a flow void is observed.

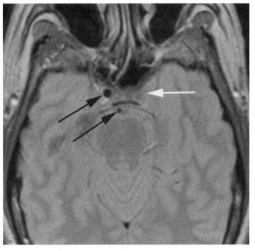

Figure 26-4. Axial PD image shows TOF losses in the right internal carotid and basilar arteries (*black arrows*); however, no TOF loss or "flow void" is seen in the left internal carotid artery (*white arrow*). Patient had left internal carotid artery occlusion.

Example

Suppose that the slice thickness $\Delta z = 1$ cm and TE = 50 msec. What is the velocity at which flow void is observed?

Using the above formula, the velocity should be at least

$$v_m = \Delta z/(1/2\ \text{TE}) = 1\ \text{cm}/(25\ \text{msec})$$
$$= 1000\ \text{cm}/25\ \text{sec} = 40\ \text{cm/sec}$$

which is seen in an artery.

Therefore, v_m is larger for thicker slices and smaller TEs, and vice versa (see Fig. 26-4 for an example).

N.B.: Remember that TOF losses only apply to SE imaging and not to GRE imaging

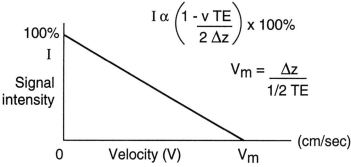

Figure 26-3. A plot of signal intensity versus velocity. The higher the velocity, the more the signal loss.

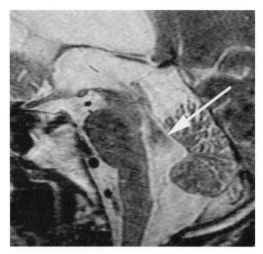

Figure 26-5. Sagittal 1.5-mm T2 image of the brain shows signal loss inferior to the aqueduct of Sylvius (*arrow*). This was due to high velocity of CSF and subsequent turbulent flow resulting in intravoxel dephasing. Patient had normal pressure hydrocephalus (NPH).

because, in GRE, the echo is formed via a single RF pulse and refocusing gradients (without a 180° pulse).

Turbulent Flow

In turbulent flow (with Re > 2100), random flow exists that contains different velocity components (i.e., with different speed and direction of flow). Consequently, each of these components has different phases that tend to cancel each other out and result in no signal (flow void). This result can occur with low- or high-velocity flow (Fig. 26-5).

Dephasing

There are many causes of dephasing. One important cause is the so-called **odd-echo dephasing.** This phenomenon results in signal void on the first and other odd echoes. The protons in a voxel do not move at the same velocity across the lumen in laminar flow; thus, each precesses at a different frequency and accumulates a different phase. (Also see the discussion below on even-echo rephasing.)

Another cause of dephasing is **intravoxel dephasing.** Because of laminar flow, different velocities may exist within a voxel, thus leading to phase dispersion (incoherence) and signal loss. *How to decrease intravoxel dephasing and increase SNR:*

1. Decrease the voxel size (increase spatial resolution), either by increasing the matrix (*trade-off:* will reduce signal-to-noise ratio [SNR]) or by reducing the FOV (*trade-off:* may cause wraparound).
2. Reduce the TE (e.g., use a fractional echo).
3. Add flow compensation (FC) techniques (see below).

Even-Echo Rephasing

This phenomenon is somewhat the opposite of odd-echo dephasing. It only occurs in SE imaging with symmetric echoes (i.e., when the second echo delay time is twice the first one: when TE2 = 2 TE1, e.g., 30/60/90/120 and 40/80/120/160). The result is higher signal intensity for even echoes compared with odd echoes. (We shall see later that in GRE or SE, FC techniques basically yield "even-echo rephasing" on the first echo to minimize signal losses.)

To see how this works, we first need to learn about the relationship between phase and velocity. Recall that along the readout gradient,

$$\omega = \gamma \mathbf{B}_x = \gamma G_x$$

Now, for a constant velocity *v*, the position at time *t* is given simply by

$$x = vt$$

Thus, combining the above two, we get

$$\omega = \gamma Gvt$$

Now, phase change $\Delta\phi$ and angular frequency ω are related by

$$\Delta\phi = \omega \Delta t$$

so that

$$\varphi = \int \omega dt = \int (\gamma Gvt)dt$$
$$= \gamma Gv \int t \, dt = \gamma Gv(t^2/2)$$

From this we can see the following:

1. Phase ϕ and velocity *v* are proportional.

2. A quadratic relationship exists between phase φ and time t, that is, $\phi = kt^2$, where k is a constant (k = 1/2 γGv).

On the other hand, for stationary tissue (with $v = 0$), the above relationship becomes

$$\phi = k't$$

that is, a linear relationship exists between phase and time for stationary tissues.

Now consider an SE sequence with symmetric echoes as shown in Figure 26-6. The phase changes over one cycle for both stationary tissues and flowing blood are plotted. This graph reveals that stationary tissues have zero phase on the first echo (TE) and the second echo (2TE). The situation for flowing blood, however, is different. On the first echo, the flowing blood has a positive phase. However, on the second echo, the phase is back to zero!

MATH: Let's try to prove the above fact mathematically. Assume that $\tau = 1/2$ TE. The phase gain at time TE/2 is $k\tau^2$, where k is a constant (k = 1/2 γGv). Right after the 180° pulse, the phase is $-k\tau^2$. Now, at time TE (i.e., at 2τ), the phase gain will be $k[(2\tau)^2 - (\tau)^2] = 3k\tau^2$. (The mathematically oriented reader will recognize this as the integral of $\int 2k\tau$ from point τ to 2τ.) Thus, the net phase gain will be $3k\tau^2 + (-k\tau^2) = 2k\tau^2$. Similarly, at 3/2 TE (or 3τ), that is, at the second 180° pulse, the phase gain is $k[(3\tau)^2 + (2\tau)^2] = 5k\tau^2$, with a net gain of $5k\tau^2 + 2k\tau^2 = 7k\tau^2$. Immediately after this second 180° pulse, the phase will be $-7k\tau^2$. In a similar fashion, the phase gain at the time of the second echo (i.e., at 4τ) will be $k[(4\tau)^2 - (3\tau)^2] = 7k\tau^2$. Therefore, the final net phase gain will be $7k\tau^2 + (-7k\tau^2) = 0$. That is to say, the net phase shift of flowing blood on the second echo is zero. This is illustrated in Figure 26-6.

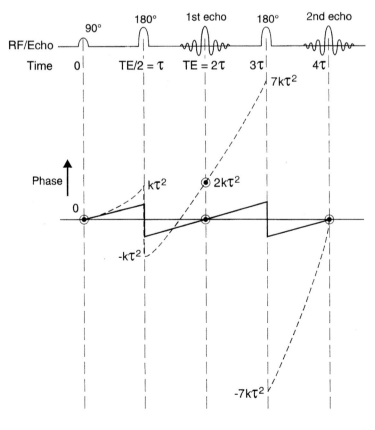

Figure 26-6. Phase accumulation for stationary and flowing protons.

Thus, protons in flowing blood lose their coherence on the first echo (causing odd-echo dephasing) and subsequently regain coherence on the second echo (causing even-echo rephasing). This pattern yields a higher signal of flowing blood on the second echo. It only works for symmetric echoes, not for asymmetric ones. (Interested readers can go through the previous math and prove this fact for themselves.)

Diastolic Pseudogating

During a cardiac cycle, blood flow is more rapid during systole and slower in diastole. Thus, in diastole, a higher intravascular signal is observed. (Remember that higher flow results in more TOF losses.) When **cardiac gating** is used, each slice is (theoretically) acquired at a fixed point in the cardiac cycle (although different slices in a multislice acquisition are obtained at different points in the cycle). Consequently, a vessel traversing several slices will demonstrate varying signal intensities at different slices. In a cardiac-gated sequence, TR must be a multiple of the heart rate (HR). For example, if HR = 60 bpm (1 beat per second = 1 Hz), then TR = 1000, 2000, 3000, etc. In general,

$$TR = 1/HR$$

with appropriate units.

Flow-Related Enhancement (FRE)

This phenomenon usually refers to the first slice that the flowing blood enters. Hence, FRE is also called the **entry phenomenon.** FRE is a type of TOF effect in which the fresh inflowing blood that enters the first slice is totally **unsaturated,** that is, the protons within it have not as yet been subjected to any prior RF pulse and thus yield full magnetization, whereas the adjacent stationary tissue remains partially **saturated** because of prior RF pulses.

Figure 26-7 illustrates the relationship between FRE and the blood velocity. This diagram demon-

strates that when $v = 0$ (i.e., stagnant blood), the protons are partially saturated. However, when the velocity is $v = \Delta z/TR$, then the unsaturated inflowing protons completely replace the previously partially saturated protons. Again, we shall give this velocity an arbitrary name v_M. The fraction of inflowing protons is then

$$v/v_M = v(TE/\Delta z)$$

Thus, the relationship between the intravascular signal intensity and velocity is

$$I \propto I_0 + (TE/\Delta z)v$$

where I_0 is the signal intensity of stagnant blood (i.e., at $v = 0$). This relationship is illustrated in Figure 26-8.

Example
At what velocity do you observe maximum FRE when $\Delta z = 1$ cm and TR = 1000 msec = 1 sec? From the previous formula,

$$v_M = \Delta z/TR = 1 \text{ cm}/1\text{sec} = 1\text{cm/sec}$$

which is consistent with a slow venous flow (Figs. 26-9 and 26-10).

Why Is Flowing Blood Bright on GRE Images? You may have noticed that on most GRE images, vessels appear bright on all the slices. There are three main reasons for this:

1. GRE imaging is usually performed in a sequential mode (i.e., one slice at a time). Consequently, every slice is an entry slice. Thus, FRE applies to every slice in the volume.
2. Due to lack of a 180° refocusing pulse and the nonslice selectivity of the refocusing gradient, TOF losses are usually not significant in GRE imaging.
3. In GRE imaging, TE is usually very short, which minimizes signal losses caused by dephasing.

See Figure 26-11 as an example.

Question: Is FRE only limited to the first (entry) slice?

Answer: The answer is no. If the velocity of flow is higher than $\Delta z/TR$ (but not too high for TOF losses to take place), then unsaturated

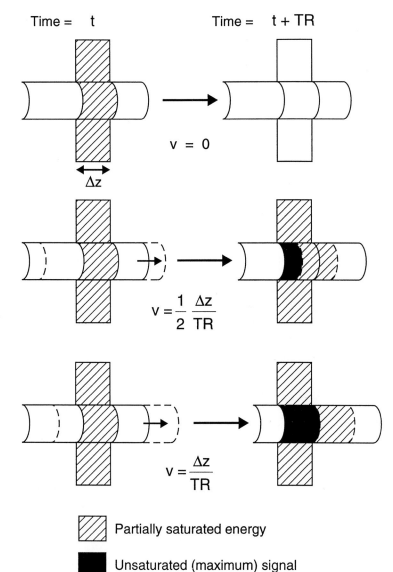

Time =   t   Time =   t + TR

v = 0

Δz

$v = \dfrac{1}{2}\dfrac{\Delta z}{TR}$

$v = \dfrac{\Delta z}{TR}$

Partially saturated energy

Unsaturated (maximum) signal

Figure 26-7. Effect of flow-related enhancement (FRE) for slow flow. Unsaturated protons produce more signals. As the velocity increases, a larger portion of unsaturated inflowing protons will replace the previously partially saturated protons, thus increasing signal intensity.

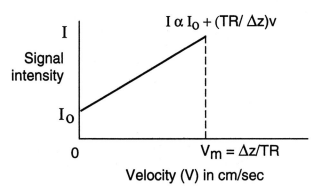

$I \propto I_0 + (TR/\,\Delta z)v$

I

Signal intensity

I_0

0          $V_m = \Delta z/TR$

Velocity (V) in cm/sec

Figure 26-8. The plot of signal intensity versus velocity in FRE.

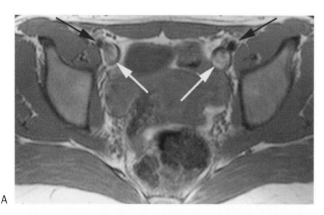

A

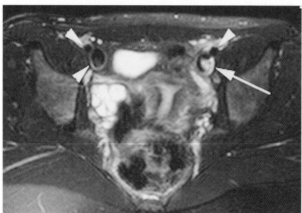

B

Figure 26-9. Axial T1 (**A**) through the pelvis shows flow-related enhancement within the slower flowing external iliac veins (*arrows*); the faster flowing arteries show time-of-flight loss. By increasing the TE in the accompanying T2 FSE image with fat saturation sequence (**B**), more time-of-flight losses are seen within the right external iliac vein in addition to the arteries (*arrowheads*). However, incomplete time-of-flight losses are seen within the left external iliac vein (*arrow*) due to a component of even slower flow within this vein.

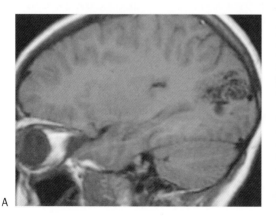

A

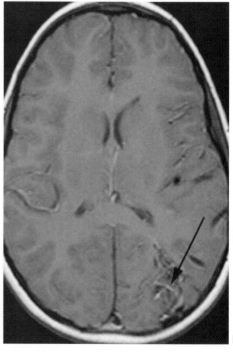

B

Figure 26-10. Sagittal T1 image (**A**) of the brain demonstrates a tangle of flow voids in a patient with an arteriovenous malformation (AVM). However, an axial T1 image (**B**) shows some vessels with flow-related enhancement (*arrow*). This demonstrates the phenomenon of in-plane saturation of protons (the sagittal image) yielding signal void and out-of-plane unsaturated protons in the axial image resulting in flow-related enhancement.

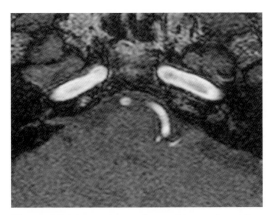

Figure 26-11. Gradient-echo axial image from 2D time of flight shows bright signal from flow-related enhancement in the internal carotid and vertebral arteries. The patient also has an ectatic course of his left vertebral artery, accounting for his left hemifacial spasm.

protons can penetrate adjacent slices and yield FRE. Obviously, as these inflowing protons travel through the imaging volume, they are subjected to more and more RF pulses and become more and more saturated. Thus, FRE is always maximum at the entry slice and becomes gradually fainter in deeper slices (a good distinguishing point from an intraluminal thrombus). Now, how far FRE can penetrate the imaging volume has to do with the direction of flow and the direction of slice excitation.

Cocurrent and Countercurrent Flow. The **slice-excitation wave (SEW)** is the direction of successive 90° excitation pulses. If flow is perpendicular to the slices, then flow is either in the direction of the SEW (called **cocurrent**) or against it (called **countercurrent**). Intuitively, in a countercurrent setting,

the flowing protons are subjected to fewer 90° pulses than in a cocurrent setting (Fig. 26-12). Consequently, FRE demonstrates deeper penetration in a countercurrent setting (Figs. 26-13 through 26-15).

Combined Flow Phenomena. What would happen if very high-velocity flow enters the entry slice? Although FRE affects the entry slice increasing intraluminal signal, TOF signal losses will also have an effect, thus somewhat offsetting FRE. In other words, in reality, flowing blood demonstrates a combination of flow phenomena, and the intensity of blood is, in the final analysis, determined by the phenomena that predominate.

Gradient Moment Nulling (Flow Compensation)

Gradient moment nulling (GMN) is one method of minimizing flow motion artifacts. It is based on the principle of even-echo rephasing. Even-echo rephasing is accomplished by adding extra gradient pulses to produce the even-echo rephasing effect on the first echo (thus eliminating first-echo dephasing). You can therefore achieve rephasing without having to use a double-echo sequence. There are several synonyms for GMN (Table 26-2).

Figures 26-16 and 26-17 demonstrate FC for both GRE and SE imaging. In both cases, protons in flowing blood will have a net phase of zero at the center of the echo. The mathematics is similar to the one for even-echo rephasing (see previous section), and the interested reader may wish to go through the exercise. The extra gradients associated with FC are referred to as gradient **lobes.** For instance, for GRE, the relative gradient strengths of these

Table 26-2		
Manufacturer	**Acronym**	**Description**
GE	FC	Flow compensation
Philips	FC	Flow compensation
Siemens	GMR	Gradient-motion rephasing

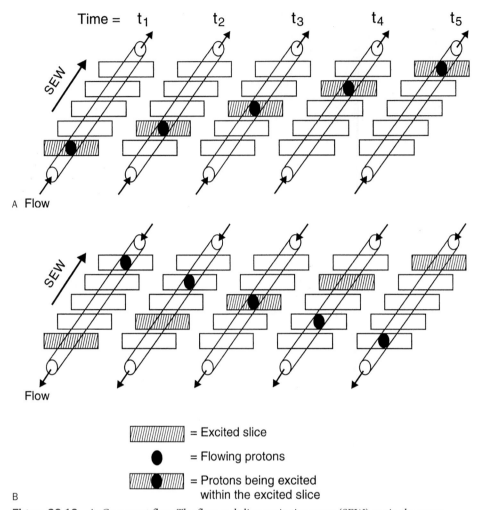

= Excited slice

= Flowing protons

= Protons being excited
within the excited slice

B

Figure 26-12. **A:** Cocurrent flow. The flow and slice-excitation wave (SEW) are in the same direction. **B:** Countercurrent flow. The flow and SEW are in opposite directions.

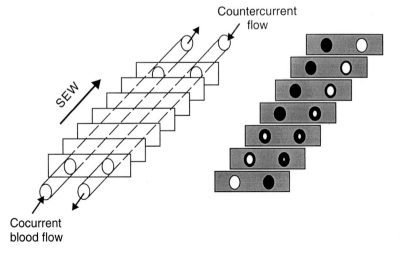

Figure 26-13. FRE penetrates deeper in countercurrent flow than in cocurrent flow.

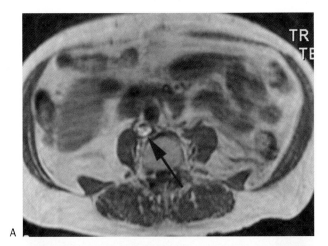

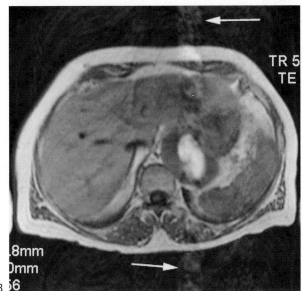

Figure 26-14. Axial T1 image of the abdomen (**A**) shows bright flow-related enhancement (FRE) in the IVC (*arrow*) on only the most inferior three cuts in this sequence, consistent with countercurrent flow-related enhancement. Comparison T1 image (**B**) at the superior slice shows no signal within the IVC; however, there is FRE within the aortic aneurysm secondary to slower flow within the aneurysm. There is also motion artifact on image **B** in the phase-encode direction (anteroposterior) from the aneurysm (*arrows*).

lobes demonstrate a ratio of 1:2:1. Remember that this type of FC only corrects for first-order[1] (i.e., constant velocity) flow. To correct for higher order motion (e.g., acceleration or jerk), additional gradient lobes are required (Fig. 26-18).[2] As you can see, the addition of these extra lobes lengthens the cycle, thus lengthening TR and minimum TE (thus reducing the number of slices).

FC can be applied along each and all the three coordinates x, y, and z.

---

[1]Zero-order motion is stationary ($v = 0$). First-order motion ($v = dx/dt = $ constant) is constant velocity. Second-order motion ($a - d^2x/d^2t$) is acceleration. Third-order motion ($j - d^3x/d^3t$) is jerk motion or pulsatility.

[2]For a more complete discussion, refer to Stark DO, Bradley WG, eds. *Magnetic Resonance Imaging*, 3rd ed, vol 1. St. Louis: Mosby; 1999.

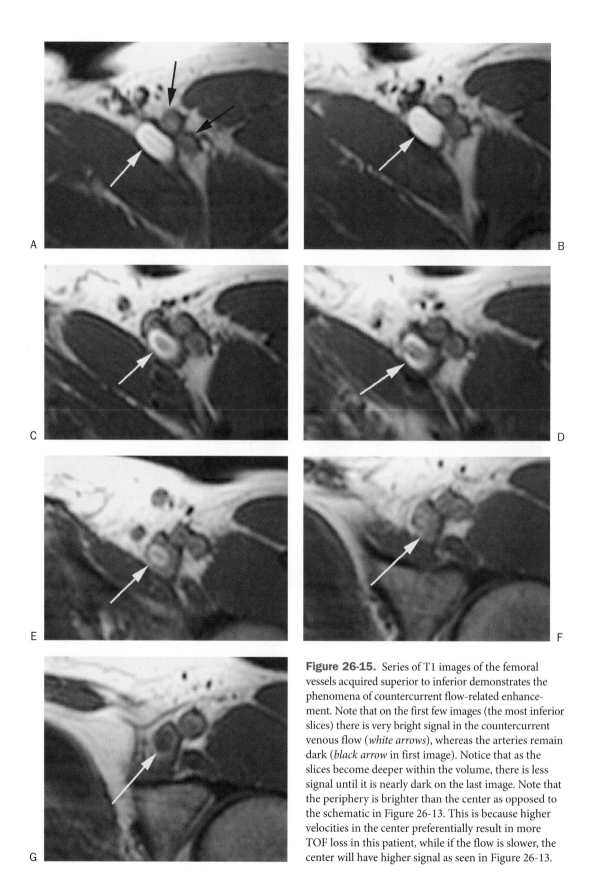

Figure 26-15. Series of T1 images of the femoral vessels acquired superior to inferior demonstrates the phenomena of countercurrent flow-related enhancement. Note that on the first few images (the most inferior slices) there is very bright signal in the countercurrent venous flow (*white arrows*), whereas the arteries remain dark (*black arrow* in first image). Notice that as the slices become deeper within the volume, there is less signal until it is nearly dark on the last image. Note that the periphery is brighter than the center as opposed to the schematic in Figure 26-13. This is because higher velocities in the center preferentially result in more TOF loss in this patient, while if the flow is slower, the center will have higher signal as seen in Figure 26-13.

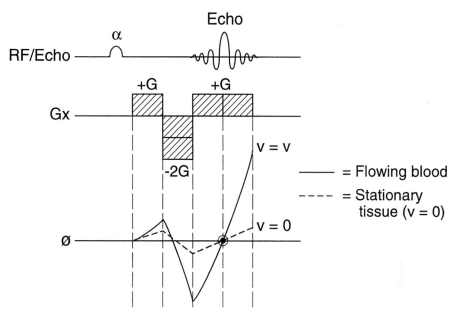

Figure 26-16. Flow compensation in GRE. With this scheme, flowing protons (with constant velocity) are in phase (i.e., zero phase difference) at the center of the echo.

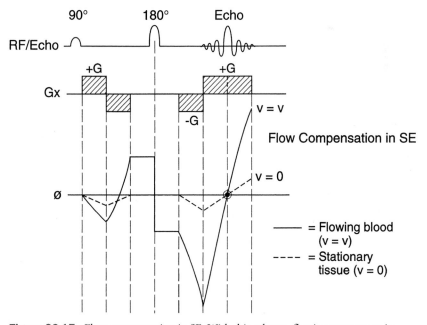

Figure 26-17. Flow compensation in SE. With this scheme, flowing protons are in phase at the center of the echo.

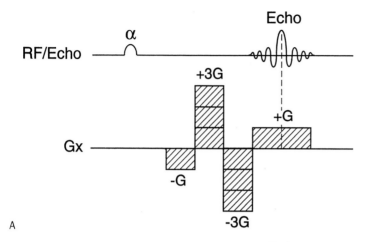

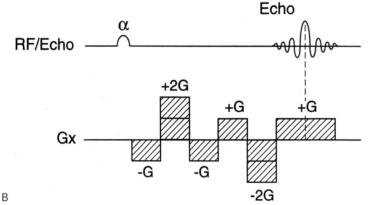

A

B

Figure 26-18. A: Second-order flow (acceleration compensation). With this scheme, protons with second-order flow (i.e., acceleration) get in phase at the center of the echo. **B:** Third-order flow (jerk) compensation. With this scheme, protons with third-order flow (i.e., jerk) get in phase at the center of the echo.

Key Points

1 Several types of flow exist: laminar flow, plug flow, turbulent flow, and flow separation/ vortex flow.

2 Intravascular flow is usually laminar, that is, it has a parabolic profile.

3 Turbulent flow occurs distal to stenoses and on vessel turns.

4 The Reynolds number can predict laminar versus turbulent flow.

5 Most flow effects can be attributed to one of two phenomena: TOF or motion-related phase changes.

6 TOF can cause either signal loss (TOF loss) or signal gain (FRE).

7 Causes of intravascular signal loss include high velocity, turbulent flow, and dephasing.

8 Causes of intravascular signal gain include FRE, even-echo rephasing, and diastolic pseudogating.

9 Dephasing may be caused by intravoxel dephasing or odd-echo dephasing.

10 FRE is based on the entry phenomenon. FRE is the basis for TOF MR angiography (MRA).

11 FRE penetrates deeper slices when flow is countercurrent to the slice-excitation wave (SEW) rather than when it is cocurrent.

12 Even-echo rephasing causes bright intravascular signal on the second echo (when the echoes are symmetric).

13 Even-echo rephasing is the basis for FC (GMN). GMN, however, is accomplished via gradients that cause rephasing of flowing spins on the first echo and thus increased signal.

Questions

26-1 Normal intravascular flow is usually:
(a) turbulent flow
(b) plug flow
(c) laminar flow
(d) all of the above
(e) none of the above

26-2 T/F Turbulent flow is expected proximal to a stenosis.

26-3 T/F FRE is synonymous with the entry phenomenon.

26-4 T/F Time-of-flight effects only cause signal loss.

26-5 Causes of intravascular signal loss include
(a) high velocity
(b) turbulent flow
(c) dephasing
(d) all of the above
(e) only (a) (b)

26-6 Causes of intravascular signal gain include
(a) FRE
(b) even-echo rephasing
(c) diastolic pseudogating
(d) all of the above
(e) only (a) and (c)

26-7 T/F The Reynolds number (Re) can predict laminar versus turbulent flow.

26-8 T/F FRE penetrates deeper slices when flow is cocurrent rather than countercurrent.

26-9 T/F FRE is only observed in the first (entry) slice.

26-10 T/F Even-echo rephasing is the basis for flow compensation techniques.

26-11 Laminar flow is given by the formula:
(a) $v(r) = V_{max} (1 - r^2/R^2)$
(b) $v(r) = V_{max} (1 - R^2/r^2)$
(c) $v(r) = (1 - r^2/R^2)/V_{max}$
(d) There is no formula for such a flow.

26-12 Plug flow is given by the formula:
(a) $v(r) = V_{max} (1 - r^2/R^2)$
(b) $v(r) = V_{max} (1 - R^2/r^2)$
(c) $v(r) = \text{constant} = V_{ave}$
(d) none of the above

26-13 TOF effects can lead to
(a) signal loss   (b) signal gain
(c) both   (d) none of the above

26-14 T/F Given the parameters TR 2000, TE1 20, TE2 80 msec, even-echo rephasing would occur.

26-15 T/F Laminar flow has a parabolic profile.

26-16 Flow effects include
(a) time-of-flight (TOF)
(b) motion-induced phase changes
(c) both
(d) none of the above

27

MR Angiography

Introduction

In this chapter, we will discuss the topic of **MR angiography (MRA)**. As in the last chapter, MRA may at first appear very complicated, but we'll try to present the major concepts in a simplified fashion. There are three main MRA techniques:

1. TOF (time-of-flight) MRA
2. PC (phase contrast) MRA
3. CE (contrast-enhanced) MRA

TOF and PC techniques can be performed using two-dimensional Fourier transform (2DFT) or three-dimensional FT (3DFT). CE MRA is performed with the 3D technique. Thus, there are a total of five different methods:

1. 2D-TOF MRA
2. 2D-PC MRA
3. 3D-TOF MRA
4. 3D-PC MRA
5. 3D-CE MRA

Each of these techniques lends itself to a different type of clinical application.

TOF MRA

TOF MRA is based on flow-related enhancement (FRE; discussed in the previous chapter) in a 2D or 3D gradient-echo (GRE) technique. (Remember that in GRE imaging, TOF losses do not play an important role.) Usually, flow compensation is used perpendicular to the vessel lumen.

2D-TOF MRA. Figure 27-1 depicts a typical pulse sequence for 2D-TOF MRA. A presat (presaturation) pulse is applied above or below each slice to eliminate the signal from vessels flowing in the opposite direction. Usually a short TR (about 50 msec), a moderate flip angle (45° to 60°), and a short TE (a few millisecond) are used. An example is seen in Figure 27-2.

3D-TOF MRA. Figure 27-3 depicts a pulse sequence diagram (PSD) for a 3D-TOF MRA. Here, a slab of several centimeters (usually about 5 cm) is obtained that contains up to 60 slices.

Advantages of 2D-TOF MRA
1. Faster scanning
2. Maximized FRE because each slice is an entry slice

Disadvantages of 2D-TOF MRA
1. In plane saturation effects (discussed later)

Advantages of 3D-TOF MRA
1. Higher signal-to-noise ratio (SNR) because signal is acquired from a larger volume
2. Improved spatial resolution

Disadvantages of 3D-TOF MRA
1. 3D techniques more susceptible to saturation effects (see below)
2. Less sensitive to slow flow

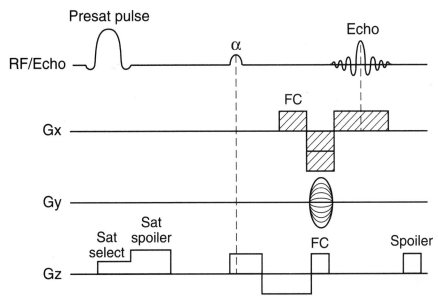

Figure 27-1. A PSD for 2D-TOF MR angiography.

PC MRA

PC MRA is based on the fact that the phase gain of flowing blood through a gradient is proportional to its velocity (assuming constant velocity). We saw in the previous chapter that phase (ϕ) and velocity (v) are related by

$$\phi = \int \omega \mathrm{d}t = \int (\gamma G v t)\mathrm{d}t = 1/2\,\gamma G v t^2$$

Therefore, knowing the phase at any point in time allows us to calculate the velocity.

The most common method to employ PC MRA is by the use of a **bipolar gradient** (Fig. 27-4A). This process is called **flow encoding.** Because the two lobes in this bipolar gradient have equal area, no net phase change is observed by stationary tissues (Fig. 27-4A). However, flowing blood will experience a net phase shift proportional to its velocity (assuming a constant flow velocity) (Fig. 27-4B). This is how flow is distinguished from stationary tissue in PC MRA. Figures 27-5 and 27-6 illustrate the PSDs for 2D-PC and 3D-PC MRA, respectively.

There are several features unique to PC MRA, as the following discussions demonstrate.

Question: What are the "magnitude" image and the "phase" image?

Answer: In PC MRA, you not only get an image of the blood vessels (**magnitude image**);

you also get an image that shows you the direction of flow (**phase map**). The phase image would tell you whether the flow is right-left, superior-inferior, or anterior-posterior. An example is determination of hepatofugal versus

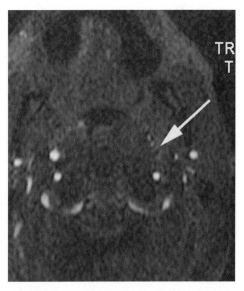

Figure 27-2. Axial source image from a 2D-TOF demonstrates no flow-related enhancement in the left internal carotid artery (*arrow*), consistent with occlusion from arterial dissection in this young patient. Normal flow-related enhancement is seen in all the other vessels.

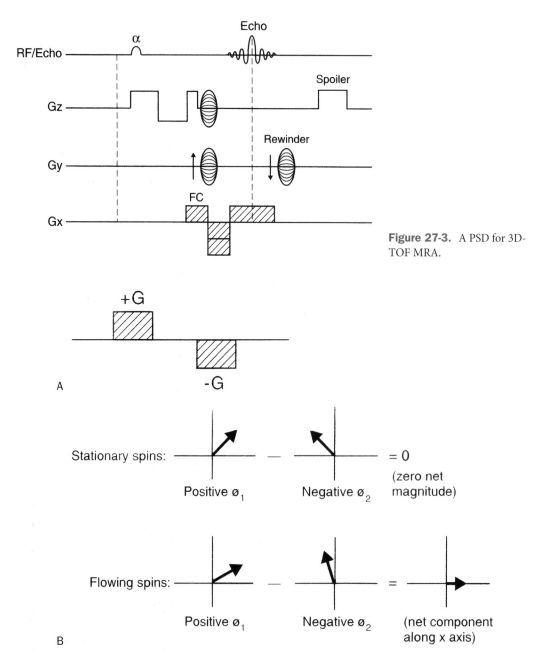

Figure 27-3. A PSD for 3D-TOF MRA.

Figure 27-4. **A:** A bipolar flow-encoding gradient. Because the two lobes have equal areas with opposite polarities, no phase change is observed by stationary spins. However, flowing spins will yield a net phase change proportional to their velocity, which is the principle behind PC MRA (**B**).

hepatopedal flow in the portal vein of a patient with cirrhosis.

Question: What is VENC?

Answer: VENC stands for velocity encoding. It is a parameter that is selected by the MR oper-ator when using PC MRA. VENC represents the maximum velocity present in the imaging volume. Any velocity greater than VENC will be aliased according to the following formula:

Aliased velocity = VENC − actual velocity

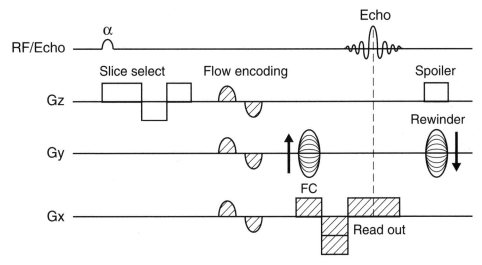

Figure 27-5. A PSD for 2D-PC MRA.

For instance, if VENC = 30 cm/sec, then a vessel with a flow velocity of 40 cm/sec will be represented as a flow of

$$v = 30 - 40 = -10 \text{ cm/sec}$$

that is, a flow of 10 cm/sec in the opposite direction (Fig. 27-7). A smaller VENC is more sensitive to slow flow (venous flow) and to smaller branches but causes more rapid (arterial) flow to get aliased. A larger VENC is more appropriate for arterial flow. Sometimes you may image the same thing with two dif-ferent VENCs—a small VENC and a large VENC—to image all the flow components accurately (an example is imaging an AVM or an aneurysm).

Advantages of PC MRA

1. The capability to generate magnitude and phase images
2. Superior background suppression
3. Less sensitive to intravoxel dephasing or saturation effects

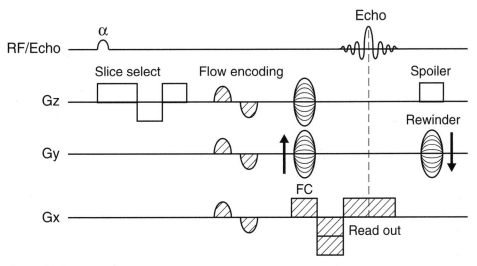

Figure 27-6. A PSD for 3D-PC MRA.

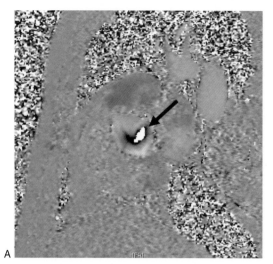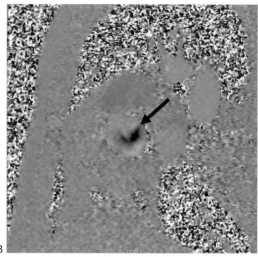

A B

Figure 27-7. Two phase contrast images (phase maps) through the root of the aorta in a patient with aortic stenosis. **A:** VENC = 150 cm/sec; **B:** VENC = 300 cm/sec. Note in (**A**) the bright central signal (*arrow*) that may indicate regurgitant flow; however, the signal is surrounded by darker signal with abrupt transition from black pixel to white pixel diagnostic of aliasing. Increasing the VENC in (**B**) eliminated the aliasing. No bright signal indicative of regurgitation was observed and an accurate maximal velocity determination was now possible.

Disadvantages of PC MRA

1. Takes longer to do
2. More sensitive to signal losses caused by turbulence and by dephasing on vessel turns (e.g., carotid siphon)
3. The need to guess the maximum flow velocity in order to select an optimum VENC

2D- versus 3D-PC MRA

1. 2D techniques are faster
2. 3D techniques have better SNR

Examples of magnitude phase contrast images are seen in Figures 27-8 through 27-10.

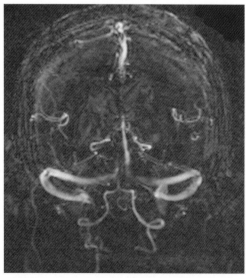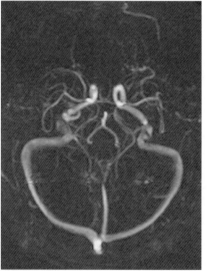

A B

Figure 27-8. Coronal (**A**) and axial (**B**) thick slab (5 cm) 2D-PC MRV (magnetic resonance venogram) of the brain in normal patients.

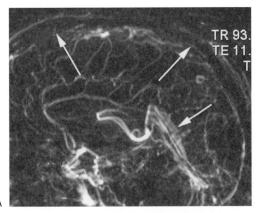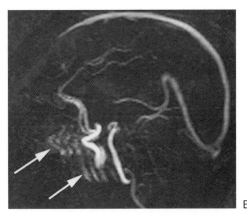

A   B

Figure 27-9. 2D sagittal phase contrast MRV (magnetic resonance venogram) (**A**) shows markedly decreased flow in the superior sagittal and straight sinuses (*arrows*) in this patient with sagittal sinus thrombosis. **B:** Normal exam. Note the phase-induced ghosting (*arrows*).

CE MRA

CE MRA is different than either TOF or PC imaging since CE MRA is primarily dependent on the T1 properties of gadolinium in the vasculature rather than the flow properties per se. This technique has been made possible due to the advent of high performance gradients (more in Chapter 30) that permit very rapid GRE imaging and the use of the paramagnetic contrast agent gadolinium. This allows imaging to be achieved

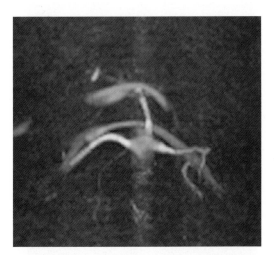

Figure 27-10. Axial 3D phase contrast MIP (maximum intensity projection) image of the renal vessels shows normal flow without stenosis. This is a magnitude image reflecting higher velocities in the renal arteries represented by brighter signal.

during the transit time and hence peak T1 shortening of the gadolinium. This technique is therefore very dependent on the precise timing of the arrival of the bolus of gadolinium in the vessel of interest. The plane of imaging is usually in the plane of the vessel (usually coronal) as opposed to 2D-TOF technique in which the imaging plane is usually orthogonal to the vessel of interest. Imaging this way increases coverage while maximizing resolution. Since this technique is more reliant on the T1 properties than any flow properties, it is very resistant to dephasing artifacts that are seen in some of the other techniques.

There are two principal CE-MRA techniques: *elliptical-centric* and *multiphase.* In the former, acquisition begins as contrast enters the artery of interest, filling the center of k-space (containing most of the SNR) first and the veins later (during filling of the low SNR periphery of k-space). This technique requires automatic bolus detection software (GE SmartPrep, Siemens CARE Bolus, or Philips BolusTrak) or a timing run to determine the time it takes the gadolinium to reach the artery of interest. The former is performed by placing a cursor over the upstream portion of the artery of interest; the latter is performed by injecting 2 cc of gadolinium and noting the time it takes the artery to turn maximally bright. In multiphase techniques, gadolinium is injected and multiple acquisitions are made, one of which is bound to be in the arterial phase. An additional benefit of multiphase acquisitions is the ability to provide pathologically delayed vessel filling of contrast material. But one important limitation to multiphase imaging is the tradeoff of spatial resolution for temporal resolution.

One approach to reduce loss of spatial resolution in multiphase imaging relies on the fact that much of the information to form an MR image is present in the central region of k-space. A faster time-series of 3D images can be reconstructed by acquiring a multiphase exam in which the central phase encoding values are acquired more often than the outer regions of k-space. This technique, time-resolved imaging of contrast kinetics (TRICKS), divides the 3D Cartesian k-space into several subvolumes located at increasing distance from the k-space center and oversamples the central region of k-space relative to the sampling rate of the outer regions. In this way, TRICKS is able to consistently capture an arterial phase free of venous overlay.

The resampling of the center of k-space results in a reduction in spatial resolution in TRICKS exams compared with single-image acquisitions acquired in the same scan time. Undersampled projection reconstruction has proved to preserve the spatial resolution and speed up the acquisition with limited streak artifacts. The combination of undersampled PR (projection reconstruction) acquisition in the k_x-k_y plane with a TRICKS encoding in the slice direction can significantly increase the temporal resolution without spatial resolution degradation.

Advantages

1. Rapid technique
2. Resistant to dephasing (e.g., from turbulent flow)
3. Large field of view with good resolution
4. Excellent SNR

Disadvantages

1. Dependent on timing (artifacts or venous contamination may occur)
2. Requires intravenous injection for administration of gadolinium
3. No directional information

See Figures 27-11 through 27-14 for examples.

Table 27-1 contains a summary of some of the major clinical applications of the five methods of MRA discussed above.

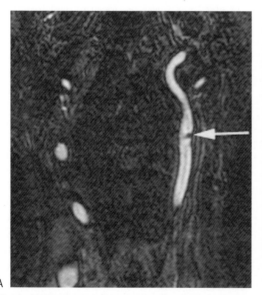
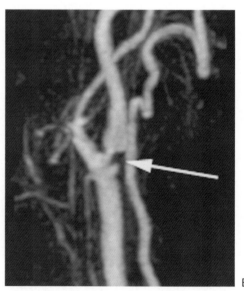

A   B

Figure 27-11. Coronal source image (**A**) and selected MIP (maximum intensity projection) (**B**) of the left carotid artery from a CE MRA shows focal high-grade stenosis at the origin of the left, internal carotid. Notice that on the source the entire course of either artery is not seen secondary to the thin slice.

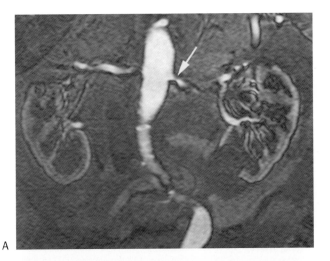

A

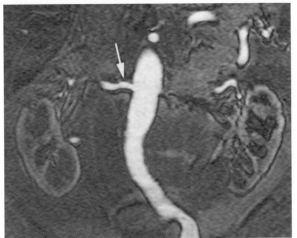

B

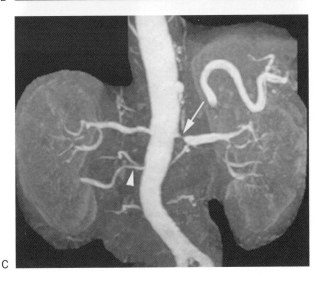

C

Figure 27-12. Coronal source images (**A** and **B**) show a focal high-grade stenosis of the left proximal main renal artery (*arrow* in **A**), whereas the origin of the right main renal artery is normal (*arrow* in **B**). Note that because these are thin slices, the images do not usually show the entire vessels. The MIP (**C**) image in this patient shows the left renal artery stenosis (*arrow*) and an accessory right renal artery (*arrowhead*).

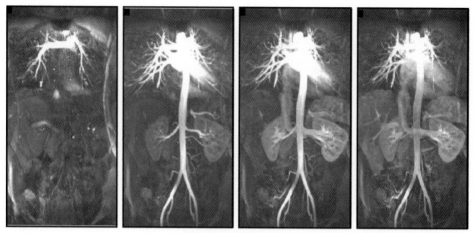

Figure 27-13. TRICKS imaging of the renal artery.

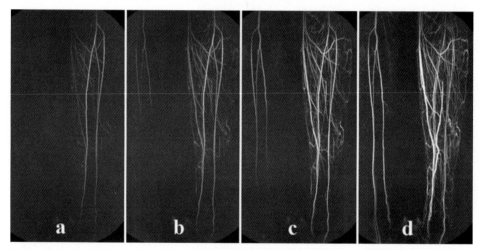

Figure 27-14. Asymmetric filling of the contrast agent is demonstrated with PR-TRICKS acquisition with a high spatial resolution of $1.1 \times 1.1 \times 1.5$ mm^3 and temporal resolution of 3.8 sec per frame.

Table 27-1

Technique	Clinical Applications
2D-TOF MRA	Carotid and vertebral arteries in the neck
	Venous structures (due to slow flow)
3D-TOF MRA	Intracranial vasculature (circle of Willis)
	Intracranial vascular malformations and aneurysms
2D-PC MRA	Portal vein
	CSF flow study
	Localizer for determining VENC (velocity encoding)
3D-PC MRA	Intracranial vasculature
	Intracranial vascular malformations and aneurysms
3D-CE MRA	Carotid and vertebral arteries of the neck
	Aortic arch, renal arteries, and upper or lower extremity runoff

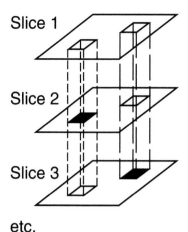

Slice 1

Slice 2

Slice 3

etc.

Figure 27-15. Maximum intensity projection (MIP). A channel of similar pixels in every slice is selected, and the pixel with the maximum intensity (provided its intensity is above a certain threshold) is projected onto an image. This process is repeated for all pixels to form an image.

Maximum Intensity Projection

We can finally explain how we can image just the blood vessels (in a way that looks 3D) and not the stationary tissue. This imaging is accomplished via an algorithm called **maximum intensity projection (MIP)**. MIP can be used as a noun, verb (the raw data are mipped), or adjective (mipped image). Mipping is done as follows: because flowing blood in MRA techniques has high intensity, the intensity of a pixel in a slice is compared with the corresponding pixels in all the other slices (as in a channel), and the one with maximum intensity is selected. For example, pixel (1,1) in slice 1 is compared with pixel (1,1) of all other slices. This process is repeated for all the pixels in the slice. In other words, the high-intensity dots in space are connected to generate an MRA image. Thus, the mipped image represents the highest intensities (hopefully all caused by flowing blood) in the imaging volume. This image is illustrated in Figure 27-15. Obviously, a certain *internal* threshold is used, below which no pixel in the channel falls. An example of a CE-MRA MIP with a comparison 2D-TOF MIP is seen in Figure 27-16.

Disadvantages of MIP

The major drawback of MIP is that bright structures other than flowing blood may potentially be included in the mipped image. Examples are fat, subacute hemorrhage, and the posterior pituitary gland (Fig. 27-17). This problem is mainly with TOF MRA and not with PC MRA.

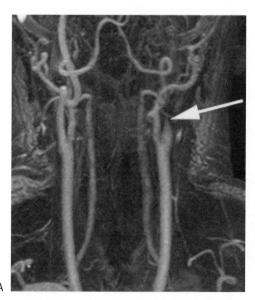

A

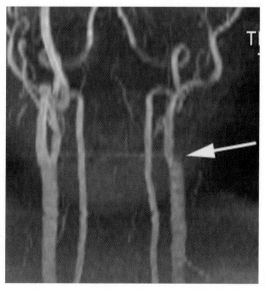

B

Figure 27-16. CE MRA MIP image (**A**) and comparison 2D-TOF MIP (**B**) show occlusion of the left, internal carotid artery in the same patient as Figure 27-2.

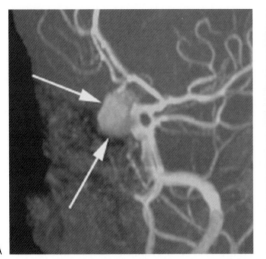

A

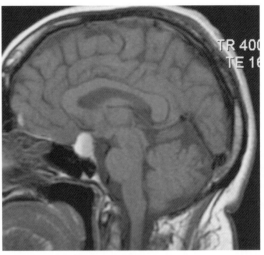

B

Figure 27-17. Sagittal MIP (**A**) image shows worrisome signal for aneurysm near the anterior communicating artery and the internal carotid terminus. Additional sagittal T1 (**B**) shows the high signal to be pituitary hemorrhage and not flow-related enhancement.

(The latter is a subtraction technique based on velocity-induced phase shifts rather than on tissue T1 and T2.)

Saturation Effects

Saturation effects refer to the gradual loss of longitudinal magnetization caused by repeated excitation radio frequency (RF) pulses. This, in turn, leads to loss of signal (and thus reduced SNR). This problem usually arises in a 2D acquisition in which flowing blood has to travel within (rather than through) a slice or in a 3D acquisition in which the blood travels through a thick imaging volume (or slab). In such a situation, saturation effects may cause the distal

portion of a vessel not to be included in the image.

There are two main causes of saturation effects:

1. Decreasing TR
2. Increasing α

Decreasing TR. As shown in Figure 27-18, a shorter TR causes less recovery of longitudinal magnetization from one cycle to the next, causing gradual loss of the $\mathbf{M}_z$ component. This effect is less pronounced with a longer TR.

Increasing α. Next consider the case of a large α. A larger α causes more loss of longitudinal

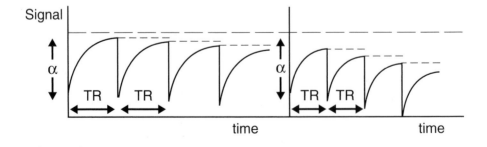

A   a) Long TR   b) Short TR   B

Figure 27-18. Saturation effects. A longer TR (**A**, for a fixed flip angle α) causes better recovery of longitudinal magnetization than a shorter TR (**B**) thus reducing saturation effects.

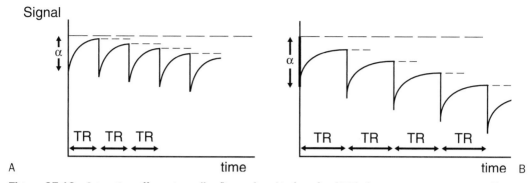

Figure 27-19. Saturation effects. A smaller flip angle α (**A**, for a fixed TR) also causes more recovery of longitudinal magnetization than a larger flip angle α (**B**) thus leading to reduced saturation effects.

magnetization. Therefore, for a given TR, there is more gradual loss of M_α with a smaller α than with a larger one (Fig. 27-19).

In GRE technique, saturation effects become problematic because very short TRs are used. The use of small flip angles counteracts this effect. These saturation effects become especially important in 2D or 3D in-plane flow or in 3D imaging in which volume imaging is performed over a slab, and signal losses might be significant from one end of the slab to the other. Multislice GRE techniques that use longer TRs decrease these saturation effects and allow for larger flip angles (which improves the SNR).

We have already discussed another mechanism for reducing these saturation effects: using a paramagnetic contrast agent, such as gadolinium (CE MRA). The use of this agent causes T1 shortening of blood. Consequently, the T1 recovery is much faster with fewer saturation effects (Fig. 27-20).

Two other techniques are available to reduce saturation effects: MOTSA (multiple overlapping thin-slab acquisition) and TONE (tilted optimized nonsaturating excitation).

MOTSA. Motsa is a combination of 2D-TOF and 3D-TOF techniques for the purpose of reducing the saturation effects associated with a *thick* slab. In this method, multiple *thin* slabs are used, which are overlapping by 25% to 50% (Fig. 27-21). The final imaging volume is created by extracting the central slices of each slab and discarding the peripheral slices (which are more affected by saturation effects). The main drawback of this technique is the potential for **Venetian blind** artifact at the points where the slabs overlap. See Figures 27-22 and 27-23 for examples.

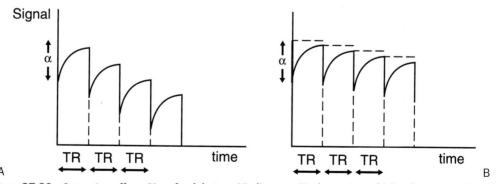

Figure 27-20. Saturation effects. Use of gadolinium (Gad) causes T1 shortening, which reduces saturation effects. **A:** Without Gad. **B:** With Gad.

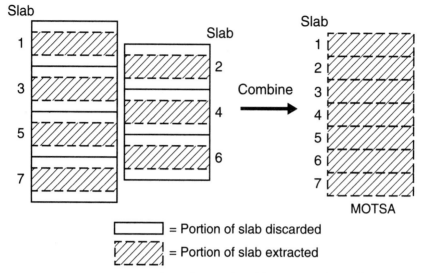

= Portion of slab discarded

= Portion of slab extracted

Figure 27-21. MOTSA (multiple overlapping thin-slab acquisition). To reduce saturation effects in deeper slices, multiple thinner slices are processed (in this example, 7). Next, the peripheral slices in each slab are discarded and the remaining slices are extracted and combined to form an image.

TONE. In this scheme, the flip angle α is increased progressively as the flowing spins move into the imaging volume by using increasing RF pulses. Recall that a larger α yields a higher SNR. Thus, increasing α counteracts saturation effects of slowly flowing blood in deeper slices. This allows better visualization of distal vessels and slow-flowing vessels. This scheme is illustrated in Figure 27-24 in which a **ramped** flip angle excitation pulse is used. In this example, the center flip angle is 30° and the flip angle at each end varies by 30% (i.e., 20° at the entry slice and 40° at the exit slice).

> **There are five main ways of reducing saturation effects:**
>
> 1. **Decreasing the flip angle α**
> 2. **Increasing the repetition time TR**
> 3. **CE MRA**
> 4. **MOTSA**
> 5. **TONE**

Question: How does magnetization transfer (MT) affect MRA?

Answer: **Magnetization transfer (MT)** saturation was discussed in Chapter 25. MT is based on suppression of the off-resonant protein-bound water protons (e.g., brain tissue). This technique, combined with TOF MRA, helps to suppress the background signal (e.g., it can reduce the signal from brain parenchyma by about 30%), increasing conspicuity of small and distal

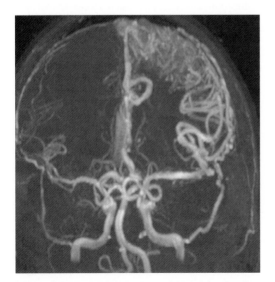

Figure 27-22. MOTSA MRA of the circle of Willis shows a left parietal lobe AVM.

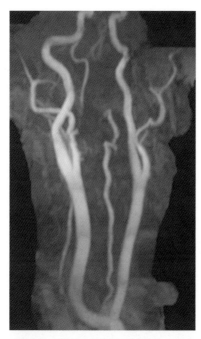

Figure 27-23. The MOTSA technique can also be used for extracranial carotid evaluation, as seen in this normal examination. The exam was cardiac gated.

branches, vessels with slow flow, and aneurysms. MT can also be combined with TONE for further visualization of small vessels.

Question: Why do MRA techniques overestimate the degree of stenosis?

Answer: Because accelerated flow through the stenotic area leads to dephasing during TE. To reduce this effect, use a shorter TE. Also, turbulent flow and vortex flow (flow eddies) as well as stream separation distal to stenosis and at vessel turns (e.g., carotid siphon) may cause dephasing and flow void, overestimating the length of stenosis (in the case of post stenosis) or mimicking stenosis (in the case of vessel turns). CE MRA minimizes these effects.

Black-Blood MRA

Black-blood MRA is a subset of TOF techniques, which accentuates the TOF losses resulting in flowing blood appearing dark rather than bright. Rapidly flowing blood (arterial flow), as discussed in the previous chapter, demonstrates TOF signal losses. Slowly flowing blood (venous flow) has higher intensity. Various flow presat pulses and dephasing methods via gradients are employed in this technique to render flowing blood black. Note that the maximum intensity projection is replaced by a ***minimum* intensity projection** algorithm.

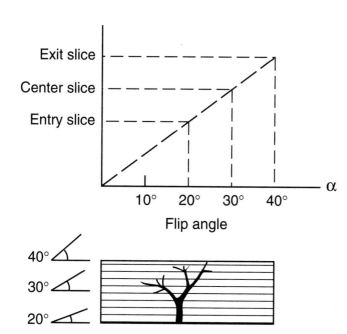

Figure 27-24. TONE (tilted optimized nonsaturating excitation). In this scheme, a ramped flip angle is used, which is larger in deeper slices. Because a larger α yields a larger transverse component in the x–y plane, this scheme would improve SNR in deeper slices, counteracting the saturation effects of slow-flowing blood.

Advantages

1. This technique does not overestimate the degree of stenosis as much as bright-blood TOF MRA.
2. Dephasing in vessel turns that mimic stenosis with bright-blood TOF MRA is not a problem here.

Disadvantages

1. Calcified plaques may also be dark and therefore invisible. Thus, this technique may *underestimate* the degree of stenosis.
2. Other black materials (such as air or cortical bone or calcification) may mimic flow.

Fresh-Blood Imaging

3D-fresh blood imaging (FBI) MRA is a new technique based on the fact that vessel signal intensity is dependent on blood flow (or cardiac phase) in T2-weighted images. The early systolic phases (0 ~ 200 msec after the *R* wave) show low signal intensity for arteries (high velocity with TOF losses) and high signal intensity for veins (lower velocities with no significant TOF loss), whereas the diastolic phases (400 ~ 600 msec after the *R* wave) show high signal intensity for both arteries and veins (no significant TOF loss). Bright-blood MRA is achieved by subtracting systolic images from diastolic images. The 3D-FBI method employs an electrocardiography (ECG)-gated 3D half-Fourier fast spin-echo sequence triggered for systolic and diastolic acquisitions. The ECG triggering time is an important factor influencing the blood signal intensity in the vessel of interest. An "ECG-prep scan" is typically used to produce 2D half-Fourier FSE single-slice images at various triggering delay times. An appropriate ECG delay time is determined for the vessel of interest and later applied in the 3D half-Fourier FSE acquisition synchronized by ECG gating for every slice encoding. An example is seen in Figure 27-25.

Advantages

1. Non-contrast technique; gadolinium not required

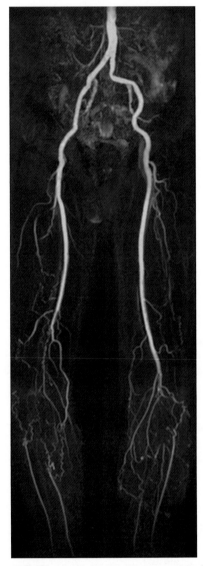

Figure 27-25. Coronal FBI MIP image of the lower extremity shows abrupt occlusion of tibioperoneal trunk, peroneal and tibial arteries, as well as geniculate collaterals.

2. Arterial and venous imaging in all areas of the body
3. Insensitive to off-resonance artifacts

Disadvantages

1. Sensitive to selection and timing of the triggered acquisitions
2. Motion artifacts and blurring
3. Longer scan time than CE-MRA

Key Points

1 Three main MR angiography (MRA) techniques exist: (i) time-of-flight (TOF), (ii) phase contrast (PC), and (iii) contrast enhanced (CE).

2 Both TOF and PC MRA can be performed in 2D or 3D.

3 TOF MRA is based on FRE.

4 PC MRA is based on velocity-induced phase changes.

5 PC MRA techniques allow acquisition of magnitude and phase images.

6 Phase images provide information regarding the direction of flow (not provided by TOF MRA).

7 VENC (velocity encoding) is a parameter that needs to be input by the operator when doing PC MRA. It represents the maximum flow velocity before aliasing occurs.

8 If VENC is too low, aliasing is more likely to occur. If VENC is too high, slow flow and small vessels are not well visualized. Therefore, low VENC is good for visualization of slow (venous) flow and small branches. High VENC is good for high-velocity (arterial) flow.

9 CE MRA is based on a rapid 3D GRE sequence that is timing sensitive and takes advantage of the powerful T1 shortening of gadolinium.

10 CE MRA is the most resistant to dephasing of the bright-blood techniques.

11 Time-resolved imaging of contrast kinetics (TRICKS) provides rapid multiphase imaging while retaining much of the SNR. TRICKS is useful for high-flow malformations or differential flow conditions (e.g., lower extremity run offs).

12 MIP (maximum intensity projection) is an algorithm used in MRA in which the highest intensity dots in space are connected to generate a three-dimensional-looking image of the vessels.

13 3D imaging is subject to saturation effects (as blood enters deeper slices).

14 Saturation effects can be minimized by several methods: (i) decreasing the flip angle, (ii) increasing TR, (iii) using gadolinium, (iv) MOTSA, or (v) TONE.

15 MOTSA (multiple overlapping thin-slab acquisition) uses several overlapping thin slices to reduce saturation effects. A potential problem is Venetian blind artifacts.

16 TONE (tilted optimized nonsaturating excitation) uses a ramped RF flip angle (small α at the entry slice and larger α at the exit slice) to reduce saturation effects.

17 TOF MRA tends to overestimate the degree of stenosis (due to dephasing effects).

18 Black-blood MRA is based on TOF signal losses. Instead of maximum intensity projection, a minimum intensity projection algorithm is used. This technique overcomes the problem of overestimating the degree of stenosis.

19 Fresh-blood imaging (FBI) is a new TOF bright arterial signal MRA technique that takes advantage of the differing velocities and TOF losses between systole and diastole.

Questions

27-1 The main MRA techniques include
(a) TOF MRA (b) PC MRA
(c) CE MRA (d) all of the above

27-2 The parameter VENC must be set for
(a) TOF MRA (b) PC MRA
(c) both (d) none

27-3 Match (i) low VENC (ii) high VENC with
(a) more sensitive to slow flow
(b) aliasing
(c) poor visualization of small branches
(d) arterial flow

27-4 **T/F** TOF MRA may underestimate the degree of stenosis.

27-5 Saturation effects can be reduced by
(a) decreasing the flip angle
(b) increasing TR
(c) using a gadolinium chelate
(d) MOTSA
(e) all of the above
(f) only (a)–(c)

27-6 **T/F** TOF MRA is based on FRE.

27-7 **T/F** MT allows better visualization of smaller vessels with slow flow in the brain.

27-8 Match
(i) ramped RF
(ii) Venetian blind artifact
(ii) deeper FRE
(iv) magnitude and phase images
(v) low VENC

with
(a) MOTSA   (b) TONE
(c) aliasing   (d) countercurrent flow
(e) PC MRA

27-9 **T/F** In the MIP algorithm, the pixel with the highest intensity is selected for each slice.

27-10 Compared with conventional bright-blood MRA, black-blood MRA
(a) uses a minimum intensity projection algorithm
(b) does not overestimate the degree of stenosis as much
(c) both (a) and (b)
(d) none of the above

28

Cardiac MRI

Introduction

Cardiac MRI is arguably the most difficult MRI examination to perform. Cardiac MRI must overcome not just respiratory motion, but also cardiac motion that cannot be suspended for the image. Additionally, there are a variety of nomenclature approaches to the pulse sequences, some of which are fairly unique to cardiac imaging while others are used in other organ systems all contributing to difficulty in understanding cardiac MRI. These different nomenclature systems are superimposed on the option of static versus cine imaging, and functional or physiologic imaging which all combine to challenge not just the patient and MRI technologist, but the MR physicist and radiologist.

Motion Effects and Compensation

Motion is a perpetual challenge to high-quality images in cardiac MRI. Body imagers are very knowledgeable of respiratory motion in abdominal imaging, but cardiac MRI has the additional challenge of cardiac motion. Respiratory and cardiac gating techniques are used frequently in cardiac MRI to compensate for motion. Gating techniques use an electrical impulse based on a physiologic marker (e.g., R wave from an electrocardiographic [ECG] or diaphragm position indicator) to accept, reject, or reorder data in k-space contributing to an image. Gating techniques fall into two broad categories: (i) **prospective** and (ii) **retrospective.** Prospective gating or

EKG- or plethysmographic-triggering uses the impulse and based on previous preset or calculated parameters determines prospectively how k-space will be filled prior to signal acquisition. On the other hand, retrospective gating runs the pulse sequence and collects the signal regardless of the electrical or pressure impulse marker, and then either "on the fly" or after the signals have all been obtained uses certain parameters to either accept or reject signals for inclusion into k-space and subsequent Fourier transformation.

Respiratory Motion. Respiratory motion can be compensated by either breath-hold imaging or respiratory gating. The average individual can breath-hold for 15 to 25 sec, while individuals with cardiopulmonary disease will be able to breath-hold for shorter periods, which limits this technique. Alternatively, respiratory gating techniques track the motion of the diaphragm either indirectly by using a **bellows** device around the chest/abdomen or directly through a **navigator-echo pulse**. Both techniques track the depth and direction of the respiration and then either eliminate or minimize k-space acquisition when the position of the diaphragm falls outside of prescribed limits.

A **bellows** device can utilize either (i) **respiratory gating (triggering)** or (ii) **respiratory compensation** (respiratory-ordered phase encoding [ROPE] or centrally ordered phase encoding [COPE]) of k-space. Respiratory gating can be either prospective or retrospective. Gating will accept signals into k-space if the bellows detects the diaphragm position at or near a predetermined position in the respiratory cycle (usually end-expiration). However, respiratory gating utilizes only about 20% of the respiratory cycle since most of the time the diaphragm position will lie outside the ideal position. Respiratory compensation (ROPE and COPE) improves efficiency by reordering the sequence of k-space filling based on the fact that the outer portions of k-space are less sensitive to changes due to motion than the central portion. ROPE gradually varies the phase-encode steps along the entirety of the respiratory cycle, while COPE acquires the lower phase-ordered steps (central k-space) around the longest respiratory cycle dwell time

(usually end-expiration) with ever-increasing higher phase steps the further away from end-expiration.

The newest respiratory gating method is **navigator-echo gating.** This technique does not require the bellows, but instead uses either a single spiral radio frequency (RF) pulse or two intersecting RF pulses, usually on the right diaphragm, to track movement. Navigator-echo gating data then usually prospectively triggers the acquisition of k-space if the object tracked is within a certain prescribed window of movement (usually 3 to 5 mm) (Fig. 28-1). Newer variants of navigator gating

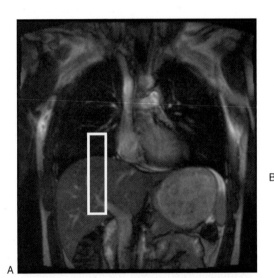

A

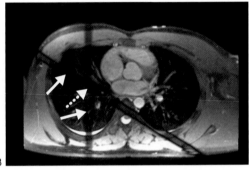

B

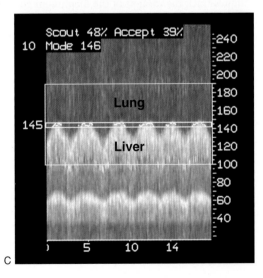

C

Figure 28-1. Navigator-echo gating. **A:** Coronal True FISP scout demonstrates column of excited tissue (rectangle) that the navigator-echo pulse will use on the right hemidiaphragm. **B:** Axial True FISP showing path of the intersecting RF pulses (*arrows*) generating the navigator-echo column at the intersection (*dashed arrow*). **C:** Tracing of navigator echo data showing the lung/liver interface and movement of the diaphragm. Time along x-axis and distance in millimeters along y-axis. Narrow window at "145" demonstrates acceptance window.

include a phase-reordered sequence that triggers the filling of the center of k-space when the diaphragm is within the ideal range while contributing to the outer portions of k-space when the diaphragm is outside the ideal range. This adaptation fills k-space during more of the respiratory cycle, resulting in a shorter scan time similar to respiratory compensation techniques. Lastly, navigator information can be used prospectively to correct for motion by adjusting the slice position if the diaphragm is detected outside the preferred window. This technique is known as **slice-tracking or motion-correction.**

Cardiac Motion. Cardiac motion is complex with various contributions from longitudinal shortening (long-axis), radial contraction (short-axis), and rotational motion. Although cardiac motion can be compensated for by using a pulse oximeter device or plethysmograph peripheral pulse monitor, ECG gating is more precise and usually yields a superior result. ECG gating allows the signal to be acquired in the same

phase (e.g., systole and mid-diastole) of the cardiac cycle, resulting in less cardiac motion. However, there are additional complexities of the cardiac cycle with resultant R–R interval variability due to (i) normal beat-to-beat variability, (ii) premature contractions, and (iii) changes due to respiration especially breath-hold. Prior to scanning, the patient's cardiac tracing is monitored and certain parameters are calculated based on the patient's R–R interval range. The R–R interval range and frequency of premature contractions vary between patients and, if significant enough, can negatively impact image quality. ECG gating approaches these limitations and variables in two fundamental ways: (i) **prospective** and (ii) **retrospective gating** (Figs. 28-2 and 28-3). Additionally, for highly variable R–R interval patients, an **arrhythmia reject window** can be used in both gating techniques that further prevents filling k-space if R waves fall too far outside expected parameters. The arrhythmia reject window length may be either symmetric or asymmetric around the expected R wave.

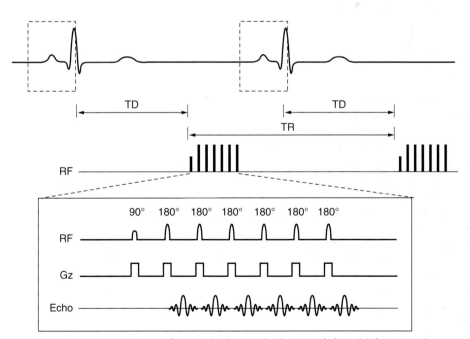

Figure 28-2. Prospective gating for a single slice/single phase (mid-diastole) fast spin-echo sequence with an echo train length = 6. Notice the long trigger delay (TD) between the R wave and the commencement of the pulse sequence with the initial 90° RF pulse. Dashed boxes around the QRS waves indicate the built-in arrhythmia reject window intrinsic to prospective gating.

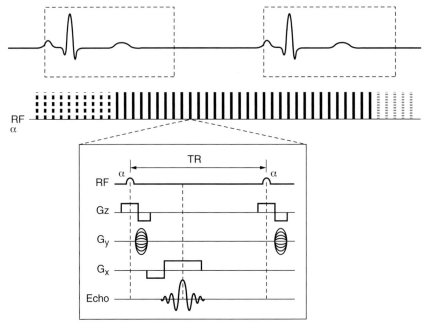

Figure 28-3. Retrospective gating for a single slice/multiphase cine sequence using a GRE pulse sequence. Notice the oversampling of the R–R interval of about 125% denoted by the different dashed or solid lines denoting a complete train of RF pulses contributing to a segment of k-space for the separate cardiac phases. There is no trigger delay as in prospective gating. Notice that the TR is much shorter in the GRE sequence than in the FSE sequence in Figure 28-2. Lastly, the dashed box represents an optional asymmetric arrhythmia rejection window (−10% to +50% expected R wave) whereupon an R wave detected outside of this box would result in rejection of the prior R–R interval's signals.

Prospective gating uses R wave detection with a variable **trigger delay** and then begins collecting k-space. The k-space is then filled over a certain prescribed percentage of the average R–R interval (usually 80% to 90% for cine imaging) whereupon no k-space is filled during the last 10% to 20% of the R–R interval. This results in a constant number of lines of k-space that are filled per R–R interval (Fig. 28-2). The last 10% to 20% of the R–R interval that does not fill k-space is designed in arrhythmia reject window that prevents acquisition of k-space during an early R wave due to beat-to-beat variability. However, this may or may not exclude premature contractions, and this can then be solved by superimposing a broader arrhythmia rejection window. Prospective gating is used in both static and cine imaging.

Retrospective gating, on the other hand, does not have any periods within the cardiac cycle where k-space is not being filled. This technique over samples the R–R interval usually at 125% and

then retrospectively goes back and based on the detected R waves determines which line of k-space corresponds with each specific cardiac phase (Fig. 28-3). This technique results in a variable number of k-space lines filled per R–R interval since the R–R interval has beat-to-beat variability and sometimes premature contractions. After the collection of signals, the computer then uses a weighted interpolation technique and determines the phase of the cardiac cycle that each signal belongs to. This technique is most commonly used in cine sequences such as gradient-recalled echo (GRE), true fast imaging with steady-state precession (True FISP, Siemens), FIESTA (fast imaging employing steady-state acquisition, General Electric), or b-FFE (balanced fast field echo, Philips) and phase contrast imaging.

If arrhythmias are too frequent, then ECG triggering can become impossible, and one can salvage the study by taking off the cardiac gating and increasing the NEX to 4. The idea behind this is that systole is typically a small percentage of most patients' cardiac cycles, and thus by increasing the NEX, it will average out the smaller percentage of the signal acquired during systole with its greater motion. If the patient's heart rate is fast, especially over 100, then this technique will be limited as well. The drawback is that scan time will increase and breath-hold techniques will be impossible, so a respiratory-gated technique must be used. Lastly, a **single-shot** technique (discussed later) can be used.

Blood Motion. Blood movement within the heart and great vessels is pulsatile with complex flow characteristics, resulting in motion-induced intravoxel dephasing from differing velocities within a voxel contributing to signal loss. Valvular stenosis and regurgitation, vessel stenosis, and cardiac shunts can all have marked effects on the blood flow velocities, direction, and subsequent dephasing and signal loss. Flow compensation or gradient moment nulling can help mitigate these problems, but at a small sacrifice of a higher minimum time to echo (TE).

Faster Imaging. The faster the imaging sequence, the less chance for any type of motion-related effects. GRE or True FISP imaging with very short TRs or half-Fourier acquired single-shot turbo spin-echo (HASTE) sequences all acquire k-space in a shorter period of time versus fast spin-echo (FSE) sequences. A motion-reducing option for GRE or True FISP sequences is to acquire the k-space in a **single-shot** mode where the entire image's k-space is acquired within a single R–R interval. HASTE sequences are by nature a single-shot sequence.

Additionally, parallel imaging can be used with any pulse sequence (see Chapter 24) and commonly reduces the time of acquisition by two to fourfold or increases spatial resolution two to four times without a time penalty. The major drawback to parallel imaging is decreased signal-to-noise ratio (SNR), so parallel imaging works best with sequences that have high SNR such as True FISP or postgadolinium imaging.

Motion in Cardiac Imaging and Solutions
  1. Gross patient movement: instruct patient to lie still, mild sedation

  2. Respiratory movement: breath-hold techniques, respiratory gating, navigator-echo gating
  3. Cardiac motion: ECG gating, pulse oximeter gating, increase NEX, single-shot technique
  4. Blood motion: flow compensation/gradient moment nulling, pulse sequences insensitive to dephasing, for example, True FISP
  5. Parallel imaging: two to fourfold decrease in acquisition time however decreased SNR

General k-space Filling Strategies

Segmented versus Single Shot. Early in cardiac MRI, only one line of k-space was filled for a single image during a single R–R interval. This was a very inefficient way of filling k-space and resulted in long scan times. Subsequently, all cardiac imaging fills k-space in a **segmented** fashion that fills more than one line of k-space for a single image during a single R–R interval. One can conceptualize k-space "segmented" into separate areas based on different R–R interval contributions of k-space. For example, if there were 160 phase-encode steps and eight lines of k-space were filled for a single image during each R–R interval, then there would be 160/8 = 20 segments of k-space. The eight lines of k-space filled per R–R interval is termed **views per segment (VPS).** If all k-space is filled in a single R–R interval, then this is equivalent to a single segment, and it is referred to as a single shot. It should be noted that a "single shot" outside of cardiac MRI usually refers to a pulse sequence where a single RF pulse tips all the required longitudinal magnetization into the transverse plane for k-space to be completely filled for a single image such as in a HASTE or single-shot EPI sequence.

Static Imaging

All of the previously described pulse sequences in this book have been or are used to produce static cardiac images. These images are usually divided into two categories: (i) **bright blood** and (ii) **dark blood.** Unfortunately, the appearance of blood as either bright or dark is a consequence of the specific pulse sequence and not a particular sequence one can select on the scanner. Blood signal has dark T1 and bright T2 signal intrinsically. Knowledge of the intrinsic signal of blood combined with superimposed time-of-flight effects (time-of-flight [TOF] loss or flow-related enhancement [FRE]) in a particular pulse sequence determines whether blood is bright or dark.

Fast Spin Echo and HASTE. Spin-echo imaging has generally been abandoned due to excessive scan times, and it is now replaced by either FSE or HASTE that provides good anatomic detail, intrinsic dark-blood signal due to TOF loss, and appropriate T1 or T2 weighting based on TR and TE. FSE with ECG gating and either breath-hold or navigator-echo gating result in good image quality; however, the drawback is lengthy scan times. HASTE sequences have shorter scan times and are usually obtained in a single R–R interval; however, the SNR will be less due to ½NEX signal averages.

Although FSE and HASTE sequences are usually dark blood, some areas of slow blood flow from physiologic, pathologic, or in plane flow can result in minimal expected TOF loss and unexpected bright-blood signal confounding interpretation. This bright signal can be minimized by using a **double-inversion recovery (DIR)** sequence. This sequence uses a nonslice-selective 180° RF pulse followed immediately by a slice selective 180° RF pulse and an appropriate T1 that is influenced by the R–R interval (T1 usually 600 msec) that nulls the signal of inflowing blood, resulting in a more robust black blood effect (Figs. 28-4 and 28-5). Due to some intrinsic changes in the position of the slice from the initial 180° RF pulses and the actual filling of k-space about 600 msec later, the slice-selective 180° RF pulse is usually twice the nominal thickness of the slice to ensure that all the myocardium is reinverted. Additionally, to allow full recovery of the longitudinal magnetization, k-space is usually filled every other R–R interval unless the patient is bradycardic.

Fast Spin-Echo Gating. Static imaging including FSE uses prospective gating. Optimal gating with minimal motion artifact is achieved when

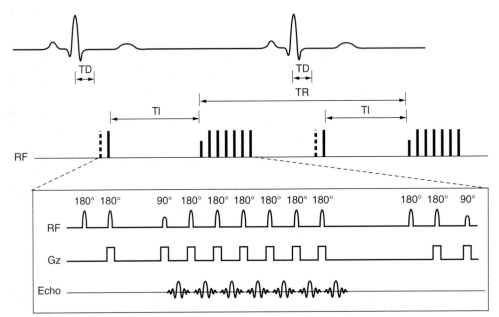

Figure 28-4. Prospective gated single slice/single phase (mid-diastole) fast spin-echo DIR sequence with an echo train length = 6. Notice the shorter trigger delay (TD) driven by the requirement to initiate the pulse sequence with the nonselective 180° inversion pulse (dashed line in pair) immediately followed by a slice-selective 180° inversion or "reinversion" pulse (solid line in pair). This schematic shows acquisition of echoes every R–R interval, which occurs only in bradycardic patients. The R–R interval is usually shorter requiring echo acquisition every other R–R interval or heartbeat.

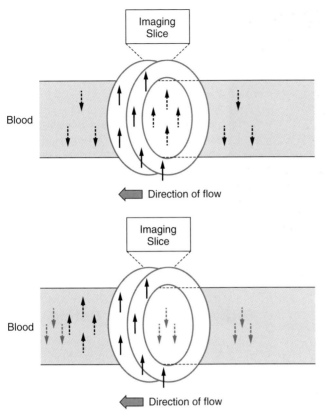

Figure 28-5. **A:** Direction of longitudinal magnetization immediately after the nonselective and slice-selective 180° RF pulses. These pulses are usually applied during late diastole immediately after the R wave is detected. *Solid arrows* represent longitudinal magnetization in the myocardium, while dashed lines represent blood. **B:** Direction of longitudinal magnetization immediately before the acquisition of echoes and filling of k-space. The TI is usually chosen to coincide with acquisition of k-space during mid-diastole. *Solid arrows* represent amplitude of longitudinal magnetization in the myocardium, while dashed lines represent blood. Notice that the *dashed arrows* that were in the imaging slice in (A) have now moved to the left with the direction of flow and will not give off signal due to their movement outside the imaging slice. The prior *dashed arrows* that were inverted have now become nearly zero in longitudinal magnetization (*gray dashed arrows*).

each image is acquired in the same cardiac phase. Static images are either acquired as a single slice/single phase (usually mid-diastole) or a multislice/single phase where multiple slices are acquired in an interleaved fashion. The single image/single phase technique fills k-space during mid-diastole and results in less motion since it minimizes changes of cardiac phase due to beat-to-beat variability; however, usually only one slice or at most two slices can be acquired during a single breath-hold (Fig. 28-2). Multislice/single phase is more efficient, but has more motion effects due to beat-to-beat variability and misregistration between slices due to the changing position of the heart at different phases of the cardiac cycle.

All FSE sequences have time of repetition (TR) that approximates or exceeds the R–R time. This requires the TR for an FSE sequence to be a multiple of the patient's R–R interval. For example, if a patient's pulse is 75 beats/min, then the R–R interval is 800 msec [(60 sec/min)/(75 beats/min) = 0.8 sec/beat], and the TR would have to be a multiple of 800 msec. A T1 FSE TR is equal to 800 msec, and a T2 FSE TR would be 2400, 3200, or 4000 msec. Faster sequences with TRs that are much shorter than the R–R interval such as GRE and True FISP sequences are not tied to this principle and thus can keep their best TR for the pulse sequence (see later discussion).

Gradient-Recalled Echo. A faster alternative to FSE imaging for static images is GRE sequences. These sequences may not give quite the T1 or T2 weighting quality of an FSE sequence, but they are acquired more quickly. Additionally, spoiled GRE sequences typically have bright-blood signal due to FRE (see TOF MRA in Chapter 27). Since GRE sequences are dependent on FRE, ultrashort TRs are not practical because the TR must be long enough to allow unsaturated protons to enter the imaging slice (Fig. 28-6). Flow compensation techniques are customarily used during bright-blood GRE techniques to maintain as much signal as possible. Postgadolinium GRE sequences can be performed, which further increase the blood

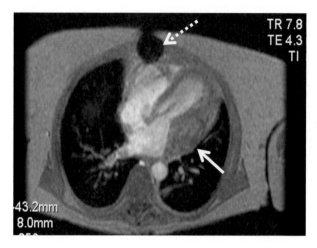

Figure 28-6. Four chamber bright-blood GRE sequence TR 7.8/TE 4.3 msec of the heart demonstrates bright-blood signal in the heart and great vessels. Area of darker signal along left ventricular free wall (*arrow*) was a pericardial hematoma. Also note the susceptibility effects from midline sternotomy wires (*dashed arrow*).

signal; however, the contrast between the blood pool and the myocardium will be decreased due to the enhancing myocardium.

True Fast Imaging with Steady-state Precession (True FISP). The current work-horse of fast cardiac imaging is the True FISP (Siemens) sequence, which is also known as FIESTA (General Electric), b-FFE (Philips), or sometimes generically as b-SSFP (balanced steady-state free precession). True FISP utilizes a high flip angle, very short TR/TE, and a completely balanced pulse sequence that preserves transverse magnetization, resulting in extremely fast T2/T1-weighted high SNR images with insensitivity to dephasing and signal loss (Figs. 28-7 and 28-8). True FISP does not rely on FRE for bright-blood effects, but rather on the intrinsic contrast difference in T2/T1 signal of blood versus myocardium. True FISP's TR/TE is usually 3 to

4 msec/1.5 to 2 msec enabling this sequence to be performed faster than most other pulse sequences.

GRE and True FISP Gating

GRE and True FISP TR times are much less than an R–R interval time, and thus their optimal TR can be used regardless of the R–R time. Prospective gating is frequently used with GRE/True FISP static imaging obtained in mid-diastole. True FISP's TRs are 3 to 4 msec allowing for a single slice/single phase image acquired in a single R–R interval, also known as a single shot. GRE sequences have longer TRs and may require two R–R intervals to create a single image during mid-diastole. Alternatively, prospective or retro-spective gating can be used for a multislice/single phase acquisition in an interleaved method. This will result in several different slices obtained at various times in the cardiac cycle.

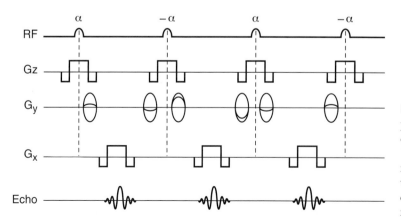

Figure 28-7. True FISP pulse sequence diagram demonstrates completely balanced RF pulses and magnetic gradients. The time to echo (TE) is exactly ½ of the time of repetition (TR).

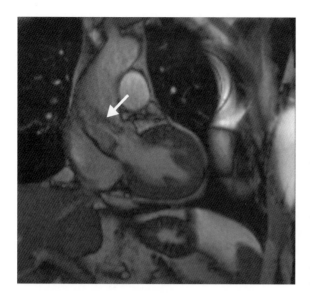

Figure 28-8. Vertical two chamber or left ventricular outlet view (same patient as in Fig. 27-7) demonstrates bright signal not only in the blood, but also within the mediastinal and abdominal fat due to the intrinsic T2/T1 bright signal. Patient had significant aortic stenosis, which is seen here as mild signal loss from marked turbulent flow (*arrow*). A standard bright-blood GRE sequence would have more signal loss.

Inversion Recovery Preparation GRE/True FISP or Delayed Enhancement Sequences

A 180° RF inversion recovery (IR) preparation pulse can be applied to a pulse sequence following gadolinium administration, usually either a GRE or a True FISP sequence, to take advantage of the fact that there are different temporal T1 post-gadolinium curves for normal myocardium versus scar. These IR-prepared GRE or True FISP sequences are frequently referred to as **delayed enhancement** or **late gadolinium enhancement** images and have proven very useful in diagnosing abnormal myocardium due to ischemic events, a variety of cardiomyopathies (CM) (e.g., sarcoid, right ventricular dysplasia, myocarditis, amyloidosis, or hypertrophic CM), or masses. These pulse sequences are performed following a 10 to 15 min delay after intravenous gadolinium that results in selective nulling out of normal enhancing myocardium while abnormal myocardium remains bright (Fig. 31-3). These IR-prepared GRE or True FISP sequences have a single IR pulse for a whole train or series of TRs (usually 20 to 25). Thus, there is a sliding time to inversion (TI) for each signal acquisition (see Chapter 21) which is analogous to the "TE effective" in FSE imaging with the central lines of k-space acquired around the desired TI (usually between 200 and 300 msec) to optimize the contrast contribution of the nulled normal myocardium at the optimal TI (Fig. 28-9). Again there is some cardiac motion during the TI; therefore, the 180° RF pulse is non-slice selective to ensure complete nulling of all myocardium. Finally, k-space is usually collected every other heartbeat allowing enough time for full longitudinal magnetization recovery.

A frequently encountered difficulty with IR-prep GRE/True FISP sequences is poor nulling of normal myocardium on later images. This is due to gadolinium continually washing out of tissues, resulting in a longer T1 times and a subsequent need for longer TI times with later images. A **phase-sensitive** version has recently been introduced to mitigate this problem. Phase-sensitive IR-prepared GRE sequences restore the polarity of the magnitude of the signal, which increases the contrast between abnormal and normal enhancing myocardium (Fig. 28-10).

Cine Imaging

Cine imaging is similar to static imaging; however, instead of getting a single image for a single slice, you obtain a series of images obtained at different phases within the cardiac cycle for a single slice resulting in a single slice/multiphase acquisition. This permits visualization of the motion of the heart, valves, and any abnormal structures within the heart. GRE and True FISP sequences

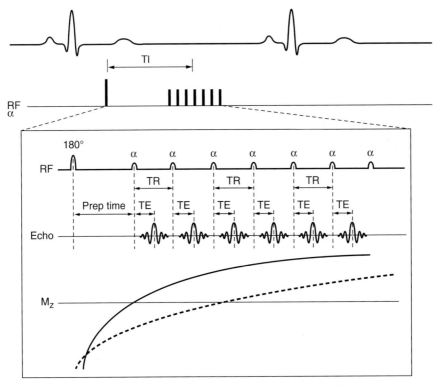

Figure 28-9. The multiple TRs in the IR-prepped GRE or True FISP delayed enhancement sequences are fewer in this example for clarity, but usually number 20 to 25; in the case of a single-shot sequence, the number of TRs would equal all the lines of k-space. The time to inversion is variable or sliding along the train of TRs; however, the nominal TI is in the middle of the TR train where the lowest phase-encode step is applied. The solid line in the longitudinal magnetization (M_z) indicates abnormal enhancing myocardium, while the dashed line reflects normal myocardium. Notice that ideally the normal myocardium crosses the null point exactly in the center of the train of TRs. Finally, there is no acquisition of k-space in the next R–R interval due to the need to allow time for longitudinal magnetization recovery.

provide this capability since FSE sequences take too long to acquire the required multiple phases per slice. In cine imaging, the user defines how many phases within the cardiac cycle per slice (usually 15 to 25) are acquired. The goal for temporal resolution between different phases should be around 50 msec. For example, a patient with an R–R interval of 1000 msec (60 beats/min) with a cine sequence with 20 phases will have a temporal resolution of 1000 msec/20 phases = 50 msec/phase. The benefit of increased phases is better temporal resolution and more precise physiologic calculations (see later discussion) with smoother cine loop viewing; however, the drawback is that it will take longer to scan. The relationship between phases, heart rate, and views per segment is given below.

Example: How long will it take to perform a prospective cine sequence using a True FISP sequence with 20 phases in the cardiac cycle, R–R interval, or time of segment acquisition = 1000 msec with a 20% arrhythmia reject window (800 msec of scanning per R–R), TR = 4 msec, and 160 phase-encode steps or views, and NEX = 1.

- 800 msec/20 phases = 40 msec/phase (temporal resolution)
- (40 msec/phase)/(4 msec/TR) = 10 TRs or 10 views/segment
- 160 views/10 views/segment = 16 segments
- Total scan time = (16 segments)(1000 msec/segment) = 16,000 msec or 16 sec

If the TR is longer (GRE for instance) or if more phases are required, then the total scan time will

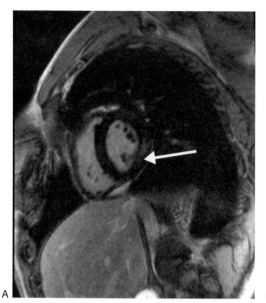
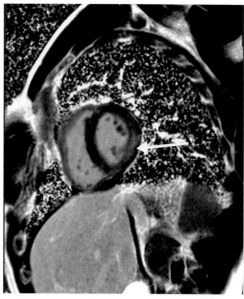

A   B

Figure 28-10. Short-axis segmented IR-prep GRE delayed enhancement imaging after gadolinium in a patient with myocarditis. **A:** Amplitude image demonstrates mildly bright midmyocardial signal in the lateral wall (*arrow*). Notice sparing of subendocardium consistent with myocarditis. **B:** Phase-sensitive reconstruction demonstrates increased contrast between the abnormally enhancing areas of myocarditis (*arrow*) in the lateral wall and the normal myocardium (compare best with interventricular septum).

also be longer which may fall outside a patient's breath-hold ability. To solve this problem, another technique known as **view sharing** can be used. View sharing is similar to the "shared echo" approach in FSE (see Chapter 19) in that echoes or views are shared between the phases. View sharing typically shares 50% of the echoes, and thus the new phases will be double minus one (Fig. 28-11).

Cine Gating Techniques

Cine imaging can be acquired with either prospective or retrospective gating. Prospective techniques are generally faster; however, they omit filling the last 10% to 20% of the cardiac cycle or late diastole and thus result in incomplete cardiac data that is especially important for determining physiologic or functional imaging (see later discussion). Retrospective gating is used when all phases of the cardiac cycle are required to be imaged.

Myocardial Tagging. An option in cine imaging used for enhanced detection of wall-motion abnormalities is the application of a tagging-prep pulse usually used with a GRE or True FISP sequence. The tagging bands are generated by a series of RF pulses separated by magnetic gradients that result in **SPAtial Modulation of the Magnetization** or **SPAMM.** The resultant image has a series of parallel dark lines or a dark grid of lines (Fig. 28-12). These lines or grid intersections are then subsequently deformed or move with contraction of the myocardium, but areas of hypo- or akinesis of the myocardium have persistent straight lines. A limitation of SPAMM is that these saturation bands fade after around 400 msec. A newer technique called Complementary SPAtial Modulation Magnetization (CSPAMM) improves the duration of the saturation bands.

Perfusion Imaging. Perfusion imaging is a subtype of cine imaging. This sequence uses a first pass of gadolinium that enters the blood pool and right ventricle initially followed very rapidly in sequence by filling of the left ventricle, coronary arteries, and perfusion of the myocardium. This is a cine technique, but due to the single pass nature of the gadolinium, a multislice/multiphase acquisition is required (Fig. 31-6). This requires very fast imaging sequences in order to achieve both the temporal and spatial resolution. Perfusion

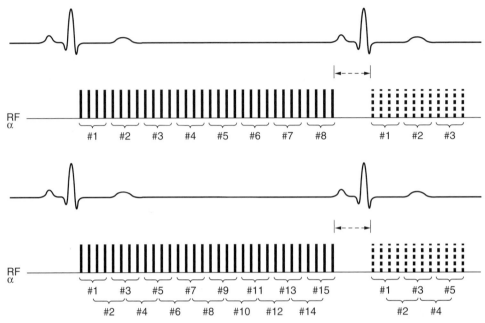

Figure 28-11. Prospective gating of GRE or True FISP sequence without and with view sharing. Notice that the trigger delay is nearly 0. The "dead" time or intrinsic arrhythmia rejection window (*dashed line*) is characteristic of prospective gating where no signal is acquired at the end of a predetermined number of echoes. **A:** Notice that with four views per segment only eight phases can be imaged without view sharing. **B:** With 50% view sharing, the number of phases increased from 8 to 15. The phase increase is double the original phases minus one for 50% view sharing.

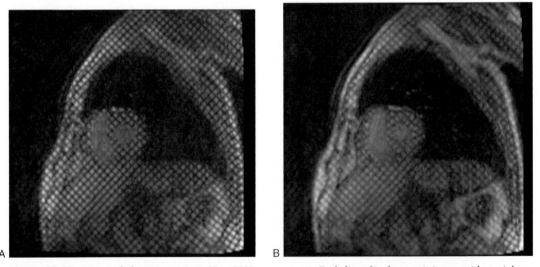

Figure 28-12. Myocardial tagging using a True FISP sequence. **A:** End-diastolic short-axis image with straight grid lines in the heart. **B:** End-systolic image with deformed grid lines consistent with movement of the myocardium. Also notice the darkness of the grid lines has decreased from (**A**) due to some T1 relaxation.

imaging is typically done both at rest and at stress (usually using adenosine) to determine areas of decreased perfusion related to ischemia. The profound T1 shortening effects of gadolinium allow for shorter TRs in GRE sequences since we no longer rely on FRE effects, but rather the intrinsic T1 shortening properties of enhancement due to the gadolinium. Fast single-shot GRE with minimum TR, a hybrid segmented GRE-EPI or True FISP sequence is used with a saturation or IR prep pulse to suppress the signal from background structures and to provide more T1 weighting.

Functional Imaging. Calculation of functional or physiologic parameters is a common request either to confirm echocardiography abnormalities or to evaluate parameters that echocardiography has difficulty with. Functional or physiologic parameters are obtained in one of two ways: (i) derived from bright-blood cine images such as True FISP, GRE, or tagged variants, or (ii) phase contrast imaging (details in Chapter 27).

A stack of short-axis bright-blood cine images are used in determining ejection fractions, myocardial mass, and volumes (Fig. 28-13).

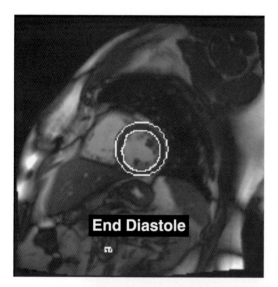
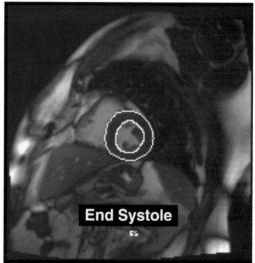

Left Ventricle - Absolute				
Cardiac Function			Normal Range (M) (MRI)	Units
Ejection Fraction	EF	47.9	56.00 ... 78.00	%
End Diastolic Volume	EDV	155.7	77.00 ... 195.00	ml
End Systolic Volume	ESV	81.0	19.00 ... 72.00	ml
Stroke Volume	SV	74.6	51.00 ... 133.00	ml
Cardiac Output	CO	6.42	2.82 ... 8.82	l/min
Myocardial Mass (at ED)		167.3	118.00 ... 238.00	g
Myocardial Mass (Avg)		163.4 ± 5.4	118.00 ... 238.00	g

Figure 28-13. Quantitative left ventricular parameters. Upper two images from short-axis True FISP cine sequence with epicardial and endocardial contours drawn. Table below indicates ejection fraction, volumes, and cardiac output. The addition of epicardial contours allowed calculation of myocardial mass as well. Notice low ejection fraction.

However, these cine images must be manipulated on a postprocessing workstation either one that comes with the scanner or a stand alone postprocessing workstation equipped for cardiac MR calculations. Identifying end-diastole and end-systole, and then delineating endocardial contours provides ejection fraction and volume measurements. Addition of an epicardial contour to the endocardial contour also provides myocardial mass and contractility measurements.

Phase contrast imaging can determine velocities, regurgitant fractions, and shunt or **Qp/Qs** ratios (pulmonary to systemic flow ratio). Phase contrast imaging by its very nature provides velocity and direction data. Determining an appropriate velocity encoding or VENC value is essential to provide the best imaging quality while eliminating aliasing. Phase contrast imaging is typically, but not always, performed orthogonal to the vessel or chamber evaluated.

Clinical Applications and Pulse Sequences

1. Infarction or cardiomyopathy: cine True FISP and delayed enhancement IR-prepared GRE or True FISP
2. Arrhythmogenic right ventricular dysplasia: cine True FISP, T1 with and without fat saturation (DIR preferred), and delayed enhancement IR-prepared GRE or True FISP
3. Mass: cine True FISP, T1 with and without fat saturation (DIR preferred), T2 (DIR preferred), T1 postgadolinium, and delayed enhancement IR-prepared GRE or True FISP
4. Coronary MRA: True FISP, GRE, or postgadolinium MRA for bright blood; DIR FSE for black blood
5. Valvular disease: GRE or True FISP, phase contrast with calculations for maximum velocity and regurgitant fraction, and DIR FSE for valve anatomy

Key Points

1 Cardiac and respiratory motion adversely impact cardiac MR images.

2 Respiratory motion is compensated for by using a bellows or navigator-echo pulse both of which track the motion of the diaphragm.

3 Cardiac motion is compensated for by ECG gating.

4 ECG gating can be either prospective or retrospective.

5 Prospective gating is faster but omits 10% to 20% of the cardiac cycle.

6 Retrospective gating is slower but covers the entire cardiac cycle.

7 FSE/HASTE sequences provide dark-blood static imaging for morphology.

8 Most FSE/HASTE sequences improve dark-blood effects by employing a double-inversion-prep pulse.

9 IR-prepared GRE or True FISP delayed enhancement sequences demonstrate infarcted myocardium and are useful in demonstrating various cardiomyopathies and even tumors.

10 GRE and True FISP sequences provide bright-blood appearance for either static or cine imaging.

11 Functional imaging can be obtained either through postprocessing of cine imaging (ejection fraction, volume, and myocardial mass) or performance of phase contrast imaging (velocity and shunt data).

Questions

28-1 Which techniques are useful for respiratory compensation?
(a) Navigator echoes
(b) Bellows
(c) Breath-holding
(d) All of the above

28-2 Which technique does not typically have "bright blood"?
(a) FSE
(b) True FISP
(c) GRE
(d) Postgadolinium GRE

28-3 Which gating technique best evaluates the entirety of the cardiac cycle in a cine sequence?
(a) Prospective gating
(b) Retrospective gating
(c) Neither, they are equivalent

28-4 To calculate myocardial mass, what contours need to be drawn?
(a) Endocardial
(b) Epicardial
(c) Both

28-5 True FISP sequences cannot produce which of the following?
(a) Cine images
(b) Static images
(c) Ejection fractions
(d) Flow velocities

28-6 Which sequence is usually obtained in a "single shot"?
(a) DIR FSE
(b) Cine True FISP
(c) HASTE
(d) Phase contrast

28-7 What feature improves temporal resolution?
(a) Lower TR
(b) Higher views per segment
(c) Shorter R–R interval
(d) Higher phase-encode steps

29

MR Spectroscopy in the Brain

Overview

Proton magnetic resonance spectroscopy (MRS) is an MR-based chemical analytical technique that can be performed on any high field magnet. Rather than providing images, it usually provides spectra consisting of individual peaks, the chemical shift of which from a universal standard helps identify the species comprising the peak. The normal spectrum from gray matter is different from the normal spectra from white matter (Fig. 29-1). MRS is the equivalent of the nuclear magnetic resonance (NMR) used in organic chemistry—only now performed on a patient in a whole-body MR magnet.

MRS is a functional technique. It can identify abnormalities not seen on conventional MRI, for example, invasion of a glioblastoma multiforme (GBM) into adjacent brain where there is no enhancement or T2 abnormality on MRI. It can distinguish between two or more abnormalities that appear the same on MRI, for example, recurrent GBM versus radiation necrosis.

As in NMR, the area under a given peak is proportional to the number of protons contributing to the peak. So, taking ethanol (CH_3—CH_2—OH) as an example, the area under the methyl (CH_3) peak would be 3 (in relative units), the area under the methylene (—CH_2—) peak would be 2, and the area under the hydroxyl (—OH) peak would be 1. Since the peaks generally have the same shape, this ratio of peak areas also holds for peak heights. In general, peak height is proportional to the concentration of a given species. MRS requires a species to be present in at least a 1 mM concentration to be seen.

The above discussion is somewhat simplified. In actuality, the protons on adjacent carbons influence the net magnetic field on each other. So the magnetic field experienced by the methyl protons in ethanol would be influenced by the adjacent methylene protons. In quantum mechanical sense, these two protons can either both point up, both point down, or one up and one down or one down and one up. When they both point up the net magnetic field experienced by the adjacent methyl protons is slightly higher than $\mathbf{B}_0$ and when they both point down, it is slightly lower than $\mathbf{B}_0$, which shifts the peaks. Up–down and down–up cancel each other and results in the same peak position as one would have without any adjacent protons. This is known as "spin–spin splitting," and it results in a big peak with area or peak height of 3 to be split into three peaks (called a "triplet") of area 1-2-1 (Fig. 29-2). Spin–spin splitting or "*J*-coupling" smears the chemical shift, making peak identification more difficult. It increases with increasing TE.

MRS in the brain is generally performed in conjunction with MRI which identifies the abnormality. For single voxel techniques, a volume of 8 cc is generally recommended at 1.5 T. A smaller voxel can be used but the signal-to-noise ratio (SNR) will be reduced (Fig. 29-3). Since peak height is generally proportional to field strength, a smaller voxel can be used at 3 T, reducing partial volume averaging. Generally, a second spectrum is acquired in the contralateral normal brain.

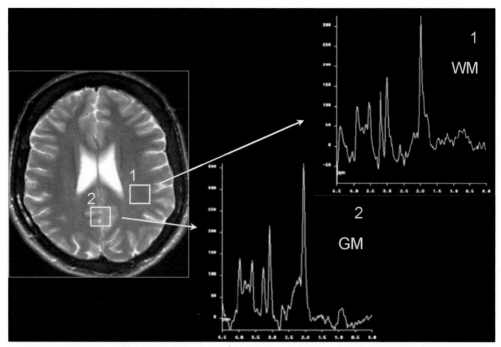

Figure 29-1. Normal spectra for white matter (*1*) and gray matter (*2*). *Note:* the higher Cho level in normal white matter (third highest peak).

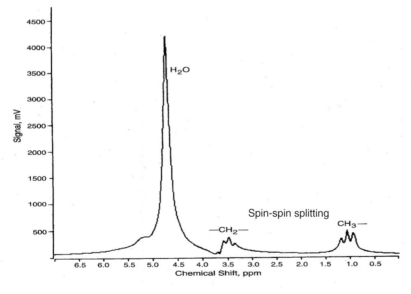

Figure 29-2. Spectrum from ethanol. *Note:* spin–spin splitting of methylene and methyl peaks.

Occasionally, the voxel is not placed on a lesion but in gray matter or white matter. Figure 29-1 shows the recommended voxel placement and resulting normal spectra. For gray matter, it is both calcarine cortices, spanning the posterior interhemispheric fissure. A standardized white matter voxel is in the high parietal lobe.

Once the voxel is placed on a lesion, the magnetic field in that voxel is made more uniform or "shimmed." Shimming results in improving the

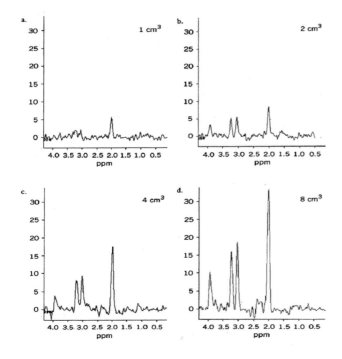

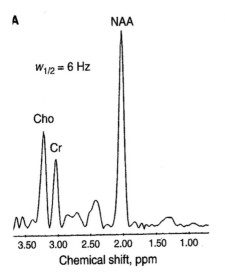

Figure 29-3. Signal-to-noise ratio as a function of voxel volume.

uniformity from 1 part per million (ppm) in the main magnetic field to 0.1 ppm inside the voxel (Fig. 29-4). For multivoxel techniques, the shimming must be performed throughout a slice, which now provides multiple 1 cc voxels.

In addition to shimming, the technologist must also suppress the signal coming from water—which has 100,000 times more signal than that coming from the metabolites compris-

ing the peaks in the spectrum. Water suppression is accomplished by exposing the voxel to an RF pulse that is 4.7 ppm from the universal standard, which, by definition, is at 0 ppm. This universal standard is TMS (tetramethylsilane). Having 4 methyl groups (12 protons) all in the same chemical environment gives it a peak height of 12! Peak position is always expressed in ppm relative to TMS because it doesn't change

A

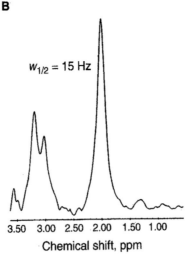

B

Figure 29-4. Effect of shimming. When full width at half maximum (FWHM or $W_{1/2}$) is 6 Hz (0.1 ppm at 1.5 T Larmor frequency of 64 MHz), Cr (3.0 ppm) can be distinguished from Cho (3.2 ppm). When the shimming is only to 0.25 ppm (15 Hz at 1.5 T), the Cr and Cho peaks start **to merge.**

between field strengths, whereas the actual frequency shift would go linearly with field strength. Thus data obtained at 1.5 T can be applied at 3 T as long as it is expressed in ppm.

MRS requires setting the repetition time (TR) and the echo delay time (TE) prospectively. The shorter the TR, the more T1-weighted the acquisition and the shorter the acquisition time, as in MRI. Choline (Cho) has a shorter T1 than the other species so it will appear relatively higher at shorter TR (Fig. 29-5). As Cho is used to diagnose cancer, it is important to standardize the TR. The longer the TE, the more T2-weighted the acquisition and the lower the SNR of the peaks (Fig. 29-6). Most institutions use a TR of 1500 msec and the shortest possible TE of 30 or 35 msec to maximize the SNR. This also allows the detection of short T2 species (like myoinositol [mI] and lipid), which would otherwise have already decayed at longer TE.

Peak width is proportional to 1/T2, thus short T2 hemorrhage will lead to peak broadening (Fig. 29-7). Peak broadening can also be seen with motion and with a poorly shimmed voxel (Fig. 29-4).

Visible Metabolites

Spectra are read from right (0 ppm) to left (4 ppm). As noted above the peaks are identified on the basis of their chemical shift (Fig. 29-1). In a normal brain, the first peak encountered is the main peak of N-acetyl aspartate (NAA) at 2 ppm. This is a marker of normal neurons. It is reduced whenever normal brain is displaced by a space-occupying lesion or in diffuse processes like dementia or diffuse axonal injury.

There are small peaks on the left-hand shoulder of NAA at 2 to 2.5 ppm (Fig. 29-1). These consist of glutamate (Glu) and glutamine (Gln) as well as some secondary NAA peaks. On commercial systems with a minimum TE of 30 msec, Glu and Gln cannot be distinguished due to spin–spin splitting so they are collectively called "Glx." Glx is elevated in ischemia and hepatic encephalopathy.

The next peak in a normal brain is creatine (Cr) at 3 ppm. It is a marker of energy metabolism and is the most constant of the peaks. Thus peak heights can be compared relative to Cr when reading spectra. Cr is reduced in near-drowning.

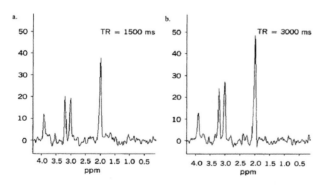

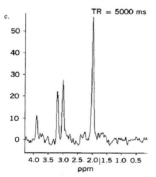

Figure 29-5. Effect of TR. At shorter TR (1500 ms), Cho is relatively increased compared to the other peaks due to its shorter T1. At longer TR (5000 ms), all the peaks have greater signal-to-noise ratio and have "caught up" to Cho similar to a proton density–weighted MR image.

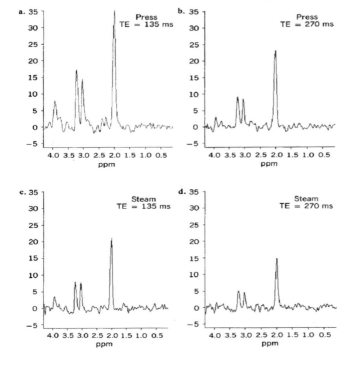

Figure 29-6. Effect of TE and technique. PRESS (based on spin echo) has twice the SNR of STEAM (based on stimulated echo) at a given TE. However, with longer TE, there is more T2 decay and lower SNR.

Cho is arguably the most important peak because it is elevated in cancer due to membrane turnover (Fig. 29-8). It occurs at 3.2 ppm.

On short TE (30 to 35 msec) techniques, mI occurs at 3.5 ppm. It is a sugar that appears to be the "prime osmolyte." Although all these species contribute to the osmolality of the brain, mI is the first to become elevated when the serum becomes hyperosmolar, limiting the amount of water shifted from the brain to the bloodstream. mI is also elevated in glial tumors compared to NAA (Fig. 29-9) as well as in Alzheimers.

Finally, there is a secondary Cr peak at 3.9 ppm. If the baseline rises on the left side of the spectrum, this is usually a sign of incomplete water suppression as water resides at 4.7 ppm.

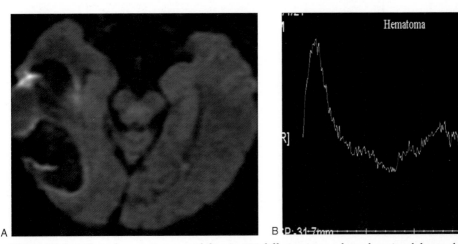

Figure 29-7. Effect of magnetic susceptibility. **A:** EPI diffusion image shows low signal due to short T2 deoxy-hemoglobin from an acute hemorrhage. **B:** Spectrum shows extreme peak broadening (FWHM is proportional to 1/T2).

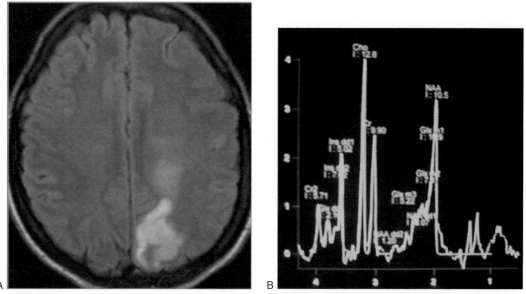

Figure 29-8. A: Nonspecific T2 prolongation in 39-year-old woman with fluctuating visual symptoms for several weeks, suggesting ischemia. **B:** MRS shows elevated Cho/NAA, suggesting tumor. Biopsy was positive for anaplastic astrocytoma.

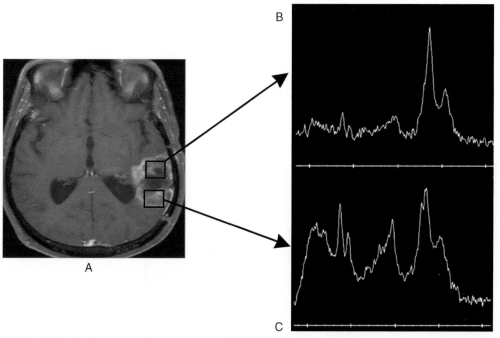

Figure 29-9. Radiation necrosis and recurrent GBM. **A:** Enhancing mass shows no elevation of Cho in anterior portion (**B**) but elevation in posterior portion (tallest peak on the left hand side of the spectra) (**C**).

(*Continued on next page.*)

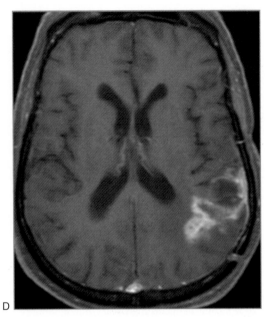
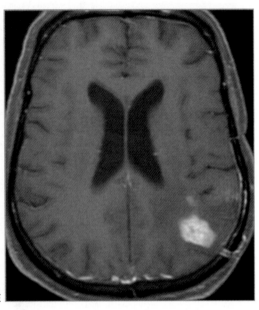

D   E

Figure 29-9. *(continued)* Four months later, the posterior portion has increased in size, supporting the diagnosis of recurrent GBM (**D** and **E**).

In certain disease states, for example, radiation necrosis, lipid is elevated due to membrane destruction (Fig. 29-9B). Since there are many lipid species, they have a range of chemical shifts from 0.9 to 1.2 ppm. Lipids also tend to have short T2s so they are only seen on short TE techniques.

Lactate is adjacent to lipid at 1.3 ppm. It is elevated in ischemia, for example, stroke (Fig. 29-10), and when anaerobic glycolysis occurs in tumors that have outgrown their blood supply (Fig. 29-11). When it is necessary to separate lactate from lipid, an intermediate TE of 135 to 144 msec can be used to flip the lactate doublet upside down using the standard PRESS (point-resolved spectroscopy) technique (Fig. 29-11B).

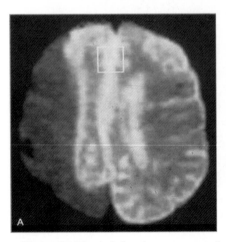
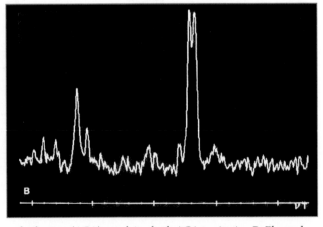

Figure 29-10. **A:** Infarct in azygous anterior cerebral artery (ACA) supplying both ACA territories. **B:** Elevated Lactate (doublet at 1.3 ppm on TE = 270 ms PRESS).

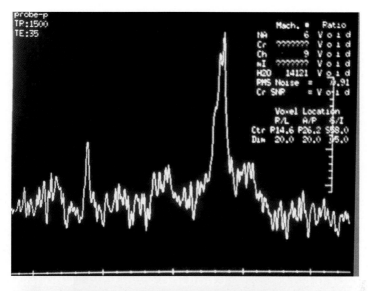

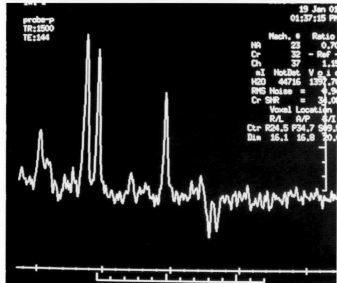

Figure 29-11. **A:** TE = 35 ms PRESS shows positive lactate doublet.
B: TE = 144 ms PRESS shows negative lactate doublet in this patient with
GBM (*Note*: elevated Cho/NAA).

Patterns of Disease

Solid tumors have elevated Cho and decreased
NAA. When they become necrotic, lipid and
lactate become elevated as well (Fig. 29-11).
Although elevated Cho/NAA is a sensitive
marker for cancer, it is nonspecific. The same
pattern is seen in tumefactive multiple sclerosis
and acute disseminated encephalomyelitis.

MRS can distinguish recurrent GBM (elevated Cho/NAA) from radiation necrosis (no
elevated Cho but elevated lipid) (Fig. 29-9B). It
can distinguish necrotic lymphoma (elevated
Cho) from toxoplasmosis (no elevated Cho).

By placing the voxel outside the area of
enhancement or T2 prolongation, MRS can distinguish a metastasis (no elevated Cho) from an
infiltrating glioma (elevated Cho) (Fig. 29-12).

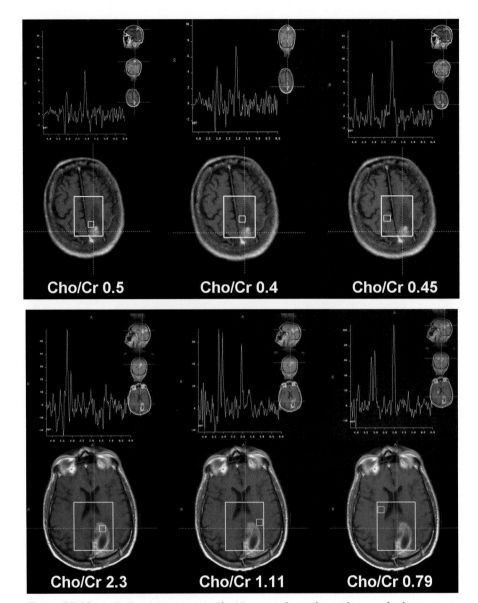

Figure 29-12. A-C: Gastric metastasis. Cho/Cr is not elevated outside area of enhancement. **D-F:** GBM. Cho/Cr is elevated both in (**D**) and outside (**E**) enhancement (Cho is the tallest peak in the spectra; compare with normal Cho/Cr in **F**). Elevated Cho/Cr in (**E**) represents infiltration of tumor outside area of enhancement.

Key Points

1 MRI images any mobile proton-containing species. MRS shows up to 10 different proton-containing chemical species, allowing more specific diagnoses.

2 MRS shows abnormalities, for example, infiltration of a GBM, not seen on MRI.

3 *J*-coupling decreases peak height linearly with TE, for example, glutamate and glutamine, which are seen jointly as Glx on the left-hand shoulder of NAA (2.0 to 2.5 ppm).

4 Species are identified based on their chemical shift in parts per million (ppm) relative to tetramethylsilane at 0 ppm (by definition).

5 In a normal brain, NAA (2.0 ppm) indicates normal neurons, Glx (2.0 to 2.5 ppm) represents glutamate and glutamine, Cr (3.0 ppm) represents energy, Cho (3.2 ppm) represents membrane turnover, and mI (myoinosotol at 3.5 ppm) is elevated in glial tumors and hyperosmolar states. Choline is elevated in all tumors and a few other states, for example, multiple sclerosis. Lactate (1.3 ppm) indicates anaerobic glycolysis seen in stroke and GBMs. Lipid (0.9 to 1.2 ppm) is seen with membrane breakdown seen in infection, radiation necrosis, and tumors.

Questions

29-1 Which of the following metabolites is normally not seen?
(a) NAA
(b) Lactate
(c) Cho
(d) Cr
(e) mI

29-2 Which of the following metabolites is not seen at long TE?
(a) mI
(b) NAA
(c) Cho
(d) Cr
(e) Lac

29-3 Which metabolite is best to distinguish recurrent GBM from radiation necrosis?
(a) NAA
(b) Cr
(c) Cho
(d) mI

29-4 Which metabolite is the best to distinguish necrotic lymphoma from toxoplasmosis in AIDS?
(a) NAA
(b) Cr

(c) Cho
(d) mI

29-5 mI is elevated in
(a) Alzheimers
(b) Hyperosmolar states
(c) Glial tumors
(d) All of the above

29-6 T/F Elevated Cho/NAA is specific for tumor.

29-7 T/F Performing MRS after giving gadolinium raises the Cho/NAA ratio.

29-8 Peak broadening in MRS is caused by
(a) Motion
(b) Short T2 hemorrhage
(c) Local metallic artifact
(d) Poor shimming
(e) All of the above

30

High Performance Gradients

Introduction

This chapter briefly discusses the new technology of high performance gradients. As you know by now, gradients have many purposes, including slice selection, spatial encoding, flow compensation (FC), and spoiling, rewinding, and presaturation. It should be fairly obvious that every time you use a gradient, you are lengthening the pulse cycle (thus increasing minimum TE).

Consider the two gradients in Figure 30-1A and 30-1B. The gradient in Figure 30-1A has half the strength of the one in Figure 30-1B but twice the duration. Thus, both these gradients have the same area (shaded area). They both achieve exactly the same result (e.g., phase shift) on *stationary* spins, but the second one is twice as fast and allows one to reduce the echo delay time TE. Therefore, the first requirement of a high performance gradient is a higher maximum strength.

When we discuss high performance gradients, not only do we want to achieve a stronger magnitude or strength, but we also want the maximum strength to be achieved in as short a time as possible (i.e., a short rise time) to minimize the duration of the gradient. Therefore, the second issue is how fast a gradient can reach its plateau (Fig. 30-2). The ratio of the maximum gradient (G_{max}) to the **rise time** (t_R) is called the **slew rate** (SR).

$$SR = \text{slew rate}$$
$$= G_{max}/t_R \text{ (in mT/m/msec)} \text{ (Eqn. 30-1)}$$

Early gradients had a G_{max} of 3 to 6 mT/m and a t_R of 1.5 to 2 msec (i.e., SR of 1.5 to 4 mT/m/msec).

> **The requirements for high performance gradients are the following:**
>
> 1. **High gradient strength (G_{max})**
> 2. **Short rise time (t_R)**
>
> i.e., a high slew rate (G_{max}/t_R).

In the mid-1980s, GE introduced shielded gradients with G_{max} of 10 mT/m and t_R of 675 μsec = 0.675 msec (i.e., SR of 15 mT/m/msec). The new high performance gradient systems (Siemens' Sonata or Symphony with Quantum Gradients, GE's Twin Speed, Philips' Intera, etc.) have G_{max} as high as 40 mT/m and t_R as low as 180 μsec with SR as high as 200 mT/m/msec .

Advantages

1. Shorter cycles are possible. As discussed previously, a stronger gradient can be applied over a shorter duration. Consider the example of FC. Figure 30-3 demonstrates two FC gradients that achieve the same thing, but the second one has higher strength ($G' > G$) and is thus applied over a shorter period ($T' < T$). (As an aside, because of the quadratic nature of phase accumulation for flowing spins, there is no linear or inverse linear relationship between gradient strength and application time, i.e., doubling the gradient strength does not halve the time of gradient application.) Higher order motion (e.g., acceleration, jerk) requires

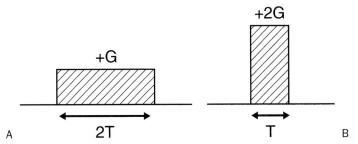

Figure 30-1. The gradient in (**B**) has twice the strength of the one in (**A**) but half the duration. Consequently, they both have exactly the same area and thus achieve the same results for stationary spins. However, the one in (**B**) has the advantage of being faster, a condition that is required for fast scanning.

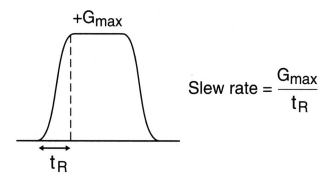

$$\text{Slew rate} = \frac{G_{\text{max}}}{t_R}$$

Figure 30-2. In reality, it takes a certain amount of time (t_R) for a gradient to rise to its plateau G_{max}. The ratio G_{max}/t_R is called the slew rate (in mT/m/msec).

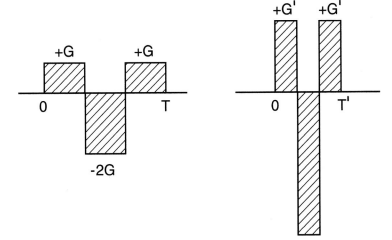

Figure 30-3. With high performance gradients, flow compensation can be accomplished faster (again because by increasing the strength and reducing the duration, the same area can be achieved).

the addition of even more gradient lobes. You can see how high performance gradients can save a lot of time during each cycle, allowing for shorter TEs (reducing dephasing) and TRs (for fast scanning).

2. Smaller field of views (FOVs) are possible. As we saw in Chapter 15, an inverse relationship exists between the gradient strength along one axis and the FOV:

$$FOV = BW/(\gamma G)$$

where G is the gradient strength and BW is the bandwidth defined as

$$BW = 2f_{max}$$

where f_{max} is the **Nyquist frequency** (see Chapter 12). Thus, increasing G allows us to reduce the FOV, leading to higher spatial resolution (an example is high-resolution imaging of a small part such as the pituitary gland). That is

$$FOV_{min} = BW/(\gamma G_{max})$$

Because spatial resolution is defined as the FOV divided by the number of encoding steps:

$$Spatial\ resolution = FOV/N$$

then minimizing FOV (while keeping N fixed) results in improved spatial resolution.

Example
For a standard high field system, the BW = 32 kHz (±16 kHz) and G_{max} = 10 mT/m. Then

$$FOV_{min} = 32\ kHz/(42.6\ MHz/T \times 10\ mT/m)$$
$$\cong 7.5\ cm$$

Now if G_{max} is increased to 25 mT/m, then

$$FOV_{min} = 32\ kHz/(42.6\ MHz/T \times 25\ mT/m)$$
$$\cong 3\ cm$$

If you reduce the BW to 16 kHz (±8 kHz), then the minimum FOV will be reduced even further to about 1.5 cm.

3. Faster imaging is possible, including faster FSE (fast spin echo), **GRASE (gradient and spin echo)**, and EPI (echo planar imaging).

4. 3D-FSE is possible (useful for 3D T2-weighted imaging in brain and spine).

5. Contrast-enhanced magnetic resonance angiography (CE-MRA) images can be acquired during the transit time of the gadolinium through the artery or vein (*first-pass technique*) or through the center of k-space (*elliptical-centric technique*)

6. Detection of very slow flow (blood or cerebrospinal fluid [CSF]) is possible via phase contrast (PC) techniques.

7. PC MRA can now be performed in a reasonable acquisition time with increased sensitivity to slow flow. (The duration of the flow-encoding gradient can be reduced, allowing for a shorter TR.)

8. High-resolution imaging of CSF flow in small shunts is possible.

9. Ultra high-resolution MRA is possible (1024 × 1024 matrix over a 22-cm FOV, resulting in 250 μm resolution!).

10. High-resolution (both spatial and temporal) dynamic MR techniques are possible because, by shortening the TE and TR, a larger matrix can be employed at a given FOV in the same acquisition time. Thus, both spatial and temporal resolutions can be improved. One application is dynamic MR study of breast cancer (turboFLASH sequence with TR = 7 msec, TE = 3 msec, 128 × 128 matrix, acquisition time = 7 × 128 = 896 msec $\cong$ 0.9 sec).

11. The minimum TE can be reduced, thus minimizing dephasing and increasing T1 contrast. For example, high performance gradients can provide high-dose gadolinium performance with the use of a single dose of gadolinium, or, alternatively, provide single dose performance with only half a dose of gadolinium.

Very fast sequential postgadolinium imaging can be performed for evaluation of decreased perfusion leading to cerebral or myocardial ischemia. Additionally, diffusion imaging is possible by the addition of diffusion-sensitizing gradient pulses to any pulse sequence. The current main clinical application is in early detection of cerebrovascular ischemia.

Key Points

High performance gradients have revolutionized MR imaging. In short, a higher magnetic strength allows a shorter duration, thus reducing the cycle time. This in turn reduces the minimum TE and TR, which shortens the acquisition time. In summary, high performance gradients allow many new and improved features, including faster scanning (including EPI, GRASE, 3D-FSE, CE MRA, etc.), improved spatial and temporal resolution, smaller FOV, high-resolution MRA (both TOF and PC) with improved visualization of small vessels and slow flow, and improved imaging of CSF flow, just to name a few.

Questions

30-1 High performance gradients require
   (a) high gradient strength (G_{max})
   (b) short rise time (t_R)
   (c) both
   (d) none

30-2 The slew rate is defined as
   (a) t_R/G_{max}
   (b) G_{max}/t_R
   (c) $\gamma G_{max}/t_R$
   (d) none of the above

30-3 Advantages of high performance gradients include all of the following *except*
   (a) faster scanning
   (b) smaller FOV

   (c) reduced chemical shift
   (d) diffusion imaging

30-4 Two gradients with different profiles but the same area (Fig. 30-1) will have the same effects (i.e., phase changes) on
   (a) stationary spins
   (b) flowing spins
   (c) both
   (d) none

31

The Many Combinations of MRI

Introduction

Thus far we have studied a vast array of MRI sequences that seem somewhat related to one another, but also, quite different. The pulse sequences that we have looked at are the basic sequences used in MRI; however, there are many more combinations of sequences that can be performed and in this chapter we will look at how these interrelate.

Basic Building Blocks

The basic elements needed to build an MRI pulse sequence can be simplified into four components: (i) **prep pulse** (optional), (ii) **radio frequency (RF) pulse,** (iii) **refocusing mechanism,** and (iv) **readout** (Table 31-1). This is obviously a fairly simplified approach and omits certain items such as the phase-encode step, which is in every sequence. It also puts in an artificial distinction between the gradient refocusing mechanism in gradient-echo (GRE) sequences and the frequency readout, which are being performed simultaneously. Additionally, the refocusing 180° RF pulses in the fast spin-echo (FSE) technique are important both for refocusing and for making multiple readouts. Regardless of the few shortcomings, this approach is useful for understanding the new sequences that the manufacturers are offering on their magnets.

Prep Pulse (Optional). The prep pulse comes temporally before the other three elements, but it is also the one component that is optional. When a prep pulse is used in a sequence, it can actually have an important part to play in the appearance of the image as the root pulse sequence. There are three basic types of prep pulses: (i) **180° RF inversion pulse,** (ii) a **fat saturation (or chemical saturation) pulse** (usually 90° RF pulse), and (iii) a **magnetization transfer (MT) pulse.** All three of these pulses have different characteristics and properties, with resultant different effects. We have discussed all these pulses in prior chapters; however, it is important to note that any of these can be used with any pulse sequence to achieve a desired effect on the image.

For instance, a 180° RF pulse is used in both STIR and FLAIR imaging with the only variables being the TI, TR, and TE (conventional inversion recovery [IR] and fast IR pathways are shown in Table 31-2; a novel application is seen in Fig. 31-1). The 180° RF pulses can also be used to suppress flow such as in a double inversion recovery (DIR) (or *black-blood*) technique that is useful in cardiovascular imaging. This technique uses a nonslice selective 180° pulse followed by another 180° pulse that is slice selective. This idea can be carried out further by adding a third 180° pulse that nulls fat (known as a *triple IR* or *fat-saturated black-blood* technique—really just a combination of STIR and DIR) (Fig. 31-2). An inversion pulse is also useful in cardiac imaging for identification of infarcted myocardium in *delayed enhancement* imaging. In this technique, gadolinium is given and the heart is imaged 10 to 20 min later using an IR-GRE technique with an inversion

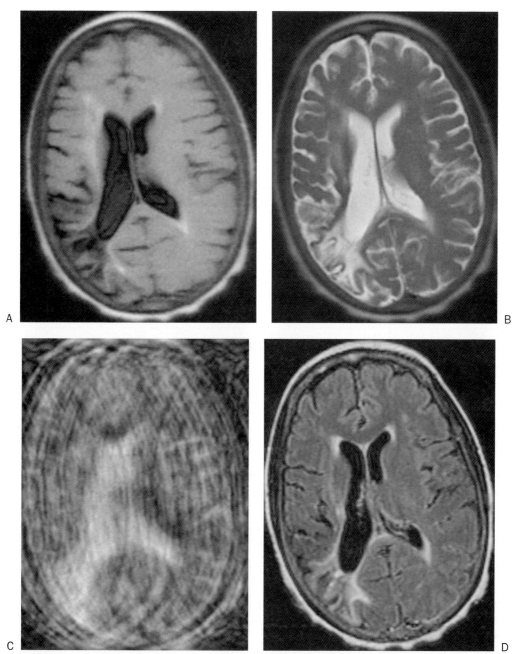

Figure 31-1. **A:** An SSFSE FLAIR image of the brain in an uncooperative patient. There are corresponding SSFSE (**B**), T2 (**C**) with marked motion, and later FLAIR (**D**) images when the patient was more cooperative. There are periventricular white matter ischemic changes and an old right parietal stroke. This example demonstrates a novel approach for newer fast imaging sequences that can be used in uncooperative patients.

Table 31-1   The Many Combinations of MR

Prep Pulse	RF Pulse	Refocusing	Readout
IR (180° pulse)	90°	180°	Single SE GRE
Fat sat (chem sat)	<90°	Gradient	Multiple (segmented) FSE EPI
MT			Multiple (single shot) EPI SSFSE

Abbreviations: IR, inversion recovery; MT, magnetization transfer; SE, spin echo; GRE, gradiant echo; FSE, fast spin echo; EPI, echo planar imaging; SSFSE, single-shot FSE; RF, radio frequency.

Table 31-2   Inversion Recovery ^{a}

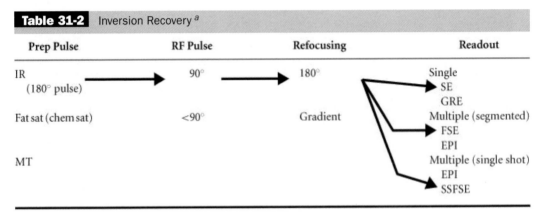

Prep Pulse	RF Pulse	Refocusing	Readout
IR (180° pulse)	90°	180°	Single SE GRE
Fat sat (chem sat)	<90°	Gradient	Multiple (segmented) FSE EPI
MT			Multiple (single shot) EPI SSFSE

^{a}For abbreviations, see Table 31-1 footnote.

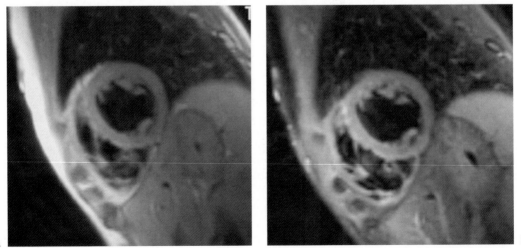

Figure 31-2. A: Short-axis DIR (double inversion recovery) or *black-blood* technique. **B:** The same slice using the TIR (triple inversion recovery) technique—notice the nulling of the fat on the TIR versus the DIR.

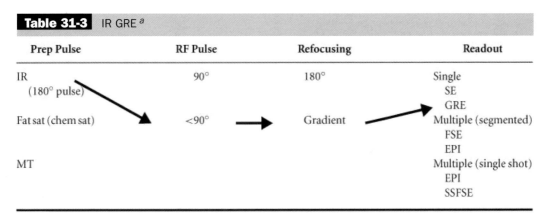

Prep Pulse	RF Pulse	Refocusing	Readout
IR (180° pulse)	90°	180°	Single SE GRE
Fat sat (chem sat)	<90°	Gradient	Multiple (segmented) FSE EPI
MT			Multiple (single shot) EPI SSFSE

Table 31-3 IR GRE [a]

[a]For abbreviations, see Table 31-1 footnote. Pathway for delayed enhancement imaging.

time of 200 to 300 msec to null normal myocardium (Table 31-3 and Fig. 31-3).

Furthermore, fat saturation (chemical saturation) is commonly used with spin-echo, FSE, GRE, and echo planar imaging (EPI) sequences, that is, any type of readout. (Table 31-4 lists some of the more common combinations and Fig. 31-4 illustrates some of these.) Thus, we have seen that the prep pulses can be added to any sequence, and any combination of prep pulses could be performed prior to the RF pulse in order to achieve a certain effect.

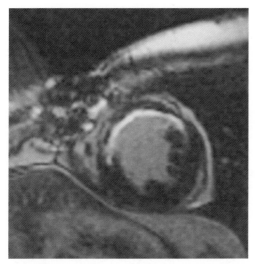

Figure 31-3. A short-axis IR-GRE delayed enhancement image showing transmural bright signal in the anterior wall and septum diagnostic of infarcted myocardium (TR 7/TE 3/TI 150 msec).

RF Pulse. The RF pulse would be the start of the sequence if there were no prep pulse. The RF pulse, as we have discussed previously, induces resonance into the system and tips the longitudinal magnetization into the transverse plane. A 90° pulse is used for the spin-echo technique, whereas a partial flip angle pulse <90° is used for GRE techniques. T1, T2, or proton density weighting is achieved by altering the TR, TE, and flip angle (for the gradient technique). Again, any of the above prep pulses can be used with any RF pulse.

Refocusing Mechanism. As we have discussed in prior chapters, the free induction decay (FID) usually comes on too early and decays too rapidly, keeping us from having enough time to encode the signal spatially and read it out (with the exception of ultrashort TE techniques currently in development). The solution to this problem is found in refocusing the spins. This is done either with a 180° pulse, which eliminates any external magnetic inhomogeneities and allows us to measure the signal on the T2 curve, or with a gradient, which can be done much faster but at the cost of measuring the signal from the steeper T2* curve. A gradient refocusing mechanism could be useful with any RF flip angle. However, the same cannot be said for a 180° refocusing pulse, which is only useful for a 90° RF pulse, but not for a partial flip angle RF pulse (see Chapter 20).

Readout. The readout is a collective concept that embodies both the frequency-encode gradient (which is also the refocusing gradient in

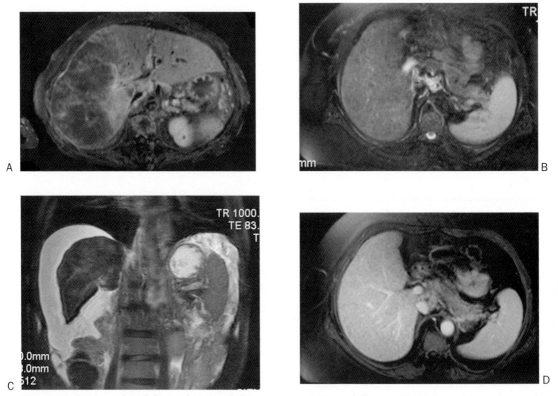

Figure 31-4. Examples of chemical (spectral) fat saturation. **A:** Postgadolinium CSE T1 image in a patient with diffuse metastasis of the right lobe (TR 467/TE 14 msec). **B:** FSE T2 image in a patient with siderotic nodules and cirrhosis (TR 4000/TE 84 msec). **C:** HASTE image (SSFSE) in a patient with cirrhosis, ascites, and multiple metastases (unusual in a cirrhotic patient; TR 1000/TE 83 msec). **D:** Postgadolinium SPGR in the same patient as **(B)** (TR 160/TE 4 msec).

GRE sequences) and any additional repetition of the readout (with its accompanying different phase-encode steps) such as additional 180° RF pulses in FSE or the alternating gradients in both the frequency and phase directions in EPI. An overarching idea is that the readout following a single RF pulse can either fill a **single** line of k-space, **multiple** lines (**segmented or multi-**

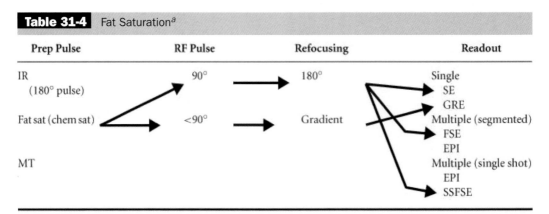

Table 31-4   Fat Saturation[a]

Prep Pulse	RF Pulse	Refocusing	Readout
IR (180° pulse)	90°	180°	Single SE GRE
Fat sat (chem sat)	<90°	Gradient	Multiple (segmented) FSE EPI
MT			Multiple (single shot) EPI SSFSE

[a]For abbreviations, see Table 31-1 footnote. Typical pathways are shown, although any combination is possible.

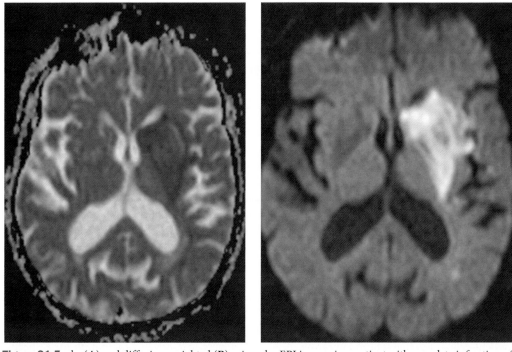

Figure 31-5. b_0 (**A**) and diffusion-weighted (**B**) spin-echo EPI images in a patient with complete infarction of the left basal ganglia from a large MCA CVA that involved the lenticulostriate branches.

shot filling of k-space), or all the lines of k-space (**single-shot** technique). Advances in gradient strengths and computers make any of these possibilities available for any technique.

For instance, we have already discussed spin-echo sequences that fill a single line of k-space versus the FSE technique that fills multiple lines of k-space versus the ½ NEX single-shot technique (HASTE or SSFSE) that fills all the lines of k-space from a single RF pulse or shot (Table 31-5 and Fig. 31-4A–C). From Table 31-5, you can also see that in typical spin-echo imaging any prep pulse and any readout (single, segmented, or single shot) can be performed. For even faster spin-echo imaging, EPI readouts could be performed, usually in a single-shot technique such as in diffusion-weighted imaging (Table 31-6 and Fig. 31-5).

Table 31-5 Spin Echo[a]			
Prep Pulse	**RF Pulse**	**Refocusing**	**Readout**
IR (180° pulse)	90°	180°	Single / SE / GRE
Fat sat (chem sat)	<90°	Gradient	Multiple (segmented) / FSE / EPI
MT			Multiple (single shot) / EPI / SSFSE

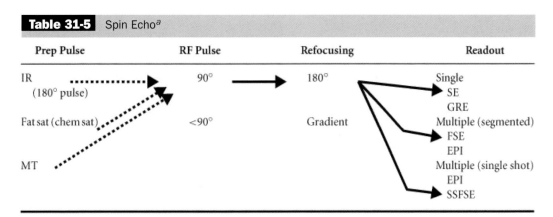

[a]For abbreviations, see Table 31-1 footnote. Dashed lines represent optional pulses.

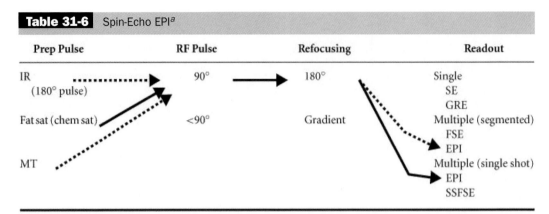

Table 31-6 Spin-Echo EPI[a]

Prep Pulse	RF Pulse	Refocusing	Readout
IR (180° pulse)	90°	180°	Single SE GRE
Fat sat (chem sat)	<90°	Gradient	Multiple (segmented) FSE EPI
MT			Multiple (single shot) EPI SSFSE

[a]For abbreviations, see Table 31-1 footnote. Solid lines represent typical diffusion-weighted image, and the dashed lines represent optional pathways. Note that EPI images are usually acquired with fat saturation due to the marked chemical shift artifacts without it.

Most gradient sequences fill a single line of k-space per RF; however, newer techniques are being implemented such as an FGRET (fast gradient-echo train) that is useful in cardiac perfusion imaging (Table 31-7 and Fig. 31-6). This is a GRE sequence with a segmented filling of k-space (four lines per RF pulse).

You can now more easily appreciate that MRI sequences (especially the newer applications) are usually a mix and match of the basic elements in a novel combination for a specific purpose.

Table 31-7 GRE-EPI[a]

Prep Pulse	RF Pulse	Refocusing	Readout
IR (180° pulse)	90°	180°	Single SE GRE
Fat sat (chem sat)	<90°	Gradient	Multiple (segmented) FSE EPI
MT			Multiple (single shot) EPI SSFSE

[a]For abbreviations, see Table 31-1 footnote. Solid lines represent GRE-EPI for FGRET sequence, and dashed lines represent other possible combinations.

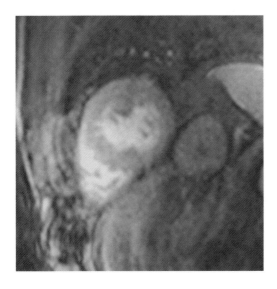

Figure 31-6. Short-axis dynamic postgadolinium perfusion study shows normal enhancement of the myocardium (TR 6/TE 1.5 msec).

Key Points

1 Each pulse sequence can be simplistically viewed as a prep pulse (optional), RF pulse, refocusing mechanism, and readout.

2 There are three main prep pulses: (i) 180° RF pulse (inversion recovery), (ii) fat saturation (or chemical sat) pulse, and (iii) magnetization transfer (MT) pulse.

3 The RF pulse is either a 90° RF pulse or a partial flip angle (<90°) pulse.

4 The refocusing mechanism is either by 180° RF pulse or a gradient.

5 The readout can either fill a single line of k-space, multiple lines of k-space (segmented), or all the lines of k-space (single shot) following the RF pulse.

6 Any of the above can be mixed and matched in any combination that is desirable for either image characteristics or speed with the exception of a partial flip RF pulse followed by a 180° refocusing pulse.

Questions

31-1 **T/F**   A prep pulse is required in every MRI pulse sequence.

31-2 **T/F**   A 180° prep pulse can be followed by a GRE sequence.

31-3 **T/F**   A 180° refocusing pulse is useful in a GRE sequence.

31-4 Which of the following sequences are not useful?
   (a) MT, 90° RF, 180° refocusing pulse, single readout
   (b) fat sat, 90° RF, 180° refocusing pulse, multiple readout (segmented)
   (c) 180° inversion pulse, <90° RF, gradient refocusing, single readout
   (d) no prep pulse, 90° RF, 180° refocusing pulse, multiple readout (single-shot EPI)
   (e) none of the above; they are all useful

31-5 **T/F**   Multiple readouts of the single-shot variety can be based either on an FSE technique or on an EPI technique.

Suggested Readings

1. American College of Radiology. *Glossary of MR Terms*. 5th ed. Reston, VA: ACR; 2005.

2. Bradley WG. Optimizing lesion contrast without using contrast agents. *J Magn Reson Imaging*. 1999; 10:442–449.

3. Bradley WG, Waluch V, Lai K, et al. The appearance of rapidly flowing blood on magnetic resonance images. *Am J Roentgenol*. 1984;143:1167–1174.

4. Bushberg JT, Seibert JA, Leidholdt EM, et al. *The Essential Physics of Medical Imaging*. 2nd ed. Philadelphia: Lippincott Williams & Wilkins; 2002.

5. Chun Y, Schmiedl UP, Weinberger E, et al. Three-dimensional fast spin-echo imaging: pulse sequence and in vivo image evaluation. *J Magn Reson Imaging*. 1993;3:894–899.

6. Edelman RR, Wielopolski P, Schmitt F, et al. Echo-planar MR imaging. *Radiology*. 1994;192:600–612.

7. Erickson SJ, Cox IH, Hyde JS, et al. Effect of tendon orientation on MR imaging signal intensity: a manifestation of the "magic angle" phenomenon. *Radiology*. 1991;181:389–392.

8. Hashemi RH, Bradley WG, Chen D-Y, et al. Suspected multiple sclerosis: MR imaging with a thin-section fast FLAIR pulse sequence. *Radiology*. 1995;196:505–510.

9. Henkelman RM, Hardy PA, Bishop JE, et al. Why fat is bright in RARE and fast spin-echo imaging. *J Magn Reson Imaging*. 1992;2:533–540.

10. Hennig J, Nauerth A, Friedburg H. RARE imaging: a fast imaging method for clinical MR. *Magn Reson Med*. 1986;3:823–833.

11. Huda W, Slone R. *Review of Radiologic Physics*. 2nd ed. Philadelphia: Lippincott Williams & Wilkins; 2003.

12. Kapelov SR, Teresi LM, Bradley WG, et al. Bone contusions of the knee: increased lesion detection with fast spin-echo MR imaging with spectroscopic fat saturation. *Radiology*. 1993;189:901–904.

13. Oppenheim AV, Willsky AS, Nawab S. *Signals and Systems*. (2nd Ed.). New Jersey: Prentice-Hall; 1996.

14. Pierpaoli C, Jezzard P, Basser PJ, et al. Diffusion tensor MR imaging of the human brain. *Radiology*. 1996;201:637–648.

15. Prince MR, Grist TM, Debatin JF. *3D Contrast MR Angiography*. Berlin: Springer; 1997.

16. Prince MR, Narasimham DL, Stanley JC, et al. Breath-hold gadolinium-enhanced MR angiography of the abdominal aorta and its major branches. *Radiology*. 1995;197:785–792.

17. Stark DD, Bradley WG, eds. *Magnetic Resonance Imaging*. Vol. 1–3. 3rd ed. St Louis: Mosby; 1999.

18. Ulug AM, Moore DF, Bojko AS, et al. Clinical use of diffusion tensor imaging for diseases causing neuronal and axonal damage. *Am J Neuroradiol*. 1999;20:1044–1048.

19. Saremi F, Grizzard JD, Kim RJ. Optimizing cardiac MR imaging: practical remedies for artifacts. *Radiographics*. 2008;28:1161–1187.

20. Lotz J, Meier C, Leppert A, et al. Cardiovascular flow measurement with phase-contrast MR imaging: basic facts and implementation. *Radiographics*. 2002;22:651–671.

21. Scott AD, Keegan J, Firmin DN. Motion in cardiovascular MR imaging. *Radiology*. 2009;250: 331–351.

22. Simonetti OP, Kim RJ, Fieno DS, et al. An improved MR imaging technique for the visualization of myocardial infarction. *Radiology*. 2001; 218:215–223.

23. Foo TK, Bernstein MA, Aisen AM, et al. Improved ejection fraction and flow velocity estimates with use of view sharing and uniform repetition time

excitation with fast cardiac techniques. *Radiology*. 1995;195:471.

24. Srichai MB, Lim RP, Wong S, et al. Cardiovascular applications of phase-contrast MRI. *Am J Roentgenol*. 2009;192:662–675.

25. Huber AM, Schoenberg SO, Hayes C, et al. Phase-sensitive inversion-recovery MR imaging in the detection of myocardial infarction. *Radiology*. 2005;237:854–860.

26. Sievers B, Addo M, Kirchberg S, et al. Impact of the ECG gating method on ventricular volumes and ejection fractions assessed by cardiovascular magnetic resonance imaging. *J Cardiovasc Magn Reson*. 2005;7:441–446.

27. Mukherji SK. *Clinical Applications of MR Spectroscopy*. Wiley-Liss: New York; 1998.

28. Salibi N, Brown MA. *Clinical MR Spectroscopy: First Principles*. Wiley-Liss: New York; 1998.

29. Danielsen ER, Ross B. *Magnetic Resonance Spectroscopy Diagnosis of Neurological Diseases*. Marcel Dekker: New York; 1999.

30. Majos C, Aguilero C, Alonso J, et al. Proton MR spectroscopy improves discrimination between tumor and pseudotumoral lesion in solid brain masses. *Am J Neuroradiol*. 2009;30:544–551.

APPENDIX

B

Answers

Chapter 1

1-1 (a) See Figure 1-17

(b) See Figure 1-18

1-2 $e^{i(x+y)} = e^{ix}e^{iy}$. So $\cos(x+y) + i\sin(x+y) = (\cos x + i\sin x)(\cos y + i\sin y) = (\cos x \cdot \cos y - \sin x \cdot \sin y) + i(\cos x \cdot \sin i + \sin x \cdot \cos y)$

1-3 $\operatorname{sinc}(0) = \sin(0)/0 = \lim_{x\to 0} d/dx (\sin x/x)$

$= \cos x/1 \big|_{(x=0)} = \cos 0/1 = 1/1 = 1$

1-4 (a) $e^{-1} = 0.37$ **(b)** $e^{-2} = 0.14$

(c) $e^{-1} = 0.37$

1-5 $d/dt(Ae^{-t/T}) = A(-1/T)e^{-t/T}$, which is $-A/T$ at $t = 0$. This is the slope of the line tangent to the curve at $t = 0$ that crosses the t-axis at $t = T$.

1-6 $\ln(e^x) = x = \ln 8 = \ln 2^3 = 3\ln 2 = 3 \times 0.693 = 2.079$

1-7 (a) 0 **(b)** 0.5 **(c)** 1

(d) 0 **(e)** 1 **(f)** 0.5

(g) 0 **(h)** −1

Chapter 2

2-1 (a) 14.9 MHz

(b) 21.3 MHz

(c) 42.6 MHz

(d) 63.9 MHz

(e) 85.2 MHz

(f) 127.8 MHz

2-2 T

2-3 F (only mobile protons)

2-4 F

2-5 T

2-6 F (speed of light)

2-7 T

2-8 F

2-9 F

2-10 T

2-11 T

Chapter 3

3-1 T

3-2 F

3-3 T

3-4 T

3-5 T

3-6 F (twice)

3-7 T

Chapter 4

4-1 (a) T **(b)** F **(c)** F **(d)** T

4-2 b

4-3 d

4-4 F (by T2*)

4-5 c

4-6 (a) i **(b)** ii

Chapter 5

5-1 (a) 1.56 **(b)** 90 msec

(c) 0.72 and 1.05

(d) 1.28, 50 msec, 0.88 and 1.28

(e) 2.10

5-2 H_2O/fat = 0.25 and 1.63; CSF/GM = 0.41 and 1.40

5-3 b

5-4 c

5-5 (a) $N(H)e^{-TE/T2}$ (i.e., ideal T2W)

(b) $N(H)(1 - e^{-TR/T1})$ (i.e., ideal T1W)

(c) $N(H)$ (i.e., ideal PDW).

5-6 (a) ii **(b)** i **(c)** iii **(d)** iv

367

Chapter 6
6-1 T
6-2 (a) iii   **(b)** i   **(c)** iv
      (d) i   **(e)** ii
6-3 T
6-4 (a) i   **(b)** ii   **(c)** iv

Chapter 7
7-1 Setting $1 - 2e^{-t/T1} = 0$, we get $e^{-t/T1} = 1/2$ so $-t/T1 = \ln(1/2) = -0.693$ so $t = 0.693\, T1$
7-2 $S\alpha N(H)\ (1 - 2e^{-TI/T1})\ (1 - e^{-TR/T1})$ and $N(H)\ (1 - 2e^{-TI/T1} - e^{-TR/T1} + 2e^{-(TR+TI)/T1}) \cong N(H)\ (1 - 2e^{-TI/T1} - e^{-TR/T1} + 2e^{-TR/T1}) = N(H)\ (1 - 2e^{-TI/T1} + e^{-TR/T1})$
7-3 (a) ii   **(b)** i
7-4 T

Chapter 8
8-1 (a) $N(1 - e^{-TR/T1})e^{-TE1/T2}$ and
          $N(1 - e^{-TR/T1})e^{-TE2/T2}$
     (b) $N(1 - e^{-TR/T1})\,e^{-TE1/T2^*}$
     (c) 0.61 and 0.37
8-2 (a) i   **(b)** iii   **(c)** ii
8-3 F (not that due to spin−spin interactions)

Chapter 9
9-1 T
9-2 (a) F   **(b)** F
9-3 T
9-4 T

Chapter 10
10-1 (a) 4.7 mT/m   **(b)** 1 mm
10-2 f
10-3 T
10-4 T

Chapter 11
11-1 (a) i   **(b)** iii   **(c)** ii
11-2 T
11-3 $360°/128 = 2.8°$
11-4 (i) d   **(ii)** a
11-5 T

Chapter 12
12-1 b
12-2 c
12-3 T

12-4 $F(1/\sqrt{BW})$
12-5 d
12-6 F

Chapter 13
13-1 T
13-2 F (phase-encoding gradient)
13-3 T
13-4 T
13-5 T
13-6 F
13-7 F (there is *conjugate* symmetry)
13-8 F

Chapter 14
14-1 a, d, e
14-2 (a) 512 sec = 8 min, 32 sec
      (b) 5120 sec = 85 min, 20 sec = 1 hr, 25 min, 20 sec!
14-3 b

Chapter 15
15-1 (a) 15 cm (reduces the minimum FOV)
15-2 b
15-3 61°
15-4 d
15-5 F (increases)
15-6 b
15-7 a

Chapter 16
16-1 T
16-2 (a) T   **(b)** F (cycles/cm)
16-3 T
16-4 d
16-5 (a) T   **(b)** T
16-6 T

Chapter 17
17-1 (a) 384 sec = 6 min, 24 sec
      (b) 3840 sec = 64 min = 1 hr, 4 min
      (c) 6 min, 24 sec
17-2 10 slices
17-3 (a) SNR is increased by $\sqrt{2}$
      (b) Chemical shift is doubled.
      (c) Coverage is reduced since $T_s = N_x/BW$ is doubled
17-4 c
17-5 b
17-6 a

17-7 g

17-8 f

17-9 d

17-10 c

17-11 c

17-12 e

17-13 a

17-14 e

17-15 f

17-16 d

17-17 **(a)** ii   **(b)** i

Chapter 18

18-1 e

18-2 **(a)** In terms of number of pixels

	0.2 T	0.5 T	1.0 T	1.5 T
50 kHz	0.15	0.38	0.76	1.15
10 kHz	0.76	1.91	3.82	5.73
4 kHz	1.91	4.77	9.54	14.31

(b) In terms of mm

	0.2 T	0.5 T	1.0 T	1.5 T
50 kHz	0.14	0.36	0.72	1.07
10 kHz	0.72	1.79	3.58	5.37
4 kHz	1.79	4.48	8.95	13.43

(c) The narrower the BW or the stronger the main magnetic field, the greater the chemical shift.

18-3 **(a)** 51.2   **(b)** 256/51.2 = 5

(c) fewer ghosts

18-4 b

18-5 d

18-6 F (the other way around)

18-7 a

18-8 T

18-9 d

18-10 **(a)** 48 pixels or 7.5 cm

(b) 2 ghosts

18-11 c

18-12 c

18-13 d

18-14 F (55°)

18-15 a

18-16 c

18-17 e

18-18 T

Chapter 19

19-1 d

19-2 **(a)** 34 min, 8 sec

(b) 4 min, 16 sec

19-3 F (decreased coverage)

19-4 d

19-5 d

19-6 c

19-7 4 min, 16 sec

19-8 T

Chapter 20

20-1 T

20-2 T

20-3 T

20-4 T

20-5 T

20-6 F (more T1W)

20-7 **(a)** 15.4 sec

(b) 230.4 sec = 3 min, 50 sec

20-8 F (the opposite)

20-9 T

20-10 b

20-11 T

Chapter 21

21-1 d

21-2 f

21-3 T

21-4 T

Chapter 22

22-1 T

22-2 F

22-3 d

22-4 F

22-5 F

22-6 T

22-7 b

Chapter 23

23-1 e

23-2 d

23-3 a

23-4 T

23-5 T

23-6 F

Chapter 24

24-1 b

24-2 b

24-3 c

24-4 F

24-5 T

Chapter 25

25-1 b

25-2 a

25-3 F

25-4 T

25-5 T

25-6 e

25-7 e

25-8 T

Chapter 26

26-1 c

26-2 F (*distal* to a stenosis)

26-3 T

26-4 F

26-5 d

26-6 d

26-7 T

26-8 F

26-9 F

26-10 T

26-11 a

26-12 c

26-13 c

26-14 F

26-15 T

26-16 c

Chapter 27

27-1 d

27-2 b

27-3 **(a)** i   **(b)** i   **(c)** ii   **(d)** ii

27-4 F

27-5 e

27-6 T

27-7 T

27-8 **(a)** ii   **(b)** i

(c) v   **(d)** iii

(e) iv

27-9 T

27-10 c

Chapter 28

28-1 d

28-2 a

28-3 b

28-4 c

28-5 d

28-6 c

28-7 a

Chapter 29

29-1 b

29-2 a

29-3 c

29-4 c

29-5 d

29-6 F: also elevated in MS and ADEM.

29-7 F: since Cho has a shorter T1 than NAA, the Gd shortens the T1 relatively more for NAA, raising its signal.

29-8 e

Chapter 30

30-1 c

30-2 b

30-3 c

30-4 a

Chapter 31

31-1 F

31-2 T

31-3 F

31-4 e

31-5 T

APPENDIX

C

Abbreviations

α, θ, ϕ	Alpha, theta, phi. Symbols used to designate an angle (e.g., flip angle)
Γ	γ. Gyromagnetic ratio (in T/MHz)
$\mathbf{M}$	μ. Micron (10^{-6} m)
Σ	σ. Standard deviation
T	τ. Symbol used to designate time
ω, ω_0	Omega. Angular (Larmor) frequency (in radians/sec)
2D	Two dimensional
2DFT	Two-dimensional Fourier transform
3D	Three dimensional
3DFT	Three-dimensional Fourier transform
A2D, ADC	Analog-to-digital converter or conversion
ASSET	Array spatial and sensitivity encoding technique
B_0	Main external magnetic field
B_1	Magnetic field associated with the RF pulse
b-FFE	balanced fast field echo
b-SSFP	balanced steady-state free precession
BW	Bandwidth
CNR	Contrast-to-noise ratio
CSE	Conventional spin echo
DE	Driven equilibrium
EPI	Echo planar imaging
ESP	Echo spacing
ET	Echo train
ETL	Echo train length
FC	Flow compensation
FFE	fast field echo
FFT	Fast Fourier transform
FGR	Fast GRASS
FID	Free induction decay
FIESTA	Fast imaging employing steady-state acquisition
FISP	Fast imaging with steady-state precession
FLAIR	Fluid-attenuated inversion recovery
FLASH	Fast low-angle shot

FOV	Field of view
FSE	Fast spin echo
FSPGR	Fast SPGR
FT	Fourier transform
G_x	Frequency-encoding gradient
G_y	Phase-encoding gradient
G_z	Slice-select gradient
GE	Gradient echo
GM	Gray matter
GMN	Gradient moment nulling
GMR	Gradient-motion rephasing
GRASE	Gradient and spin echo
GRASS	Gradient recalled acquisition in the steady state
GRE	Gradient echo or gradient-recalled echo
HASTE	Half-Fourier acquired single-shot turbo spin echo, Siemens
Hz	Hertz (1 cycle/sec)
IPAT	Integrated parallel acquisition techniques
IR	Inversion recovery
kHz	Kilohertz
M_0	Initial longitudinal magnetization
MAST	Motion artifact suppression technique
MEMP	Multi-echo multiplanar
MHz	Megahertz
mm	Millimeter (10^{-3} m)
MOTSA	Multiple overlapping thin-slab acquisition
MPGR	Multiplanar GRASS
MP-RAGE	Magnetization-prepared, rapid acquisition gradient echo
MR	Magnetic resonance
MRA	Magnetic resonance angiography
MRI	Magnetic resonance imaging
msec	Milliseconds
MT	Magnetization transfer
MTC	Magnetization transfer contrast
M_{xy}	Transverse magnetization in the x–y plane
M_z	Longitudinal magnetization
NEX	Number of excitations
nm	Nanometer (10^{-9} m)
NMR	Nuclear magnetic resonance
NPW	No phase wrap
NFW	No frequency wrap
NSA	Number of signal averages
N_x	Number of frequency-encoding steps in the x direction
N_y	Number of phase-encoding steps in the y direction
N_z	Number of phase-encoding steps in slice-select direction (in 3D imaging)
PC	Phase contrast
PD	Proton density

PDW	Proton density weighting
PDWI	Proton density-weighted image
pixel	Picture element
POMP	Phase offset multiplanar
pm	Picometer (10^{-12} m)
ppm	Parts per million
PS	Pulse sequence
PSD	Pulse sequence diagram
PSIF	Opposite of FISP
RARE	Rapid acquisition with relaxation enhancement
Re	Reynolds number
RF	Radio frequency
SE	Spin echo
SENSE	Sensitivity encoding
SMASH	Simultaneous acquisition of spatial harmonics
SNR, S/N	Signal-to-noise ratio
SPGR	Spoiled GRASS
SSFP	Steady-state free precession
SSFSE	Single-shot fast spin echo, GE
STIR	Short TI (or tau) inversion recovery
T1	T1 relaxation time, longitudinal relaxation time, and spin-lattice relaxation time
T1W	T1 weighting, T1 weighted
T1WI	T1-weighted image
T2	T2 relaxation time, transverse relaxation time, and spin–spin relaxation time
T2*	T2* relaxation time
T2W	T2 weighting, T2 weighted
T2WI	T2-weighted image
T2*W	T2* weighting, T2* weighted
T2*WI	T2*-weighted image
T	Tesla; period of a periodic signal
TE	Echo delay time (time to echo)
TI	Time to inversion (inversion time)
T_0	"Overhead" (dead) time in the pulse cycle
TOF	Time of flight
TONE	Tilted optimized nonsaturating excitation
TR	Repetition time (time of repetition)
t_R	Rise time
T_s	Sampling time
TSE	Turbo spin echo
Turbo	Siemens' and Philips' prefix to denote a fast scanning mode
VB	Variable bandwidth
VENC	Velocity encoding
VEMP	Variable echo multiplanar
voxel	Volume element
WM	White matter

Index

Page numbers followed by *f* and *t* indicate figures and tables, respectively.